T·H·E
NATURAL
PREGNANCY
BOOK

Herbs, Nutrition, and other Holistic Choices

Aviva Jill Romm

Foreword by Ina May Gaskin

THE CROSSING PRESS
FREEDOM, CALIFORNIA

This book is dedicated to all of the women who have, over the centuries, kept women's wisdom alive. It is because of their courage that I am here today. And to my sister-in-law, Felicity Romm, and her children, Serenity, Caleb, and Keziah Romm, for their incredible strength. And finally, to the spirit of my brother-in-law, Chip Romm.

Copyright © 1997 by Aviva Jill Romm
Illustrations by Marna Groves
Photos by Lise Alexander, except: pp. 11, 73 and 92 by Erica George Dines; pp. 121 and 123 by Aviva Romm
Typeset in Janson Text and Gill Sans
Printed in the U.S.A. on recycled paper

Visit our Web site on the Internet at: www.crossingpress.com

For information on bulk purchases or group discounts for this and other Crossing Press titles, please contact our Special Sales Manager at 800-777-1048.

ISBN 0-89594-819-2

Acknowledgments

This book could not have been written without the unfailing support of my mate, Tracy Romm. Tracy is truly a midwife at heart, a man who understands what it means for me to leave home in the middle of the night to wipe a woman's brow, say a few encouraging words, and be honored to greet a new member of our human family. He has joyfully played with, fed, read to, and nurtured our four children during the numerous hours it took to write this book. And he has encouraged me to keep writing because he cares so much about those who might benefit—the next generations, as well as our own.

I am also overjoyed by and thankful for the presence of my four children—my son, Iyah Khalil, my stalwart supporter and ardent encourager, and my three daughters, Yemima Shanti, who said, "Mom, you're an awesome woman!" and Forest Grace and Naomi Shoshannah, who have played the most magical games by my side, as I have typed away on these keys. These four people have shared me generously with the world, and I am honored to be their mom.

I would like to thank all of the midwives, herbalists, and healers who have been my teachers and inspiration, including Shafia Monroe, the first midwife I ever met, Sarahn Henderson, my friend, sister, and mentor, Debbie Pulley, who has known me "since I was in diapers," Jeannine Parvati Baker, for being the brilliant and radical woman that she is and for welcoming me into her circle of friends, and Susun Weed, Ina May Gaskin, Elizabeth Davis, Rosemary Gladstar Slick, David Hoffman, Snowbear (Steven Taylor), Michael and Lesley Tierra, Valerie Appleton, Anne Frye, Nancy Wainer Cohen, Gayle Peterson, and so many others. I am also grateful for the support of Lesley College, and particularly, my academic advisor and now friend and colleague, Dr. Deborah Piper, for her input into the manuscript, her vision of education, her commitment to women's health, and her ongoing encouragement, and to Dr. Richard Clofine for careful review of this manuscript and budding friendship.

My deep thanks goes to Cindy Gomez and Rick Spiers (and their kids), Lizzie McDaniels-Feigenbaum, Mark Miller, Marcial Rodriguez Arenal, and all of the other folks around Boston who told me about herbs, midwives, and natural healing long before they were in vogue, and first showed me the world as I know it today. I honor your vision with the work that I do.

Thanks to Elaine Gill and the staff at The Crossing Press for recognizing that creating a book is very much like a pregnancy and for midwifing the process along the way.

Finally, I am always grateful to the families that have welcomed me into the sacred space of their pregnancies, and who have called me, with joy, their midwife.

Contents

Foreword

by Ina May Gaskin

When I was pregnant for the first time back in 1965, I naively supposed there must be a book that would answer the questions that continuously bubbled up in my mind. How was I to stay within the twelve to fifteen pound weight gain allowed by my obstetrician and not be constantly hungry? Why was this weight limit necessary? What should I expect when I went into labor? How was I to learn how to take care of a baby? How did maternal instincts develop? (I thought I was sadly lacking in this department, because I hadn't played with baby dolls as a child.) I searched both the university and public libraries in my town for the book I wanted, but came up with nothing.

My obstetrician was little or no help in answering my questions, because he always seemed to be in a hurry—even though I never saw anyone else in his waiting room. In fact, for all I knew, I was the only pregnant woman in that small midwestern town where I was attending graduate school. Not once during this pregnancy did I talk to anyone (besides my obstetrician) who was either pregnant or claimed to know anything about pregnancy. Obtaining a midwife was totally out of the question—in fact, doing that never once occurred to me, because I was unaware there was any such being in all of the United States.

It was at my last prenatal visit before going into labor that my obstetrician informed me that since this was my first baby, I would be having a forceps delivery. When I protested, he interrupted to tell me that a natural birth of a first-time mother was likely to result in a brain-damaged baby. Unconvinced, I decided the best strategy for avoiding a forceps delivery (I knew from reading historical novels that forceps could cause brain damage) was to be the quietest woman ever to have a baby in that hospital.

It didn't work. My baby was pulled out by forceps, despite how silently I labored. She wasn't brain-damaged, but she and I were both negatively affected for many years by the psychological separation that stemmed from our physical separation for nearly twenty-four hours after her birth, and I felt that her birth had been something that had happened to me instead of something that I had done.

Young mothers these days do not have to worry about unnecessary forceps deliveries, because this fashion in obstetrics, once so widely and uncritically accepted in our country, is now as extinct as the pterodactyl. There are now far more books available on pregnancy and childbirth than most women have time to read or money to buy, and childbirth classes are available to probably the majority of women in the United States. Husbands, partners, family members, and even friends are allowed in the labor and delivery rooms of most hospitals, and it is a common, if mistaken, perception that childbirth is now handled in the best way possible.

The reality is far less reassuring. For one thing, not all of the books are that helpful. Many contain misleading information or even misinformation. As for interventions in the process of pregnancy, labor, and birth, it is now possible—even likely—for American women to have unnecessary ultrasonography during pregnancy, unnecessary inductions, unnecessary intravenous feedings, unnecessary electronic fetal monitoring, and unnecessary anesthesia during labor. Needless cesarean sections reached epidemic proportions in the United States during the 1970s and have remained at historically high levels ever since, despite the strenuous efforts of consumer organizations such as the International Cesarean Awareness Network (ICAN) to lower them and despite the repeated recommendations by the obstetricians' own professional organization, the American College of Obstetricians and Gynecologists (ACOG).

Because, after forty years of concerted efforts to revive the profession of midwifery in the United States, there are still only a few thousand midwives available to attend the four million births that happen annually, not every woman is going to be able to find a midwife to provide her prenatal care and to attend her birth.

Regardless of whether you have a midwife, or if you are one of the women who cannot obtain midwifery care, Aviva's book is going to be a comfort to you. She understands as a mother and as a midwife what you are going through, and she has an uncommon gift of writing down her knowledge in a way that is accessible and graceful. Read it and be nurtured.

Preface

This book was conceived nearly ten years ago, in the kitchen of a dear friend's home. At that time she and I, both midwives and each the mother of a young child, were beginning a lifetime journey of uncovering and rediscovering a great wealth of information about childbearing and child raising. We were gleaning information from a variety of sources: anthropological research, medical and lay texts, our work as mothers and midwives, the experiences of other midwives and mothers, and most significantly what we were learning from our intuition, from each other as women friends, from our partnerships with our mates, and from our babies. We had seen that pregnancy did not have to be ten (lunar) months of drudgery, discomfort, and exhaustion. We were finding that pregnancy and motherhood could be highly creative times, filled with confidence, perceptiveness, awe, and appreciation for the beauty of our changing physical shape, and the extension of this in the form of our growing children.

Standing in the doorway of that kitchen on an early spring day, a moment ripe for beginnings, I found an inspiration and made the commitment to carry this inspiration inside me, to gestate and nurture my discoveries, until, like a baby after a full-term pregnancy, a book would be ready to emerge—to be born—a book to share the joy and strength I was gaining from my experiences. That so many women see pregnancy as a burden to be endured, a time fraught with insecurity and doubt, seemed a great loss. Aware of the transformative potential of the written word, I became determined to contribute a positive, supportive narrative about pregnancy by a woman and mother, for women.

I now have four children. I've had healthy pregnancies, strong labors, and beautiful births. I've nursed and deeply enjoyed each of our children. Each pregnancy has reaffirmed my conviction that natural health care is the bedrock of my continuing wellness and that of our children. In addition to my own pregnancies, I have had the honor to know and assist many women and families on the mostly joyous, sometimes tumultuous, and occasionally painful path of pregnancy.

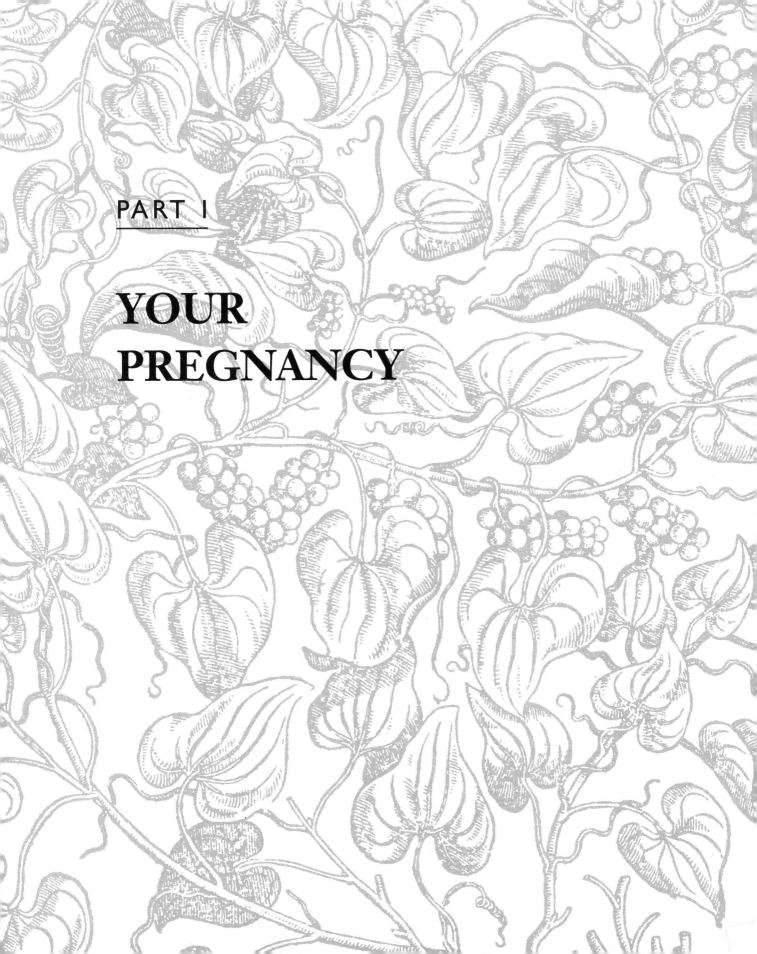

PART I

YOUR
PREGNANCY

The Basics

WHO THIS BOOK IS FOR

The Natural Pregnancy Book is written for all women, regardless of how extensively they want to use natural remedies. Women who simply wish to have a relaxed and healthy pregnancy and to be knowledgeable about this process can gain a great deal from the sections on nutrition, movement, and relaxation. Women with jobs outside the home can learn how to stay healthy and well nourished. Women who choose to forego careers in order to be with their children full-time will find support and validation for that choice. Women who are not yet pregnant but would like to be can use this book as part of their preparation for entering pregnancy in optimal health.

Grandmothers, aunts, sisters, friends, and partners of pregnant women can read this book to recreate the support systems that women have relied upon for generations, both during pregnancy and after the baby is born. This book will enable these women to be a positive and nourishing influence for the pregnant woman.

Women who are interested in what is known in our country as "alternative healing," "holistic medicine," "complementary medicine," or "natural health" will find this book one they turn to again and again for practical methods of relieving common pregnancy discomforts and promoting optimal health in pregnancy.

Most of this book is addressed to women, because pregnancy, although it offers a transformational experience for their male partners, is a woman's experience, one that a woman can, and I believe should, claim as her own. With this ownership of pregnancy, hopefully will come a sense of pride and self-respect that will give women the confidence to make choices and be the creative agents of their prenatal care. It is my profound hope that our culture will evolve to respect the rich potential for growth also available to men through their participation in pregnancy, and that men will respectfully

The open heart, freed from fear, experiences the world in all its mystery and brilliance. All of us need to practice awe-robics, like Lilly Tomlin's character, Trudy.

—Diane Mariechild

avail themselves of this possibility. Ideally, men will become cooperative partners, with a healthy respect for the primacy of the needs of the pregnant women and their babies. Optimally a partnership emerges in which both partners are finely attuned to each other's needs, with everyone benefiting including the child. Pregnancy is an opportunity for both partners to join together on the joyous path of building a lasting family.

Pregnancy is a time rich in possibility for relationship building between the parents and baby, even while the baby is still gestating. Hopefully, involved partners will read much of this book. Chapter 13 is written specifically for fathers. I also mean it to include partners in nontraditional relationships. Due to my lack of experience with lesbian couples, I cannot speak directly to their needs. To these women I apologize and hope that this book is still valuable to them.

A BRIEF HISTORY OF BIRTHING PRACTICES

Approximately 4 million women in the United States give birth every year. Of these women, the majority (96 percent or about 3,840,000 women) choose physicians to attend them. (Not accounted for in this figure of 4 million are those women who miscarry or choose an abortion. They too overwhelmingly choose physicians for their care.) Only 4 percent (about 16,000 women) receive care from midwives and only 1 percent (1,600) women choose home births.

Prior to the 20th century in the United States, home birth and natural childbirth were the norm. After that time the midwife's role was usurped by medical doctors with final control assumed by obstetricians. The idea was conveyed that doctors and hospitals were safer and more desirable than midwives

and home births. However, the fact is that in those days there was greater danger of women dying in childbirth in hospitals due to puerperal fever, primarily because physicians failed to wash their hands between patients.

With this shift toward hospitals and obstetricians, women became more passive, and less active in giving birth to their babies. Technology encouraged such passivity, for instance, with the standard obstetric tables with the stirrups high in the air, wrist straps to hold the woman immobile, twilight sleep to keep them unconscious, and excessive use of forcep deliveries and cesarean sections.

In the late 1960s, prompted in part by the Civil Rights and Women's Rights movements, women began to demand equality. At the same time, various methods (Leboyer, Dick Read, and Lamaze) were promulgated, emphasizing a more natural approach to birth. Women began to ask their partners to participate in their pregnancies and births, and it became commonplace for men to do so. Nevertheless, with all these advances, women were still cast in stereotypical roles, compliant as before.

In the 1970s and 1980s, technology became more emphasized in obstetrical care. Due to legal and financial considerations on the part of many doctors, hospitals, medical supply houses, and insurance companies, prenatal and intrapartum testing became requisite for all pregnant women, rather than optional for those at higher risk. Women as a whole did not question this growing number of interventions or their consequences.

Well into the 1980s, most women were still not informed about pregnancy and birth, and obstetrics all but absolved them of their responsibility. They were still patronized, frequently drugged, strapped down for birth, and subject to isolating and inconsiderate treatment. Babies, directly after birth, were still held upside down and slapped, and whisked away from their mothers. Few women breastfed their babies.

Despite some gains in equal rights in the workplace and home, women were still not decision makers in their pregnancies and birthing experiences. Women lost the political control over childbearing that existed when it was a private, women's experience, and have instead let the medical establishment become the authority.

Never before have pregnant women been expected to subject themselves to the level of prenatal testing, screening, and diagnosis as now. Because of our tendency to believe unquestioningly in medical experts, we allow ourselves and our babies to undergo practices that we are told are safe, but which medical literature often cites as harmful. This book offers suggestions for a different model of care, but also documents medical techniques that women might choose or need. This book is a compilation of the best that the tradition of midwifery has to offer in noninvasive methods for promoting and maintaining pregnancy wellness. It is a woman to woman guide to pregnancy care.

I believe that pregnancy is a natural process of which our bodies are perfectly capable, and that pregnancy is a process of initiation and growth into a value system that respects and honors women's creative power.

This book is woman-centered and feminist for two reasons. First, I firmly believe that women are the only true authorities about the female reproductive cycle. It is through the voices and experiences of women, the true authorities, that we gain the most valuable knowledge about pregnancy, birth, and mothering. I aim to bring attention to these women's voices and experiences. Second, as feminists we are puzzled as to how we can keep women's rights in childbearing without tying women to a false view of reproduction as a biological imperative. Devaluing childbearing in the effort to prove women's equality to men is harmful for all women. This may seem irrelevant to many women who do not consider themselves feminists, but such values have deeply affected all women to the point where many shun the idea that pregnancy, birth, and mothering are valuable experiences.

It is essential to acknowledge the importance of the pregnancy experience for the growth of not only the baby but for the woman as well. This book invites women to claim our bodies' processes as a part of our strength, not of our weakness, and to work together for the empowerment of women. I believe that reclaiming pregnancy should be part of our collective effort for broad-reaching social changes in all aspects of women's health care.

While this book offers many alternatives to conventional medical care, it is not anti-medical, anti-hospital, or anti-obstetrician. As a midwife I have seen truly necessary medical interventions and have been thankful for their skillful employment, have met dedicated and caring physicians, nurses, and nurse-midwives, and have seen great improvements in hospitals. What I take issue with is the inappropriate use of technology and the attitude that pregnancy is an illness.

I wish to create a new view of pregnancy. Pregnant women are viewed, culturally, as weak (they are discouraged from physical work), girlish (evidenced by childish-looking maternity clothes and the patronizing attitudes of some doctors), and irrational (demonstrated by strange food cravings and heightened emotional sensitivity). This book strives to help women reframe their thinking in order to regain their natural authority. Through the development of our own voice and story, trust in our ability to understand common medical rationale and practices, and confidence in our capability for competent decision making, we can feel more fully empowered to transform the cultural stereotypes that undermine the potential for positive growth and transformation inherent in the pregnancy experience.

The Natural Pregnancy Book is devoted not only to helping women gain trust and respect for their birthing abilities, but to planting the idea that babies are sensitive and aware in the womb. The physical nourishment and emotional caring that babies receive in the womb lays the foundation for their physical as well as their emotional and social health. Children who feel cared for and wanted have a greater likelihood of developing into confident and caring adults. If babies can hear and respond to music while in the womb (this has been scientifically documented), then certainly they can sense love or rejection. So it is that from early in gestation we can begin to teach our children to trust and respect their bodies, by setting the example of doing so for ourselves.

It is my sincerest hope that those who read this book will be inspired to listen to and respect their bodies, and in doing so, find a sense of well-being and confidence that will assist them throughout their lives. May this be a gift that we pass onto our daughters and sons, that they too may respect themselves, and each other.

WHAT I MEAN BY NATURAL

With the popularization of "natural childbirth" through such childbirth education methods as the Lamaze method, it has become common to consider any birth that occurs vaginally (as opposed to a Cesarean-section) as a natural birth, regardless of whether there have been interventions or the use of medications. While it is a disservice to a woman to feel guilty if she ultimately decides to have an epidural, to call such a birth "natural" trivializes the common use of drugs and interventions during both pregnancy and birth, and dilutes the likelihood of women recognizing that it is possible and empowering to experience a pregnancy and birth free of unnecessary intrusions or interventions. When I use the word natural, I am referring to untampered-with and unhindered biological processes, techniques that support such healthy biological functioning, and substances that are primarily derived from unrefined sources.

A natural approach to pregnancy necessitates that you respect the forces of your body—those that cause conception to occur and that also cause your baby to grow in your womb—and that you try to work in harmony with those forces by bringing elements from the natural world (for example, foods in their natural state and herbs) into your pregnancy experience.

ALTERNATIVE CHILDBIRTH AND THE RESURGENCE OF MIDWIFERY

In the mid-1970s, a small but determined number of women began to question the type of treatment they were receiving from the medical profession in their pregnancy and birth experiences. Coincident with the rise of the women's self-help movement and the so-called back-to-the-land movement, women began to turn to a more traditional and natural approach to pregnancy and birth, relying more on trust in natural cycles for reassurance of their wellness than on medical advice and testing. There began a resurgence in midwifery care, home birth, and the use of practical self-care. Some of the earliest pioneers of this movement include Ina May Gaskin, Sheila Kitzinger, Jeannine Parvati Baker, Elizabeth Davis, Raven Lang, Nan Koehler, Suzanne Arms, and Rahima Baldwin, as well as the midwives who founded the Childbirth Providers of African Descent—Shafia Monroe, Sondra Abdullah Zaimah, Ayanna Ade, and Rashida Mujtabah—and countless other women whose persistent and courageous efforts have kept natural birth options open for all of us.

With the growth of this alternative childbirth movement, midwives and mothers had available to them both the best natural traditions and best advanced obstetrical knowledge on which to draw. In fact, many midwives were women who wanted to provide other women with the type of care that they wished they had received during pregnancy. Women began to teach childbirth education classes, and some of them, such as sociologist and anthropologist Sheila Kitzinger and midwife and educator Rahima Baldwin, founded international organizations to inform and empower pregnant women. A handful of supportive physicians also provided assistance for those desiring a more natural approach to pregnancy and birth.

By the 1980s the alternative childbearing movement had gained momentum, and though less than 1 percent of all women chose home births, midwifery was no longer a thing of the past. With the resurgence of midwifery came a resurgence of the prejudice against women healers and the attendant persecution of midwives. In many areas of the United States traditional midwives have been arrested, harassed, faced with restraint-of-trade charges, and have endured emotional and economic hardships as a result of court cases and legal fees. Of course, the families of these practitioners have suffered greatly as well. Even certified nurse-midwives, fully trained and sanctioned by the medical establishment, are forced to practice strictly under the auspices of an obstetrician. It is determined by individual obstetricians, as well as the regulating organization of nurse-midwives, just how much autonomy a nurse-midwife is allowed.

In an effort to consolidate knowledge and create internal midwifery standards, as well as to provide a consistent forum for education, in 1982, midwives across the United States formed the Midwives Alliance of North America, an organization that now has an international membership and is working to foster public acceptance and recognition of independent midwifery not only as a respected profession, but also as an option available to a greater spectrum of women. This is in keeping with the belief that midwifery is political and social work that extends beyond small circles of "back-to-nature" women who choose to have babies at home. Midwives are committed to the care of pregnant women and are working to create a political environment in which all women have the option of receiving the kind of care and support midwives offer—professional care that is nurturing, designed to meet the needs of individual women.

The alternative childbirth movement has had a significant impact on women's experiences of childbirth, even for those choosing to give birth conventionally and in the hospital. Practices such as rooming-in, the presence of fathers, friends, and children at births, and the development of birthing suites and birthing centers are all testimony to the efforts of the alternative childbirth

Midwives are committed to the care of pregnant women and are working to create a political environment in which all women have the option of receiving the kind of care and support midwives offer—professional care that is nurturing, designed to meet the needs of individual women.

—A. J. R.

movement. The growing popularity of organic foods during pregnancy, exercise and yoga for prenatal relaxation and toning, and attention to holistic and spiritual health, including the use of herbs, massage, and meditation, also reflect the influence of the alternative birth movement on mainstream pregnancy and birthing practices.

LOOKING TO THE FUTURE

Even though changes can be seen in how our country views pregnancy, most women still hand over that responsibility to the medical profession, awaiting validation at regular intervals that their bodies are—or are not—working. We wait for confirmation of pregnancy from a doctor or a home pregnancy test because we have lost trust in the sensations and messages that arise from within us. We think we need someone to tell us that we're pregnant, that our babies are growing, that our pelvis is big enough, etc. Despite the enormous contribution and progress of the women's self-help movement, most women have no idea what their cervix looks or feels like, what nutrients they need for a healthy pregnancy, or what their uterus does to help the baby get born. We have so thoroughly externalized information about our bodies, and have become so doubtful of our bodies' abilities, that we see pregnancy and birth as fully medical events—almost as if it is the ultrasounds, alpha-fetoprotein tests, and chorionic villi samples that make the baby healthy. Yet ultrasounds have not been proven safe for babies, alpha-fetoprotein tests have an exceptionally high false positive margin, and chorionic villi sampling has resulted in babies with missing limbs.

I am not suggesting that we abandon all prenatal testing. I do question the routine use of invasive testing and the way such testing affects the ability of a woman to form a strong, intuitive connection with her baby. I also wonder how a woman can give birth naturally or trust herself to be a mother if she can't trust her body to grow a healthy baby. At a time when a woman should be developing into a confident parent, the medical profession in general deals a severe blow to that developing confidence by making her dependent upon its experts for guidance.

Further, women who choose to forego such invasive prenatal testing are frequently subjected to guilt, especially if a problem does arise. All women should be encouraged to trust their bodies' ability to nurture a child and should be free to request or forego medical interventions during pregnancy without emotional coercion. True freedom means being able to say no, as well as being able to say yes.

I propose that women consider what it would be like to regain confidence in ourselves, beginning with the experiences that our bodies present to us through our reproductive cycles, if not before. Regaining confidence in our bodies, it seems to me, is the most challenging aspect in overcoming what we have lost in our complex history of childbearing.

It is within our grasp as women and mothers to determine what pregnancy and prenatal care will be as we move into the twenty-first century. Will we become so convinced that technological intervention is wiser than our bodies' natural processes? Or will we welcome these processes and come to view our bodies—indeed, ourselves—with respect for our strengths, power, and beauty?

Becoming Body Centered

HOW OUR CULTURE DEFINES OUR BODIES

On TV and in other media, our culture can be seen as body-image-centered, not body-centered. Most of us therefore relate to our bodies not by what we feel but by how we think we look to others. We base our feelings about our bodies on our appearance. This often leads to dangerous patterns. Dieting, for example, has become a major focus for many women. Studies report that in the 1980s and 1990s there has been an explosion of eating disorders, particularly in teenage girls. An estimated eight million American women are reported as anorexic, bulimic, or compulsive dieters.

Commercials and advertisements offer an array of products that will make our bodies cleaner, more convenient, and more pleasant smelling. What are the effects on our psyches of such an implied contempt for the female body and the view of its functions as fundamentally dirty? It is only when we decide not to sanitize our bodies in order to make them conform to external standards that we become capable of understanding the language of our bodies.

BECOMING BODY-CENTERED

According to Dr. Christiane Northrup, an obstetrician and gynecologist and a specialist in holistic health for women, "The state of a woman's health is indeed completely tied up with the culture in which she lives and her position in it, as well as in the way she lives her life as an individual. We cannot hope to reclaim our bodily wisdom and inherent ability to create health without first understanding the influence of our society on how we think and care for our bodies." How we think about and care for our bodies is the basis for how we feel during pregnancy. Therefore, it is important to look at some of the underlying beliefs and attitudes that women in our culture are exposed to and too often internalize. By understanding and redefining your relationship with your body, you will be improving the likelihood that you experience pregnancy as a positive and magical process.

Not only does popular media cause us to distrust our bodies' natural processes, the medical profession, into whose hands most of us were literally born, has conditioned us to rely on its experts for answers to our questions about our bodies. Conventional medicine subordinates our subjective knowing, emphasizing that our ability to heal is not an innate human capacity, but a result of medical training and techniques. We are taught that normal processes such as birth, menopause, and death are processes that require medical supervision and intervention. It is not encouraged, or even acknowledged, that we have the ability to be healthy without constant medical assistance. We learn that fatigue, hunger, sadness, stress, headaches, menstrual cramps, the sensations of childbirth, and most other physical feelings that are uncomfortable or unpleasant can be suppressed. We are not taught that these feelings are the language of our bodies, and that our bodies speak to us more and more strongly until we are finally forced to sit up and listen. This happens usually when we ignore little messages until they turn into discomforts, then symptoms, then outright diseases. But we can change this conditioning by listening to our bodies.

LEARNING TO LISTEN TO YOUR BODY

Each of us receives messages daily from our body, informing us when, what, and how much to eat, when to sleep, when to exercise our muscles, when to have a bowel movement, etc. Your body is quick to detect, through cellular responses of assimilation and rejection, when you are nourishing yourself and when you are harming yourself. This is true of not only foods and substances that you ingest, but also situations in which you find yourself, and thoughts and feelings you have. You can feel these responses, if you pay attention, in your nerves and muscles. For example, you may find that areas of your body tense up in a stressful situation, or that you sneeze in a room where a cat has recently been, if you are allergic to cats.

The concept of being body-centered is not meant to imply separation of the body, mind, and emotions. In fact, all of these faculties are inextricably connected and interwoven in the organism we call a human. On a literal and biological level one cannot say that the mind begins here and ends there, as if the mind were only the brain, and the body everything below the brain. Actually, nerve pathways, hormones, and genetic messages course throughout the body, connecting the messages of the brain throughout the body, and vice versa, from the entire body to the brain—the brain is part of the whole body. Feelings occur when internal, physiological processes trigger various emotional responses, as well as when external situations trigger biological and emotional reactions.

Becoming body-centered is in no way meant to imply that you shouldn't exercise your intellect—quite the contrary. However, it is possible for your thoughts to subvert your emotions and physical sensations in a culture where we are taught to do so. Being body-centered means unlearning the process of subverting your body, while still using your intelligence. You can learn to override and transform the culturally imposed and inauthentic voices that tell you how you should think and how you should be, so that you know and accept who and how you truly are.

All women would benefit by listening to their bodies, and ideally women will learn this skill prior to pregnancy. However, if you are new to this idea, pregnancy is a particularly ripe time for learning to do so, because it is a time when your body manifests many new and noticeable messages.

Learning to listen to your body, like learning any language, takes time, commitment, and practice. People who are fluent in numerous languages often comment that the best way to learn a new language is to be totally immersed in hearing it, such as by spending time in a foreign country, or at least by surrounding oneself with native

with an opportunity to be around other women who are also trying to understand the language of their own bodies. Women who have already had children, "native speakers" if you will, are often eager to share their experiences. Spending time with women who have had natural and healthy experiences may help you gain comfort and confidence listening to the unique language of your own body.

Pregnant women not only experience dramatic physical transformations, but also emotional and social transformations, as our perceptions of ourselves as mothers grow, and as our social roles and responsibilities

speakers of that language. Pregnancy, though not separate from the continuity of a woman's life, is a unique experience permitting a time of total immersion in the language of the body, with many heightened physical sensations. Women are also apt to speak more freely with one another about their bodies when they are pregnant than they are at any other time, providing you

change. However, unless we reflect about our attitudes toward our bodies and make a commitment to loving and trusting our bodies, we run the risk of carrying harmful patterns into our pregnancies. For example, a woman with an eating disorder may not allow herself and her baby to gain enough weight to nurture herself and her baby for a healthy pregnancy, birth, and postpartum.

It's amazing what fears float around in our society about birth. At times it takes a grand effort to swim past the worries. I try to stay focused on my love for my baby and my desire for him or her to be born in pure gentleness. In general I have a deep and underlying faith in my body wisdom and the baby's as well.

—A. J. R.

A woman who feels she is fat or not beautiful may become very depressed when her body seems to be getting bigger as pregnancy progresses. This depression, unpleasant in itself, can also lead to physical problems such as poor dietary habits, bad posture, and further problems such as constipation or lower backache. This is just a simple example of how poor self-image, based on comparing oneself to a cultural ideal, may be harmful during pregnancy.

Perhaps the most practical way to begin listening to your body is to pay attention to the most common messages you receive daily: hunger, thirst, fatigue, and elimination. Try to notice when you begin to feel the sensations that alert you to eat, drink, rest, or go to the bathroom. What are these sensations? When do you notice them? And most important, how do you respond to them? For example:

- Do you eat when you're hungry, or do you think about whether you should eat, and then skip a meal, afraid that if you eat too much you might get fat?

- Do you urinate when you feel the urge to, or like so many women, do you wait until a more convenient time or until you just can't wait any longer? Many women do the latter, not realizing that this can cause urinary tract infections, which women are especially susceptible to during pregnancy.

- Do you allow yourself to rest or sleep when you feel fatigued, or do you keep pushing yourself to do more until you collapse at the end of the day? Or do you push your body further with the help of coffee, chocolate, or sugar? Do you get down on yourself for being tired, thinking that you should be getting more done?

- Do you recognize that you may be feeling weepy, irritable, nauseous, faint, cold, and clammy, or that you have a headache because your blood sugar is too low and you need to eat a solid meal?

- Did you know that particular food cravings are your body's way of calling out for specific nutrients? For example, you may be craving sweets because you need more energy, but your body really needs more protein, which will provide you with more lasting energy.

Like many women you may realize that you are not listening to your body. Just by deciding to be more alert to your own needs, you'll find yourself recognizing and responding to your body's signals more readily, and you will feel better for doing so. Keeping a journal can be a useful method for charting specific urges or sensations, as well as your responses and reactions. Remember that it takes time and patience to learn any language, but that you and your baby both deserve optimal care and loving attention.

FEELINGS AND FEARS ABOUT YOUR BODY

Another aspect of being body-centered is to admit to yourself how you truly feel about your body. If you stand before a mirror unclothed do you find yourself criticizing parts of your body? Do you criticize your nose, breasts, thighs, or buttocks? Try to understand where those critical messages came from—were you criticized as a child, as a teenager by other kids, or do you compare yourself to the images on magazine covers? Try to replace those old, critical voices with positive messages called affirmations—for example, "I love my body for growing my baby so well" or "I love these breasts which will provide my baby with warm and nourishing milk." You can create not only a greater appreciation of your body by doing this, but can actually improve your health by giving yourself positive affirmations about your inherently miraculous, beautiful, and unique self.

It is also helpful to acknowledge fears that you have about your body—for example, if you carry an undercurrent of fear that you won't be able to breastfeed, or are afraid that your cervix won't dilate adequately in labor. All of us have heard stories of such problems, and sometimes we internalize other people's experiences. Being in a constant state of low-level fear can directly affect wellness and increase the likelihood of that problem occurring. If you harbor fears, or suspect you might, talk to your body in a loving way, saying something positive instead. Give yourself permission to accept and love your body just as it is, and trust that your body is perfectly designed for health. For example, if you fear that your cervix won't dilate adequately in labor, one of the things you can do is to tell yourself daily, "My cervix will soften and open to birth my beautiful baby." You can visualize your cervix as a flower bud, gently and steadily opening, and you can put visual reminders of your opening cervix around your home: photographs of fully opened blossoms, or of the planet Saturn with its wide rings encircling the round planet much the way your cervix will eventually open around your baby's head.

The basic idea is that if you have a negative body image you can work actively to transform yourself into someone who feels genuinely good about herself and her abilities. You can use a journal for writing loving affirmations to your body. Expressive artwork, such as drawing, is also a way to create positive images for yourself.

The most useful skill any of us have for responding to the messages that arise is *feeling*. From our earliest experiences we are taught to squelch our emotions ("it's not nice to be angry," "don't cry"—sometimes followed by "or I'll give you something to cry about," or "you're a scaredy-cat") and to follow our intellect. We have also been taught that unpleasant physical sensations are a nuisance, and have been encouraged to suppress such sensations with medication or by putting on a happy face. We were not taught that emotions are both a signal of our comfort or discomfort in a given situation or environment, and that our physical sensations let us know what is going on in our bodies. We were also never taught that our physical sensations can reflect our emotions. The best way to regain this knowledge is simply to stop and feel. If you have a headache coming on you don't have to reach for the aspirin, or even herbs, nor do you have to analyze why you have a headache. By becoming very still and relaxed, and paying attention to your body from this still place, you will find that you can gain an awareness of exactly what you need to do for yourself—perhaps eat, drink water, rest, or remove yourself from a stressful situation. Perhaps an herbal remedy will help, or speaking with a friend or health care provider. However, first you need to get in touch with that part of you that is your best authority. Try paying attention to how you feel emotionally about the sensations or discomforts you are having, and see what information you get from allowing yourself to feel your feelings. No one knows you better than you!

MOVING YOUR BODY JOYOUSLY

Becoming body-centered requires us to be oriented to our physical needs, and this includes spending time enjoying and nurturing our bodies. Bodies need to be moved, sometimes slowly and gracefully, sometimes quickly and with some force.

Activities such as yoga, dance, swimming, walking briskly, volleyball, tennis, cross-country skiing, horseback riding, Tai Chi, you name it (as long as it is safe if you are already pregnant) are all ways to move your body joyously and exuberantly. They fill your body with vitality, stimulate your circulation (which improves cardiovascular functioning), oxygenate the body, enliven your mind, and lift and prevent depression. You not only improve your health and prepare your body for the very physical work of birth, but you enrich your body awareness and self-esteem.

Regular massage is also a way to get in touch with and enjoy your body as you let tension melt away. In addition, massage is a form of passive exercise for the recipient, with many of the benefits of physical exercise, such as improved circulation and removal of waste products from the muscles. Scheduling problems and the high cost for professional massage need not prohibit you from exploring this possibility for nurturing your body. Your mate or a friend can give you a massage. Even as little as twenty minutes of massage on an occasional basis will be beneficial. See Chapter 7 for further discussions and explanations of both movement and massage techniques for pregnancy.

As you learn to release tension from your body and develop appreciation and respect for your body, you will gradually find yourself better able to respond to and nourish yourself. And you will discover that as you take better care of yourself, you will feel happier and healthier, and that your self-esteem and positive body-image will come from within. You will like yourself just for being who you are.

RECLAIMING WOMEN'S WISDOM

Women's wisdom is a term used to encompass the practices and beliefs that women have developed over centuries, and that still benefit women today. Among these are midwifery, nourishing and therapeutic methods of food preparation, herbalism, healing touch, and many other kinds of healing that can enrich our lives. Women have often been the primary physicians for their families, tribes, and villages. These are the main healing modalities which I draw upon in this book.

Women's wisdom is also based on the stories that women tell about their lives and what we can learn from these stories. Women's wisdom allows us to bring our whole selves into the treatment, rather than fragmenting parts of ourselves. Likewise, in women's ways of healing there is the awareness that healing must occur in the person's life, not just in her body, and that physical healing alone cannot occur until the underlying factors of illness and discomfort are addressed. These factors may be as simple as finding more time in your own life, say thirty minutes twice a week, to nurture yourself in whatever way suits you.

Women's wisdom also embraces our subjective knowledge based on feelings and personal experience. This intuition may include dreaming about your baby before conception and sensing who the child will be, and transpersonal knowing, such as having abdominal cramps only to discover that your best friend or sister is in early labor. These are all without logical explanation, they are sympathetic experiences that allow us to realize the psychic aspects of our connection to our bodies and to each other.

These experiences remind us that there is more to life than what meets the eye, and that there really is no separation between the mind, body, and spirit.

Women have always been considered more psychic, more closely related to the mysterious aspects of life due to menstruation, pregnancy, and ability to birth our young. Our culture has discredited this multi-sensory awareness, considering it unreliable, even nonexistent. Women's wisdom, like much of the work that women do, is based on the human aspects of life and valuing emotional and sensory experiences. Women have long recognized the deep psychic connections between a mother and child, knowing, for example, even from thousands of miles away when a child is well or in danger. Breastfeeding mothers are all too familiar with the experience of having their breasts begin to leak milk while they are at work, only to find out later that their baby had awakened from a nap at the same time and was crying for her. This kind of intuitive awareness is too common to be dismissed as coincidental and too valuable for us to dismiss as fallacious.

To reclaim women's wisdom is to put feminine modes of intuition and intelligence into their respected places among the many options available to us for our health care. To reclaim women's wisdom we have to proclaim that we are the true authorities about ourselves, and we have to reinstate traditionally feminine methods of healing as part of a sensible approach to medicine and wellness.

One of the ways that I and other women have chosen to reclaim what is rightfully ours is to replace the word vagina with the word "yoni." Vagina literally means a sheath, and is obviously a reference to the fact that our sexual organs exist only in relationship to men's needs. The word yoni, however, is a Sanskrit word for the female genitalia, and refers to the sacredness of a woman's sexual self. In this book you will often see the word yoni used where you might commonly use the word vagina.

PELVIC CROSS-VIEW

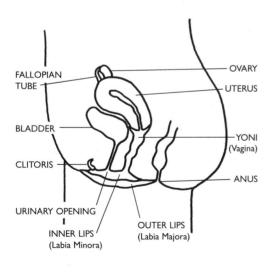

FALLOPIAN TUBE
OVARY
UTERUS
BLADDER
YONI (Vagina)
CLITORIS
ANUS
URINARY OPENING
INNER LIPS (Labia Minora)
OUTER LIPS (Labia Majora)

PELVIC FRONT VIEW

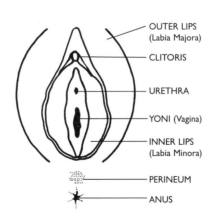

OUTER LIPS (Labia Majora)
CLITORIS
URETHRA
YONI (Vagina)
INNER LIPS (Labia Minora)
PERINEUM
ANUS

Learning to trust and recognize our intuition and body messages is particularly valuable for pregnant women. Pregnancy is a time when you and your baby are experiencing many increased nutritional demands, as well as a greater need for nourishment in other areas, such as massage, exercise, rest, and relaxation. Our body awareness alerts us to our needs, and our intuition can help us to name exactly what we need to do to meet these. One example of using intuitive guidance occurred with a very young couple having their first baby, with whom I worked long ago. The woman, actually still a teenager, had a very poor diet, consisting in large part of pizza and candy bars. I felt that she needed to recognize what her body told her she needed to eat. I taught her and her partner the following exercise: I had them sit facing each other, holding hands. I suggested they ask the baby what he or she needed right now for optimal nourishment. They were both completely silent for a few moments, waiting for a response from the baby. When they both become quite still, I told them to open their eyes and voice what they heard. Simultaneously, both the father and the mother said, "Carrots, the baby needs more carrots." So the mother ate more carrots, practiced this exercise more often, improved her diet greatly, and gave birth very easily (after a three-hour labor) at home to a healthy baby.

Today, as we try to ensure the healthy development of our babies during pregnancy we can look beyond the conventional prenatal care offered by a typical obstetrician. Exploring your intuitive connection with your baby and trusting your inner wisdom can help you grow a healthy baby.

As you explore the various healing options available for supporting pregnancy health, I invite you to reacquaint yourself with your women's wisdom, and discover the techniques that can best nourish you, your baby, and your family.

The Baby Inside You

For me conception rings a bell of immediate awareness in the center of my being. I know as soon as I conceive. Within days my body tells me that I am no longer just myself, but have a new companion. With each child the experience is a bit different.

With my first I could see an imaginary door open above me and light begin to pour through as my mate and I came together, with my second I had vivid dreams of seeing a magnificent seashell in the ocean, too deep for me to reach, so my husband dove for it. The shell he handed me had a deep pink, shimmering lining that in waking consciousness reminded me of my womb's lining. At my third child's conception my husband and I felt a breeze come over us, as if a door opened, and with my fourth baby, somehow, I just knew she was with me. With the first couple of babies I did home pregnancy tests (one of which was negative, though I was pregnant) to confirm what my body and spirit already knew, but after that I chose just to trust my gut feelings and my subtle physical sensations. This was part of my personal commitment to trust my body to tell me what I needed to know. As soon as I felt that I had conceived, I treated myself as if I was definitely pregnant, eating extra well, resting, and avoiding anything that might be harmful to my newly growing child. From the onset this was my child, not an embryo or a fetus with potential defects or a pregnancy with potential complications, but my child. I truly believe that it is partially this attitude that has nurtured health in each child. But had one of my babies not been perfectly healthy, that baby would still have felt loved and accepted from the beginning.

Later in this book you will find a discussion of the various prenatal diagnostic tests that are commonly offered to pregnant women. There are times when these tests are medically warranted; however, routine use of such testing can prevent a woman from developing and trusting her connection with

It is my sincerest hope that those who read this book will be inspired to listen to and respect their bodies, and, in doing so, find a sense of well-being and confidence that will assist them throughout their lives.

—*A. J. R.*

her baby. The real connection between a mother and her baby pre-exists a connection that is fostered by seeing the baby on a screen, knowing whether the baby is a boy or a girl, or hearing the baby's heartbeat by electronic amplification.

While it is true that you may feel more confident in your pregnancy after receiving some objective measure of your health or the baby's health via a prenatal diagnostic test (keeping in mind that many tests of fetal well-being are inaccurate), you will have to decide for yourself at what point you draw the line between a natural experience and a technological experience. Therefore it is up to you to be well-informed as to the benefits, risks, and necessity of such testing, and to choose for yourself what you do and don't want done. Developing a strong prenatal connection with your baby, as well as trusting in your inner knowing will enable you to make the most appropriate use of technology during birth, your children's early years, and possibly later.

While the intention of this chapter is to facilitate your inner awareness of your baby, having a clear visual idea of how babies generally develop can help make the conscious connection with your baby more tangible. As a midwife I am so aware of feeling babies' arms, legs, little bottoms, and heads while still in their mamas' wombs, that a baby in the womb is almost as tangible to me as a baby in arms. However, pregnant women often sense that their baby is inside, kicking, rolling, and playing, yet the wholeness of this actually being a baby, a real person that will one day be in their arms, is often overlooked. The same goes for the dads. Therefore at each prenatal visit I show the parents or mother how to feel and massage her baby so that this awareness is strengthened. This chapter will be devoted to the development of the baby, and the impor-

tance of the prenatal environment for your baby, as well as communicating with your baby prenatally.

YOUR GROWING BABY

The following discussion of a baby's development begins at conception, this being "week one." However, most health care practitioners measure pregnancy from the first date of the last menstrual period, which is generally two weeks prior to conception. This comes out to ten lunar months—also the way that women in many traditional cultures counted their pregnancies and determined when they were due—ten lunar months from their last period. If you are trying to compare the following information with how far along you are in your pregnancy, count the weeks from conception which is generally two weeks fewer than the number of weeks you are figured to be pregnant by your physician or midwife. This will also vary slightly according to the length of your menstrual cycles. For example, if your period occurs every five weeks you will likely be a week further behind. And of course, each baby has an individual growth rate. If you want a general idea of what stage of growth your baby is in, read about the development of a week before and a week after your week's gestation.

— Conception —

Conception occurs and pregnancy begins when the sperm and ovum unite. This brings both parents' genetic potential into contact and creates the physical foundation of a new life—your baby. Fertilization generally occurs in the fallopian tube and then over the next five days, as the "zygote" divides into a cluster comprised of numerous cells, it makes its way toward the uterus, where by about the sixth day it attaches to the uterine lining. The process of implantation is complete by about the tenth or eleventh day after conception. By the end of the first two weeks the placental formation has begun and the cells of the baby are beginning to differentiate. The first two weeks are known as the pre-embryonic phase.

— Weeks Three Through Seven —

From week three through week seven the developing baby is referred to as an embryo. It is during this remarkable period of development that all of the baby's essential features and body parts will be formed. Because it is the most vulnerable phase of development for the baby, it is important for pregnant women to avoid all substances such as alcohol and drugs (including many prescription and over-the-counter medications), and environmental contaminants such as pesticides, chemical fumes, and cigarette smoke, which could harm the baby.

By the fifteenth day after conception when you might be expecting your period to start, you may notice breast tenderness and a feeling of fullness in your abdomen. You may find that your hair is hard to manage. This is the way you would normally feel before your period. If you tried to conceive, you may have already begun to take special care of yourself even before you missed your period. If your period is late then it is sensible to treat yourself as if you were pregnant until it becomes evident that you are not. This will afford your baby optimal protection for healthy development.

During week three the shape of the baby begins to take form.

During week four the heart begins beating and by the end of this week the embryo has assumed the appearance of a salamander. There are arm and leg buds, facial and neck structures, and small pits that will later become the ears. By the end of this week your baby is less than 1/4 of an inch long.

The fifth week brings extensive growth of the brain and head and the beginning development of the eyes. Because a baby's growth occurs from top to bottom, the head is large in relation to the body.

During the sixth week since conception, the nose, mouth, and palate take shape, and the eyelids have formed. By this time the arms and legs make rapid development so that by the seventh week the baby has clearly defined wrists, elbows, knees, fingers, and toes, etc. The baby is now about 1/2 inch long.

In the seventh week the baby's urogenital system is developing, the neck area is established, and the external ears are visible. By the end of this week the baby clearly looks like a human baby. The end of the seventh week is also the end of what is called the embryonic period.

At this point all of the baby's essential structures, both internal and external, have been formed and require only further growth and development. By now the baby can respond to touch: if it were possible to touch the baby's palm, the baby's hand would close. The baby can touch his or her own face, as well as make other gentle movements.

— Week Ten —

At ten weeks the baby will begin to have both hair and fingernails and one can begin to differentiate boys from girls.

— Week Twelve —

By twelve weeks the baby is about 3 3/4 inches long and weighs about an ounce. The baby is able to make facial expressions, and the lips can make sucking motions. In fact the baby can now swallow amniotic fluid and

20 weeks

24 weeks

28 weeks

pee it out, too. The eyes are almost fully developed and the lids fused closed while the rest of this development occurs. By this time your uterus is about the size of a large grapefruit and you are already entering the second trimester of your pregnancy. If you have been nauseous and uncomfortable, you will soon begin to feel much better.

— Week Fourteen —

At fourteen weeks the baby is covered with lanugo, downy hair that grows in whorls over the body, and the baby has fingerprints. Nipples appear, and the back, which has been curved, straightens. The bones are hardening and the baby, who fills your womb, is now becoming more active. You may even notice movement, particularly when you are resting.

— Week Sixteen —

By sixteen weeks the baby measures about 7 or 8 inches in length and weighs about 4 ounces.

— Month Five —

At five months the legs reach their full length and toenails form. By now you are likely to notice some subtle fluttering movements or even some obvious "kicks and pokes." If you've not yet noticed movement it is likely that you will soon. The baby also hiccups occasionally which you will feel as a series of rhythmic "knocks" in your belly. Your baby can suck his or her thumb, can grasp the umbilical cord, and can even scratch his or her face. There is more hair on the head and eyebrows are formed. The eyes are still fused shut. The body is now covered with vernix (which literally translates as "cheese"), a creamy substance that protects the baby's skin while surrounded by water. The heart-

beat may now be audible by fetoscope and will usually range between 120 and 160 beats per minute. The baby's ears are now fully functional, and because water conducts sound so well (when we are underwater sounds are muffled because we have air in our ears, but babies have no air in theirs while in the womb), the baby hears sounds all of the time—the rhythms of your heart and breath, the placenta, and your digestion, as well as all of your speaking, singing, crying, yelling, praying, and so on. The baby is able to hear and respond to music and will also respond to your emotions with more or less gentle movements. It is therefore optimal to surround yourself with beautiful and soothing music, as well as making your own sounds as peaceful, joyous, and comforting as possible. Through sound the baby begins to learn about the world. Your baby is now about 10 or 12 inches long and weighs about 8 ounces.

— Month Six —

At six months the skin is wrinkled, translucent, and appears red due to the blood being visible through the skin. Permanent tooth buds are present and hair growth is obvious. The eyes are open again and the baby can make both crying and sucking motions. Strong arm and leg muscles have developed and if the foot is tickled the baby will respond by planting the foot downward. You may notice that the baby responds to your touch with movements. The baby is 12–14 inches long and weighs about 1 1/2 pounds.

— Month Seven —

At seven months the lungs, though not fully mature, could function minimally outside the uterus. The baby would have a good chance of survival if born prematurely at this point. The baby now sees sunlight through your abdomen and will turn away from very bright light. He or she is about 15 inches long and weighs 3 to 4 pounds. The baby will gain about 1/2 pound a week.

— Month Eight —

During the eighth month the baby begins to put on fat and the wrinkled skin begins to smooth out. Vernix and lanugo still cover the baby except for the face, but these will gradually lessen in quantity by birth. The eyes are open and the lungs are much stronger. The baby is between 16 and 18 inches long and may weigh between 4 and 7 pounds.

— Month Nine —

At nine months the lanugo and vernix have begun to disappear and the baby is reaching full maturity, ready for life outside of your womb. All of the sense organs are well-formed and the rest of the organs are ready for extra-uterine life. The wrinkles have disappeared and the baby's head will begin to settle into your pelvis, ready for birth. The baby is now 19–21 inches long and on the average weighs between 6 and 9 pounds.

CREATING A NOURISHING PRENATAL ENVIRONMENT

During pregnancy you are quite literally your child's environment. So how can you create a home for your baby that is stable, nourishing, comfortable, and soothing? Well, in truth, you cannot do this 100 percent of the time, nor is this necessary. Every pregnant woman will experience some stress, whether it be a car that won't start or a toddler who spills things fifty times a day, or important deadlines that must be met, or

clothing that doesn't fit. These stresses are temporary, and if you can deal with them without internalizing the stress to the point that you skip meals or lose sleep, your baby is unlikely to be affected. Even anxieties caused by financial issues, marital tensions, or housing problems, for example, can be resolved without upsetting your baby, provided that you take care of yourself responsibly and that you maintain communication with your baby, letting her or him know that yes, there is stress occurring right now in your life, but you still love and welcome the baby, and will in time resolve the stress. While the baby might not intellectually understand the exact reasons for the tension, she or he will have a sympathetic sense of your emotional state, as your state of mind influences the hormones, oxygen, and blood flow the baby receives. When you feel tense the baby receives tension signals, and when you relax, so can the baby.

There are, however, situations that can cause both temporary and extended emotional impact to babies, and this may be of either a physical or psychological nature, or both. Some situations that occur are unpredictable and are part of the challenging experience of being human, for example, the death of someone you love, the loss of a job, an accident, or other misfortune. Such experiences challenge the soul and if they cause ongoing grief they can cause the mother to withdraw from nourishing herself as well as providing the baby with emotional attention. It will take great will and strength of spirit to overcome such adversity and maintain the focus on creating a healthy environment for the baby.

Fortunately most of us do not experience traumas of such magnitude during pregnancy. Nonetheless, we can let the stresses of our lives consume and preoccupy

32 weeks

36 weeks

40 weeks

We can nourish our babies so that they may enjoy prenatal wellness and be prepared to meet the inevitable challenges of the world.

—A. J. R.

us to such an extent that the results are similar—we withdraw our attention from physically and emotionally nourishing ourselves and our babies. In addition, our emotional reactions, such as depression, anger, or sadness, and the reactions and expressions of others, especially our mates, can have a profound effect on the baby's well-being. The hormones you produce during such stressful times can reduce the flow of oxygen and nutrients to the baby; babies will react to intense and unpleasant emotional outbursts with vigorous kicking. Extended stress can result in failure to thrive and emotional insecurity. Such behavioral patterns that are established in the womb can persist as life-long patterns of physical and emotional illness to varying degrees depending on the intensity of the situation.

Furthermore, habits of the mother such as smoking cigarettes and drinking alcohol or using other drugs, all of which have notably harmful physical effects, may also have adverse psychological effects on the baby, as the baby lives in a constant state of negative expectancy, never knowing when the mother will again engage in the behavior that causes the baby to be poisoned or asphyxiated or have other harmful physiological responses. Listening to rock music has also been shown to cause an adverse reaction in the baby, leading to violent kicking. Even rushing around all day, day after day, can cause a baby to become overstimulated and affect his or her development.

Of course all of this places a great responsibility on the woman to act wisely. This responsibility should not be shouldered by mothers alone, but shared by fathers and the culture in general. Women should be supported in appropriate ways so that they have the time to eat well, rest, exercise, and engage in activities that nourish

their body and spirit. No woman should have to worry about an abusive husband, how she will feed herself or her children, or whether she will be fired from her job for taking days off to care for herself. Unfortunately, that type of support does not always exist in our homes or in society. As mothers we must work together to create such changes. The choice is ours: we can nourish our babies so that they may enjoy prenatal wellness and be prepared to meet the inevitable challenges of the world, or start them with emotional and physical difficulties that leave them less prepared to succeed in this complex world.

How we respond to stress is up to us. None of us has to have a drink or a cigarette—these are personal choices. When you fully grasp the importance of the connection between you and your baby, the choices become more apparent—you'd never give your baby a beer or a cigarette. Similarly, when your awareness extends to the effects of your emotional state on your baby, and how these can adversely or beneficially influence your child's sense of security, belonging, confidence, and emotional health, it becomes most important to surround your child with a sense of well-being, even in the midst of a struggle. As many mothers of young babies have experienced, if the mother can stay calm even in the midst of chaos, the baby is more likely to do so, and if you are very upset, the baby will likewise become fussy and irritable. The next section explores how to communicate well-being to your baby throughout your pregnancy. These skills learned now will help you deal with stresses that sometimes arise during parenting while still letting your daughter or son know that she or he is loved, safe, and is a welcome member of your family. In turn your child will also learn to make use of these skills.

COMMUNICATING WITH YOUR BABY

Communicating with your baby, as with anyone, is a two-way exchange—that is, you can communicate with your baby and he or she can communicate with you. It is quite possible for this communication to begin even before pregnancy occurs through dreams and extrasensory awareness. For example, before I conceived my second child I had a vivid dream, which I recorded in my journal, of being in a snowstorm with a close woman friend. In the dream she went into a room and I assisted her at the birth of her child, a girl, and then I went into an adjacent room and birthed my own baby, also a girl. Several months after this dream my friend conceived a baby, and in the following month I too conceived. Later I assisted her—in the midst of a snowstorm—at the birth of her daughter, and weeks later I birthed my baby, also a daughter.

It has been my experience as a woman, a mother, and a midwife, that babies need our love for their health as much as they need food. They have a genetic and biological imperative to be loved and touched, talked to and soothed, long before birth. And loving our babies prenatally not only nourishes them, it feeds us in return, for all of the spiritual forces that help to grow our babies return the gift of love to us. We become infused with grace and light. The connection we build is one that can never be severed. Unlike the tangible, physical umbilical cord that becomes detached after birth, the deep connection we build deliberately with our babies will prevail, preventing detachment from ever developing. Many mothers feel this even though they didn't build a prenatal bond with their babies. We are even more blessed with empathy for our children when we open our hearts to them from the beginning. Fathers, too, can develop and benefit from such prenatal bonding.

— Talking to Your Baby —

It is not hard to speak to your baby. Talk to the child inside of you throughout your day, sharing even mundane tasks, the music you love, your musings about the beauty of the world around you. When you feel sadness or anger, talk to your baby about it. Although the child may not intellectually understand your concerns, he or she will feel the calm and soothing nature of your voice which will reassure the child that you are both okay. Massage your baby during the day by rubbing and patting your belly, and also each morning when you rise or each evening before you sleep. During these relaxed times put a little oil on your hands and rub deeply, actually massaging the parts of the baby's body that you feel. This cannot hurt your baby, and babies respond positively to such caring both during the pregnancy with excellent growth as well as after birth. Babies that have been regularly massaged prenatally will love to be massaged throughout childhood. This is an excellent technique for the prevention of illness as well as a remedial treatment. Talk to your baby as you massage her or his body or sing a special, beautiful song. Chances are the baby will continue to be soothed by this song after birth and will quickly learn to sing it once she or he learns to speak.

Some mothers enjoy reading verses of poetry or even children's books to their babies even before birth. These books will probably become your child's all-time favorites, as babies definitely have exhibited preferences from their prenatal time.

If you listen to your baby and be very quiet, you may "hear" your baby telling you something important.

—A. J. R.

Speaking affirmations to your child can foster your confidence as well as nourish the baby's growth with ideas that reinforce his or her well-being. For example, as you massage your baby you can repeat a few times, rhythmically, "You are so welcome and wanted here, we love you so," or "You are a strong and healthy baby," or "I welcome you for whoever you are." These positive statements can also be used to help you dispel anxieties that may creep into your mind about the baby's health or normal development. As you get closer to the birth you can say things like: "We are so ready for you to be born, we welcome you into our open arms," or "It is safe to be born, and we look forward to holding and caring for you, dear baby."

—Listening to Your Baby —

Listening to your baby takes inner trust and quiet. Each day when you take time to quietly rub your baby, become silent and ask your baby, either in your mind or aloud, what he or she needs, and how you can best serve your child's needs. Ask if there is anything the baby wants you to know. Then just listen very quietly and you may be surprised at what you hear. You may not hear a baby's "voice" but in time you may feel a message coming through to you.

Many women find themselves experiencing an intense need to be near their mates during pregnancy, odd desires for foods, and even yearnings to be in certain environments such as at the beach or in a forest. While we cannot assume that all of our emotions and desires stem from the baby, the baby does make his or her will and desires known through the mother. If you find yourself having feelings, thoughts, or desires that are unfamiliar, you may try to take the view that the baby may be trying to communicate with you.

Dreams are another vehicle for your baby to communicate with you. Many women dream that their baby is already born and is a child of three years old or so. When you dream of your baby, try to talk and listen. However, it is not necessary to take all birth dreams literally. Many women

will have disturbing dreams of a deformed baby or other problems, yet these dreams are most often not really premonitions. They frequently are simply a landscape in which women can safely explore their anxieties. Women who work out these anxieties prenatally often experience smooth births and have healthy babies. If you have particularly disturbing dreams, discuss this with your midwife or a trusted friend.

THE NATURAL PREGNANCY BOOK

— *Creative Insights* —

Keeping a journal of your insights about your baby or dreams can be a delightful way to preserve these experiences for both of you to cherish for decades to come. Make a note of the words to the songs you sing, stories you read to the baby, or particularly magical places you visit during your pregnancy.

One of my favorite forms of receiving insight about my baby is through artwork. I am not a professional artist, nor am I artistically gifted. I just enjoy the experience of creating so I'll sit down with a blank paper and supplies, and let my body talk through whatever medium I am using. I find that colored chalks and oil pastels reflect the subtle energy of pregnancy in that lines and colors can be blended to create a smooth, soft image. Many supplies are available inexpensively at an art supply store. You can therefore enjoy yourself without spending a fortune. I've found myself creating images of angels' wings surrounding babies, mothers holding babies, buds opening, and so on. Let your body speak to you. Go deep within yourself to find the reservoir of creativity that resides in your womanplace, and express yourself from there. Artwork can open and release blocked creative energy and be highly therapeutic, but only if you do it for enjoyment and don't judge your results.

The joyous welcoming of your child into your life sends messages to your child that will help him or her to thrive and develop a sense of self-esteem long before birth. None of us can be happy 100 percent of the time, but we can choose to stay in close touch with the messages we are sending our babies. How we treat them prenatally can set the tone for how they will treat themselves and expect others to treat them for much of their lives. While prenatal influences are not the only influences that emboss patterns on our psyches and emotions, they do hold great sway over us. We can help a whole generation of children to feel loved. And this will sow the seeds of loving each other and creating a just world coming from our most evolved awareness.

CHAPTER 4

Prenatal Care

WHAT IS PRENATAL CARE?

The most significant prenatal care a woman receives is the care a woman gives herself—ultimately it is this care that all other forms of prenatal care should nurture.

When most people refer to prenatal care they mean prenatal medical monitoring. Focused on detecting and reducing problems such as premature delivery, birth defects, and infant mortality, conventional prenatal care neglects to place adequate emphasis on nutrition, exercise, emotional, social, and psychological health, all of which are essential to mothers and babies. The key to excellent prenatal care is individual care rather than routine procedures that ignore the unique needs of mother and baby. To restore a healthy balance to prenatal care in this country, we need to place more emphasis on projects that give all women access to healthy foods, reduced stress, and other necessities of prenatal health, rather than narrowly directing our resources to the

research and development of sophisticated methods of prenatal testing. An ultrasound cannot help a baby grow—food does!

Prenatal care also includes the care a pregnant woman receives from others besides her health care provider—be it her mate, children, mother, friends, or childbirth educator. A back rub, some help with older kids, a kind word, or nurturing and informative classes with a knowledgeable childbirth educator can enhance the care you are able to give yourself.

Again, none of this can replace the need for you to take care of yourself optimally, but it can contribute to your wellness by creating a very effective support network for you.

CHOOSING YOUR PRENATAL CARE PROVIDER

The purpose of prenatal care is to support the mother, her baby, and her family so that a healthy pregnancy can ensue, followed by a healthy birth, baby, postpartum, and integration of the baby into the family. This means working with a care provider who is sensitive to women and their families and knowledgeable about their needs, including optimal nutrition, exercise, mental and emotional well-being, and spiritual growth. In addition, this care provider should understand what compromises a healthy pregnancy for both the woman and baby, and have the ability to identify both health and health problems. The care provider must be sensitive, considerate, responsible, and professional yet warm. She must help the mother to become educated, well-informed, and confident about her body. She must also maintain an excellent relationship with other health care practitioners so that she can help the mother to receive the care she requires.

I generally refer to prenatal care providers as women throughout this book. I believe that women are the most appropriate care providers for pregnant women. While there are sensitive male obstetricians and male nurse-midwives, I strongly believe that it is women's rightful place to provide prenatal and birth care. This is how it has been throughout history until the recent past, and this is how I believe it should be again. However, many women still take comfort in a male physician. If you do choose a male care provider, choose one who truly respects women.

Most practitioners (obstetricians, certified nurse-midwives, or traditional midwives, certified or not) see pregnant women on generally the same prenatal schedule, once a month until 32 weeks of pregnancy, then bimonthly until 36 weeks, and weekly until the birth. Many of the same procedures are done—for example, checking urine, determining the position of the baby, checking the blood pressure, and so on (see "Prenatal Visits", p. 32). However, the way

a practitioner has been trained greatly affects her/his philosophies and perspectives, and thus, your care. This section provides an overview of the main types of care providers currently in the United States. Of course these descriptions are generalizations, and any practitioner may be more or less holistically or medically oriented. You will have to decide which approach you are looking for and then choose an appropriate care provider. Many practitioners offer a free consultation.

When choosing a health care practitioner always ask questions that are important to *you* that will help you choose. Here are several essential questions to ask midwives:

- What training and experience do you have? Are you involved in continuing education?
- Can you handle both complications and emergencies?
- Do you have medical backup or a contingency plan for emergencies? What will be your role in an emergency? Will you continue to be with me during the emergency?
- What kind of equipment do you carry? Do you know how to use this equipment?
- Do you intend to see me with an assistant or by yourself? What about births?
- Is there a backup care provider should you be ill or otherwise unavailable at any point during the pregnancy or the birth?
- Do you have clear protocols and, if so, are these protocols rigid or flexible? For example, what happens if I go into labor prematurely or if I go past my due date? What if my baby is breech, etc.?
- What are your fees and what do they cover? Are any expenses covered by medical insurance? Am I entitled to any reimbursement in the event that I need to transfer out of your practice, for instance, if there is an emergency and a planned home birth becomes unreasonable?

"It's like growing food—if you take care of the soil, the food will grow. Cluck over the mother, nurture her."
—Candace Fields-Whitridge, CNM

• What are your philosophies about birth? Are they consistent and harmonious with my own?

If you are interviewing an obstetrician you will want to ask:

• What are your credentials?

• What is your cesarean rate?

• What is your episiotomy rate?

• What is the rate of medicated births in your practice?

• How many women in your practice request rooming-in with their babies?

• How many women in your practice breastfeed their babies?

• What are your feelings about natural birth?

• How much time do you spend with women at prenatal visits?

• Will you be at my birth or will another physician attend (and if so, who will that be)?

• What are your policies for women who go past-due, who have had previous cesarean sections, for permitted length of labor and pushing (or any other concerns or questions you might have)?

• Do you encourage women to participate actively in prenatal care and the birth?

You must be honest and comfortable with your care providers if you are really to meet your needs. It is of utmost importance that you work with someone you trust, whether this be a practitioner with an unconventional training, or a formally trained physician. If you aren't comfortable, seek another practitioner. This is your pregnancy and your decision to make. Ideally, your mate should feel comfortable with this person as well. The practitioner should respect you as an equal and talk to you with respect, answer your questions directly, and never treat you in a condescending way. If you feel that you are being treated in a way that makes you uncom-

fortable find another practitioner with whom you do feel comfortable. In birthing it is essential that you can be open, both literally and figuratively, and that your confidence in yourself be nurtured and reinforced.

— Midwives —

Midwives come from a philosophy that honors the importance of the pregnant woman in the entire childbearing experience. At all times the woman is treated with respect and sensitivity for the intelligent adult that she is. Midwives also maintain respect and sensitivity for the needs of the baby. Perhaps the central belief that unites midwives is that pregnancy and birth are natural processes for which women are inherently and biologically capable, and that with the participation of the woman in caring for herself and with the assistance and guidance of the midwife, the woman will enjoy a healthy experience. Midwives honor childbearing as a rite of passage and therefore encourage full participation by the mother during pregnancy and birth, and support her in this transition, helping her to grow in confidence and ability to nurture herself and her baby both before and after birth.

Midwives mainly attend home births. However, many presently have birthing centers or clinics where they provide prenatal care and birthing services. Midwives (with occasional assistance from a physician or nurse-midwife) have been fighting the battle to keep alive the right to birth at home with a skilled attendant. This right to birth at home has been challenged in most states, to the point that many midwives have been arrested or harassed. While I cannot discuss this issue at length in this book, I encourage you to read books such *The American Way of Birth* and *Immaculate Deception*, as well as other titles found in the appendix.

Midwives, who are variously referred to as traditional midwives, lay midwives, or direct-entry midwives, maintain advanced levels of knowledge and understanding about the normal physiological processes of childbearing, as well as variations and deviations from normal. They are also knowledgeable about both preventing and treating problems that can arise during pregnancy, birth, and the postpartum period. Midwives have incorporated conventional knowledge, skills, and techniques for assessing both pregnancy health and complications, and complementary healing modalities such as dietary awareness, herbalism, and massage. Many of the innovations and progressive changes that have occurred in hospitals in recent years have been inspired by the kind of intimate, professional care provided by midwives.

Most midwives train as apprentices under the tutelage of other experienced midwives, gaining extensive clinical experience by attending numerous women throughout pregnancy, birth, and afterward. Midwives also engage in extensive independent academic study, familiarizing themselves with both conventional and traditional theories, techniques, and procedures for providing women with optimal health care. There are also several schools in the United States that provide formal midwifery training. The national midwifery organizations—the Midwives Alliance of North America (MANA) and the North American Registry of Midwives (NARM)—have developed a national certification process for those midwives who demonstrate their proficiency by passing an eight-hour written examination and an equally lengthy clinical examination. This certification (which confers the title of Certified Professional Midwife, or CPM) has been fostered in order to gain validity in state governments so that midwifery care can be made accessible to a broader range of women. The primary disadvantage of the certification and legalization processes is they make midwives subject to external protocols that might be more limited in scope than those adopted by strictly independent midwives.

Studies indicate that in midwife-assisted births, even in high-risk women, there is a reduction of maternal and infant morbidity and infant mortality. Other countries which rely primarily on midwifery care have the lowest infant mortality rates in the world. (The United States ranks 25th in international infant mortality ratings; many other developed countries have a lower infant mortality rate.) At present in many states midwives are illegal. Midwives can generally be found, however, with a bit of effort, by contacting local childbirth educators and La Leche League leaders, natural foods stores, or by contacting MANA, or other organizations found in the "Resources" section of this book.

As with all professions, midwives vary in their skills and integrity. It is therefore up to you to determine the level of skill you want your midwife to possess (including the type of equipment she carries to births) and to explore her references and documentation of her training. To some women seeking a midwife, a midwife's skills at handling complications may be less significant than their personal relationship with her. It is your birth and if you choose a midwife with minimal experience because you feel that your relationship with her is the most important factor, that is your right; however, this choice must be based on honest information provided by your midwife, and it is your responsibility to arrange access to a practitioner or facility capable of handling an emergency should one arise beyond the capability of you or your practitioner. It is

"Pregnancy is a great time to have sex—you can't get pregnant!"

—*Ina May Gaskin*

unfair to you and your baby, as well as your midwife, to expect her to be able to help you should an unexpected complication arise for which she lacks the necessary skills.

Midwives, because they are independent professionals, are able to provide mothers and their families with individual care. They are not bound by the regulations of hospitals or the time limitations of a medical office. In addition, most midwives have borne children and loved the experience. As women and mothers they are uniquely capable of understanding pregnant women. They have firsthand knowledge of what they teach and do. Because midwives consider themselves your partner in your health care rather than *in charge* of your health care you will usually find that you will be comfortable expressing your needs and desires, and they can help you achieve these. Most independent midwives provide prenatal care in their own homes, providing you with a comfortable and informal atmosphere. They will also do at least one prenatal visit at your home prior to the birth.

Because most midwives rely on low-tech diagnostic techniques using their common sense, intuition, and sensitivity, many midwives are uniquely able to detect and avert pregnancy problems without the use of invasive (and expensive) procedures. Because midwives tend to choose their profession out of their deep caring for mothers and babies, they will provide you with excellent continuous care, seeing you from the time you initially contact them to the first months after your baby is born. Unlike other practitioners, most midwives make themselves readily available to their clients by phone for questions and concerns, in addition to being on call by pager for urgent situations. However, because midwives are not recognized as members of the medical profession in most states, nor are they trained to perform certain emergency medical procedures, your midwife is unlikely to be able to continue to provide you with treatment should an emergency arise and transport to the hospital become necessary. Most midwives will, however, accompany you to the hospital and continue to serve as a support person and advocate for you and the baby.

In the states where midwives are treated with hostility, your midwife might not be able to accompany you to the hospital, or if she does, may prefer to accompany you provided you do not refer to her as a midwife. In states where midwifery is legal, or where there are supportive obstetricians willing to serve as a medical liaison to the hospital in case of emergency, a back-up physician can be obtained before the birth. It is important that you discuss the issue of an emergency at some point during the pregnancy, and decide upon a clear course of action. Most midwives will have clear protocols that they can explain to you.

If you are working with either a direct-entry midwife or a nurse-midwife (see below), she should be able to provide you with the name of an obstetrician should you not be a candidate for a home birth or a birthing center birth, or should medical problems arise during your pregnancy. If you are at risk or have developed problems, you may need to work with an obstetrician, but you may in addition want to work with a midwife as a consultant, as problems of pregnancy and birth can often be reduced. In such cases, a team of health care providers can be ideal.

— Nurse-Midwives —

Nurse-midwives have completed the same training as registered nurses, then specialized in midwifery care. They first attend academic classes and gain clinical experience in caring for childbearing women and general gynecological care. They then begin midwifery training. Their ability to practice is limited by the fact that they can practice only if they have the consent of a supervisory obstetrician.

In general, nurse-midwives are more woman-centered than obstetricians and are likely to respect birth as a natural process. Nurse-midwives are very dedicated to their professions and are a great alternative for women who are seeking woman-centered medical care. However, their decisions regarding care are subject to the protocols of both their supervisory obstetrician and the hospital or birthing center in which they practice. Nurse-midwives may or may not be aware of complementary therapies that can facilitate health during pregnancy and birth. Instead, they are trained to rely on technology for information and may feel more secure by so doing. Few nurse-midwives attend home births compared to independent midwives, though there are some who do so.

— Obstetricians —

Obstetricians are physicians who, in addition to their four years of medical training, have trained four additional years in obstetrics and gynecology, preparing them to assist women through both normal and complicated pregnancies and births. They are trained to provide women with gynecological care from puberty through old age.

Unfortunately, obstetricians are trained to manage pregnancy and birth as medical events. Few obstetricians are trained to let the mother be the orchestrator of her own health care, and because of their training, may come to see all pregnant women as emergencies waiting to happen. Additionally, because they often feel it necessary to protect themselves from lawsuits, they may use routine protocol with all patients. Overwhelmingly, obstetricians require that patients give birth in a hospital setting. However, some obstetricians will help women achieve natural births in the hospital. A few courageous obstetricians do have home birth practices. These obstetricians may be ostracized by their colleagues and some have had their licenses suspended.

Because of their training, which encourages obstetricians to rely on technology, few are comfortable with personal care, opting instead for routine tests and procedures to determine the well-being of the mother and baby. Similarly, few receive training in preventive health care. If you choose an obstetrician, you'll need to get input from other sources.

Most obstetricians are men (though the rate of female medical residents is now nearing 50 percent) and may therefore carry with them, consciously or not, culturally conditioned, condescending attitudes towards women. This can greatly affect the care you receive and the way you are treated. So please take care in choosing your doctor. Please insist upon natural, woman-centered, and family-centered childbirth. This will cause changes in obstetrical practice and lead to greater choice in hospital birth experiences in the future.

Obstetrical care is the best choice for those women with a high likelihood of developing complications during pregnancy or birth, such as those with diabetes, kidney or heart disease, toxemia, hypertension, or any problem that is likely to require medical intervention or emergency care.

— *Osteopathic Obstetricians* —

Osteopathic physicians trained with a specialty in obstetrics go through medical training and a residency program nearly identical to other obstetricians, and have exactly the same privileges and rights, including permission to do cesarean sections and other surgery. Many osteopathic obstetricians hold positions on hospital staffs. Osteopathic training integrates an acceptance of holistic healing with organized medicine, making many osteopaths open to a natural approach to childbirth. You may want to consult with an osteopathic obstetrician if you prefer to have an obstetrician for your prenatal care and birth. See "Resources" for locating an osteopathic physician.

— *Self-Care* —

I present this option as the last in this list because it is the least likely choice for most American women. However, a small percentage of couples and single mothers choose to provide their own prenatal care, paying close attention to a lifestyle that supports a healthy pregnancy and prevents problems. These women recognize that excellent self-care and intuitive awareness can guide them through pregnancy and birth safely, joyously, and in optimal health. This is a very empowering experience and creates a deeply intimate atmosphere in the family. In my own family we've had three such pregnancy experiences in which my husband and I have independently cared for myself and the baby. It is important to say that I have spent nearly fifteen years as a midwife, and also have an excellent support network of other midwives and physicians

upon whom I can call for support in the event of an emergency. Nonetheless, I have found that by looking inward for the information about my wellness and my baby's health, I have developed an enduring confidence in my body as well as deep connection with my children. One need not be a midwife to achieve this level of awareness.

If you choose to provide your own prenatal care it is essential that you possess the humility that allows you to be able to ask for help, support, advice, or information at any time you want or suspect you need these, and that you be uncompromisingly committed to your well-being during pregnancy. I have seen couples so stuck on the idea of doing everything themselves that they endure unnecessary health problems which might have been easily resolved had they been willing to see a practitioner. It is important to be realistic and establish some sort of contingency plan for yourself in case a problem or emergency develops.

You may feel that you want a midwife or other experienced practitioner to support you on your independent path, but you should realize that in choosing the do-it-yourself route, you may be limiting your ability to consult with practitioners, because most practitioners, including midwives, will not want to be held responsible for you if you have not seen them regularly for prenatal care as a client, or if you have made choices with which they do not agree.

PRENATAL VISITS

Prenatal visits ideally provide the opportunity for you (and your family) to have personalized and intimate time with someone who is knowledgeable about pregnancy and birth, who can answer your questions and give you information, support, encouragement and confirmation of the baby's growth and health, as well as your own. It is also a time when a basic prenatal examination can indicate if there are any problems developing that require further assessment, treatment, or just watching. Prenatal visits should provide a chance for you and your care provider to get to know each other, developing a comfortable relationship that you can call upon for support during your pregnancy, birth, and transition to motherhood. During these visits your care provider should also help dad and siblings to feel the baby, listen to the baby's heartbeat, and so on. This helps all members of the family develop a deep prenatal bond with the baby and also lessens the difficulty of introducing a new baby to older siblings. In my experience children who have been well integrated into the prenatal care readily accept their siblings and often participate in their care. A wise practitioner will always honor the primary relationship of the parents and do what she can to foster communication between them, helping the father accept his role as an active participant.

Prenatal care can vary greatly depending upon the type of practitioner you are seeing and her personal philosophy. The setting in which your prenatal visits occur, the regulations to which your practitioner is subjected, and the extent to which you help to shape your own care also matter.

— Midwife Visits —

As discussed above, a direct-entry midwife is likely to be steeped in a philosophy that is woman-centered, based on the belief that pregnancy is a natural process. Most traditional midwives, while utilizing noninvasive methods for prenatal testing, will tailor their actions to the individual needs of the pregnant woman. Not only will she provide the same standards of pregnancy care provided by other practitioners, but she will also try to see how the pregnancy affects the woman's life and vice versa. Midwives, therefore, have to develop personal relationships with their clients. Most traditional midwives spend at least an hour per prenatal visit with their clients, often more than this. This depth of relationship is beneficial to a pregnant woman as well as her family. It can raise your sense of comfort, enabling you to relax your inhibitions and discuss personal issues that might affect your health, such as marital stress, herpes outbreaks, or parenting concerns. It can also reduce your anxiety about entering labor. You, as a woman, will be more willing to discuss intimate physical discomforts or concerns with your midwife that you might be reluctant to discuss with a male practitioner.

The setting for prenatal care is generally the midwife's home or your own home. This environment, in my opinion, also increases a pregnant woman's sense that pregnancy is a normal, everyday event—that she is a client, not a patient—and that her birth can also occur in a relaxed, comfortable, and nonmedical environment. In addition, a traditional midwife is likely to include you in all procedures, teaching you if you are interested, and encouraging you if you're not, to be an active participant in your prenatal care, learning how to perform your own prenatal tests, understanding the significance of these, and learning how to care for yourself. As most midwives are very glad to share information openly with pregnant mothers (and families), your prenatal care is a perfect chance for you to learn about how your body works, the process of pregnancy, your anatomy and physiology—in other words, how to be closely in touch with your body and baby.

When you are pregnant is a perfect time to get information about how your body works.

—A. J. R.

— Nurse-Midwife Visits —

Nurse-midwives most often provide prenatal care within the context of an obstetrician's office, and though many try to establish personal relationships with their clients—and succeed at this—they are still subject to the limitations of time allowed for visits. Frequently nurse-midwives will meet with clients for only 15 to 30 minutes. Additionally, you may not have the choice of which midwife you see prenatally (or which midwife attends your birth) if you are working with a group practice. Nurse-midwives have access to technology and medications, so if you want or need to employ tests or medications that require a prescription, you will have someone who can prescribe these, whereas most direct-entry midwives will have to refer you to a physician or lab. (If any situations arise that are beyond her scope, the nurse-midwife is obligated to refer you to an obstetrician.) The disadvantage of this is that the use of medications and procedures increases when they are easily available. You might find yourself subjected to greater levels of intervention if you work with a nurse-midwife rather than a traditional midwife. For example, if your urine sample reveals the presence of sugar, a traditional midwife is likely to first try to rule out diabetes using other noninvasive physical tests such as assessing your history, diet, and other symptoms, before recommending bloodsugar testing. A nurse-midwife might be obligated to verify that there is no diabetes by requiring you to undergo bloodsugar tests that require fasting and/or bloodsugar loading, neither of which are healthy for you or your baby. Nurse-midwives who practice independently (often found in rural areas) or who practice in their homes are often more natural in their approach to prenatal care than those working in clinics, hospitals, and most obstetrician's offices.

— Obstetrician Visits —

When you see an obstetrician, you will first be seen by the nurse who will weigh you and check your pulse, bloodpressure, and urine. She will then take you to an office where you will wait for a period of time until the obstetrician comes to examine you. While there are some excellent obstetricians who provide holistic medical care and spend time familiarizing themselves with their patients' needs, most of these office visits will be brief, with the pregnant woman sometimes seeing the doctor for only 15 minutes. The advantages of working with an obstetrician is that she or he can provide you with continuity of care in situations ranging from a normal vaginal birth to a complicated cesarean section. Neither traditional midwives nor nurse-midwives can offer this. Obstetricians are also much more likely to see birth as a medical event (you are a patient, not a client). This view of birth has its advantages and disadvantages. Moreover, since most obstetricians are men, you may find yourself inhibited in certain discussions, even to the point of enduring certain physical discomforts, such as a symptomatic yeast infection because you are too embarrassed to discuss the vaginal itching and discharge, or a difficulty in your sexual relationship for similar reasons.

When working with most obstetricians you are not likely to be involved in the medical aspects of your care, such as understanding routine tests and procedures. While some women may prefer not to take this responsibility, I believe that participating in your pregnancy empowers you as a woman. Your care provider should not be more knowledgeable about your body than you are.

PRENATAL TESTING

It is urgent that we examine the safety of routine reliance on such tests as the doppler and diagnostic ultrasound, alpha fetoprotein, chorionic villi sampling, and amniocentesis during pregnancy. All of these tests may pose risks to the baby, though the danger is often minimized. In addition to their potential physical harm, these tests externalize the mother's authority and body-wisdom, keeping her distanced from the trust she might otherwise learn to develop in herself. This is not to say that testing is always unnecessary; it can be a great relief to a concerned mother, or provide invaluable life-saving information when a problem is suspected. I am suggesting that we question the routines we have accepted blindly. (See "Further Reading" for many of the excellent books, particularly titles by Suzanne Arms, Nancy Cohen, Henci Goer, Marsden Wagner, Robbie Davis-Floyd, and Barbara Katz Rothman.)

In my practice as well as during my own pregnancies, mechanical technology has not been my focus. Rather, emphasis has been and is placed on nutritional awareness and other aspects of physical wellness, such as exercise and rest, and emotional and psychological health. Personal and social issues (such as financial stress or relationship tensions) may be disturbing the mother and may interfere with her taking care of herself. I also explore what the pregnancy means to a woman and how she is feeling. In addition, I assess the pregnant women physically with tests which are noninvasive and harmless, yet can confirm the mother's feelings of wellness or discomfort, or may reveal the development of a problem. These basic tests, the same as those that are performed by obstetricians and nurse-midwives,

include testing the urine with coated test strips (the mother does this herself), checking her pulse, blood pressure, and weight, checking the baby's growth by measuring the growth of the uterus abdominally using a tapemeasure and feeling the baby for growth, listening to the baby's heart rate, and feeling the baby's position. Midwives, as well as other practitioners, may also perform a few more tests such as checking for kidney tenderness if a urinary tract infection is suspected, or checking the hemoglobin if anemia is thought to be a problem. The pregnant woman will also be asked whether she has had any problems such as nausea, headaches, dizziness, visual disturbances, heartburn, unusual urinary frequency, and other signs which may indicate the need for further attention.

Most practitioners also require pregnant mothers to obtain complete prenatal lab tests, which usually check blood type and Rh-factor, hemoglobin, and an analysis of red and white blood cells, as well as ascertaining whether there is an immunity to rubella (German measles) and toxoplasmosis (contracted from handling infected cat feces and ingesting raw meat, both of which should be avoided by all pregnant women). You will also be tested for sexually transmitted diseases. It is also common for practitioners to require vaginal cultures to rule out the presence of gonorrhea and chlamydia.

More than ever, unreliable and invasive procedures have become routine components of prenatal care. A mere twenty years ago, many tests, such as amniocentesis, were performed only if problems were suspected, and others, such as chorionic villi sampling, were not yet developed. Because obstetricians became able to perform these tests with greater accuracy, they used these tests

It is up to each woman to become educated about the risks and benefits of the tests available to them prenatally, and to develop the confidence to agree to tests that they do want done, and to refuse the rest.

—A. J. R.

more frequently. Also if a woman gave birth to a baby who had a problem which was not detected in utero, the obstetrician may have been blamed and sued for malpractice.

Each test has advantages and disadvantages. For example, a woman knowing that she will give birth to a child with Down's syndrome, as revealed by an amniocentesis, may enable her and her partner to prepare for this, both emotionally, psychologically, and materially, and find resources, organizations, and special supplies that they will need for caring for their child. Or if they choose to abort the child, they will avoid the stress that they perceive will accompany both raising a Down's syndrome child, and the stress for the child in a society which is often discriminatory. However, the amniocentesis procedure can also cause damage to an otherwise perfectly healthy fetus, or even cause the miscarriage of a normal baby. It is up to each woman to become educated about the risks and benefits of the tests available to them prenatally, and to develop the confidence to agree to tests that they do want done, and to refuse the rest.

Following are explanations of the purpose, procedure, risks, and benefits of several of the most common prenatal tests that might be considered invasive. I use the term invasive to mean that these tests require penetrating the body, either directly or by sound waves, or that they have the potential for harmful effects. Prenatal testing is an important issue in prenatal care, particularly if you are working with a medical practitioner, and I therefore encourage you to read *Pursuing the Birth Machine*; *The Encyclopedia of Childbearing*; *Research Myths vs. Research Realities*; *A Guide to Effective Care in Pregnancy and Childbirth*; and *Immaculate Deception* (see "Further Reading").

— Doppler Ultrasound —

The doppler is an electronic device used routinely at a prenatal examination, by both doctors and nurse-midwives, and occasionally by midwives, to hear the fetal heartbeat. It can detect the fetal heartbeat as early as 8 weeks into the pregnancy. The doppler works by directing a continuous sound wave at the baby, which is then received by the amplification device, and makes the heartbeat audible to those in the room. Many women enjoy hearing their baby's heartbeat amplified, but do not question the safety of the doppler. In fact, the doppler has not been conclusively proven safe for use in pregnancy; not enough long-term evidence is available. Nor has the doppler been proven more effective or accurate in assessing fetal heart tones over the completely benign use of the fetoscope, a fetal stethoscope. One minute of exposure to doppler has been estimated as equivalent to 35 minutes of imaging ultrasound exposure. The doppler is very useful for hearing the fetal heartbeat when it is difficult to hear it manually. In a threatened miscarriage in early pregnancy if you are trying to hear the baby's heartbeat, and in other medically indicated situations, its use is warranted. You may want to request that your care provider use the fetoscope in place of routine use of the doppler, reserving its use for medical necessity, such as when the safety of the fetus is of concern, and the heartbeat is inaudible with a fetoscope (i.e., threatened miscarriage, lack of normal fetal movement).

Diagnostic Ultrasound — (Ultrasonography, Sonography) —

Imaging ultrasound employs a similar technology to the doppler ultrasound, but produces a screen image of the fetus and the placenta, which can be evaluated diagnostically. It is used routinely—most pregnant American women can expect to have at least one, and frequently several, ultrasounds. It too has not been proven safe for use in pregnancy.

While pregnant women find it exciting or reassuring to see a picture of their baby, imaging ultrasound is more appropriately reserved for use when there are medical indications such as suspected fetal demise, suspected placenta previa, a significant size/dates discrepancy, and determination of fetal position if it is difficult to determine it with palpation alone. If you do require an ultrasound, you can request that it be done by a technician with a lot of experience in order to reduce the amount of time that you are exposed.

Maternal Serum Alpha-fetoprotein Testing — (MSAFP) —

Alpha-fetoprotein (AFP) is a substance produced by the liver of the fetus, minute quantities of which appear in your bloodstream. The level of AFP rises progressively throughout pregnancy. Maternal blood levels are assessed for the amount of AFP present; an abnormally low or high level may indicate the presence of fetal anomalies. This test may be performed routinely without your knowledge, at the time of your initial prenatal lab screening.

MSAFP is not a harmful test; however, it has a high rate of false positives. When a woman is determined to have abnormal AFP levels, she is then referred for further testing, usually an amniocentesis. Frequently, then, the woman will be anxious until the amniocentesis is performed. She will then be exposed to tests with higher risks for the mother and baby. The optimal time to have the MSAFP test performed is between 15 and 18 weeks, gestation, as the test is thought to be the most accurate when done during this time.

When a fetus is determined without a doubt to have anomalies, the only choices are to have the baby or abort.

— Amniocentesis —

To perform an amniocentesis, a doctor inserts a long, sterile needle through your abdominal and uterine walls into the amniotic fluid. This test is done with an ultrasound in order to view the fetus and placenta. The amniotic fluid that is collected contains fetal cells that will provide information on fetal well-being and can indicate whether the fetus has certain birth defects (such as Down's syndrome), hemolytic anemia (destruction of the red blood cells that occurs from Rh disease), and many diseases, including carbohydrate, fat, and amino acid metabolism disorders, and cystic fibrosis. It can be used to determine lung maturity when a premature labor is occurring, or if a pre-term Cesarean-section is necessary.

Risks include puncturing the umbilical cord, placenta, or uterus, or causing infection or miscarriage. In addition, if an insufficient amount of fluid is collected, or if the culture of the fetal cells doesn't grow, the test will need to repeated.

If the baby is determined to have a disorder, you must then choose whether to keep the baby or abort. Amniocentesis cannot screen for all possible fetal disorders, and it can potentially damage a normal fetus. You must weigh the risks and benefits of having this test done, especially if you plan to keep the baby no matter what the problem is.

We have become so highly acculturated to accepting birth as a technological and medical event that we must unlearn the cultural conditioning.

—A. J. R.

— *Chorionic Villi Sampling (CVS)* —

To perform this test (at between 9 and 11 weeks gestation), tissues are removed from what will develop into the placenta. The tissue is obtained by going through either the abdomen or cervix, and using an instrument to remove the tissue while directly looking at the area. This test can check for chromosomal abnormalities, but cannot detect all of the problems that can be picked up by amniocentesis.

Risks of this test include damaging the embryo (damage can be as severe as the loss of a limb), damage to the cervix and uterus, infection, hemorrhage, and miscarriage. This test should not be done in the presence of a vaginal infection, Rh sensitization, or multiple gestation. I deeply question the potential problems we've not yet discovered, as disrupting the placenta is a significant interruption of what nature intended.

As with other diagnostic tests, you must evaluate the risk/benefit ratio. If you plan to abort the baby if there is a problem, CVS can provide you with quick (results are usually available in 24 hours) and early diagnosis. If you plan to keep the baby if there is a problem, you must keep in mind that an otherwise healthy baby can suffer severe damage as a result of this procedure.

CHILDBIRTH EDUCATION CLASSES

Ultimately, our bodies know how to birth and need very little instruction. However, there are three main aspects of childbearing in our modern culture that make childbirth education classes useful. We have become so highly acculturated to accepting birth as a technological and medical event that we must unlearn the cultural conditioning that can undermine our efforts to birth naturally. Second, we have lost our connection to the elders of our communities who share with us the information and wisdom that facilitates these transitions that we must make in becoming mothers, fathers, families—we must learn on our own by trial and error, a task that is both difficult as well as fraught with stress. Third, we have become so isolated in nuclear units, thinking that our problems are unique, unusual, or worse than those of other families. This can lead to unnecessary stress, shame, confusion, and in the long run, if not addressed, depression, exhaustion, and divorce. For example, many couples experience sexual tension during pregnancy (one partner may want more physical intimacy than the other), or confusion and anger over unmet expectations (pregnant women may want their mates to be more involved in touching the baby or buying baby clothes than the partner cares to be). Many pregnant women experience similar physical and emotional challenges, and many men feel unsure in their new role.

Childbirth education classes provide a forum for parents to explore such issues under the guidance of a childbirth educator, usually a woman (or a couple) who has knowledge about pregnancy and birth through both study and personal experience. While midwives can provide excellent prenatal education which can often substitute for prenatal classes, the opportunity to share and learn with other couples is very valuable, particularly for first-time parents. In an obstetrician's office, rarely is there time allocated for prenatal education. Classes in this case are also necessary if you are to have any understanding of the birth process, or of hospital procedures and protocols.

There are numerous childbirth education organizations, offering their own philosophies, material, and educational styles. Classes offered in hospitals are nearly always geared toward a hospital birth. While natural childbirth might be a term that regularly pops up in the discussion, you are also likely to receive complete information on the drugs of choice for pain relief, full preparation for a cesarean section, and minimal information that would truly support you in achieving either a natural pregnancy or birth. If a truly positive and natural experience is your goal, you will want to seek a childbirth teacher who is well versed in positive, natural birth and who orients classes toward home birth or home and hospital birth. Whether you are planning a home or hospital birth, it is imperative that the classes educate you about medical procedures commonly used during birth, so that you can discriminate between necessary procedures and hospital policies, protocols, which might expose you to unnecessary testing and intervention that the hospital requires in order to reduce its insurance liabilities. It is your right to exercise authority over your own body.

Ideally, classes should begin in early pregnancy in order to address the needs of pregnant mothers, couples, and families. For example, there should be discussion of nutrition and common discomforts during each trimester, there should be discussion of emotional issues that are likely to arise, and there should be preparation for the experience of pregnancy and parenting of which birth is just a part (albeit a very profound part). Classes that encourage you to focus mainly on breathing techniques will distract you from finding your own strength, and in a subtle way promote a fear of birth. Such classes may stress the necessity of avoiding the pain or intensity of labor. You will know what to do. A good class will help you identify your inner resources for birth and prepare you for parenting and

breastfeeding. A good class will help you find confidence in your abilities, while welcoming the intensity of birth and parenting.

In "Resources" you will find organizations that offer childbirth education services with trained teachers around the United States, Canada, and Europe. Midwives will often offer classes to their clients, and so do hospitals. If not, they can recommend childbirth educators in your area.

There is much literature available on pregnancy, birth, and parenting. You can learn a lot by reading either on your own or with your mate (some men are very reluctant to read pregnancy and birth books, so

you might have to be persistent), or by joining a study group with other pregnant moms. The Birth and Life Bookstore (see "Resources") offers a comprehensive selection of titles and their catalog is well worth receiving. Local women's bookstores and even many large bookstores carry a selection of such books. Libraries often have limited book selections but may be convinced to expand their resources if enough women request that they do so.

Nutrition During Pregnancy

WHAT IS NUTRITION?

The words nutrition and nourishment both have as their root the word *nourir* which literally means "to suckle." A similar word, nurturance, means affectionate care and attention. "Nurture" is also defined as "the sum of the influences modifying the expression of the genetic potentialities of an organism." From this etymological and defined perspective it is apparent that nutrition is much more than obtaining a certain amount of vitamins and minerals. Optimal nutrition is a way of loving and caring for ourselves and others that allows us and those we serve to reach our (or their) fullest potential. Indeed this is obvious when a close relative or friend serves us a bowl of warm soup and we feel that we are being fed much more than the food itself. Excellent nutrition is more than just taking in a certain number of recommended daily allowances, it is also an awareness of how we prepare, eat, and digest our food, of how we feel about our bodies as well as our emotional,

mental, and spiritual selves, of what chemicals are in the foods we eat and how these affect not only our own health but our baby's health, and the health of our environment. Nourishment is a holistic experience that goes far beyond simply eating.

Because we live in a fast-paced and highly industrialized culture, one that places material gain and external approval over an intrinsic sense of wellness and satisfaction, many women do not take the time to nourish themselves—nor do many women truly know how. Many women entering pregnancy, for example, know very little about eating well. I've worked with highly educated women, including health care professionals, whose idea of a nutritious vegetable is canned green beans, and whose idea of a high calcium food is ice cream. Similarly, most women do not know how to relax deeply, do not know how to exercise to improve the health of their pelvic muscles, do not know how to use their Earth-given gifts of herbs to support pregnancy health, do not know how to supplement their diets with essential nutrients, nor how to prevent or reduce many common pregnancy discomforts. But many pregnancy problems, including serious complications, can be prevented with optimal pregnancy nourishment, precluding the need for testing and interventions during pregnancy and birth, and also for their newborns. An optimally healthy woman will usually feel well for most of her pregnancy, and therefore have a greater chance of enjoying the experience and looking forward to her baby's birth with joy. So many women consider the common complaints of pregnancy to be "natural." To some degree, it is likely that the changes that occur during pregnancy will cause periodic discomfort, but many common problems are a reflection of a lifestyle that did not prepare us to be healthy pregnant women. While some nausea may be unavoidable, such problems as persistent constipation, headaches, leg cramps, and exhaustion can be prevented or relieved with good nutrition.

Optimal pregnancy health not only helps to ensure that your baby is healthy, intelligent, and resistant to infections, but will ensure that you are healthy during the pregnancy and birth. This will lay a foundation of health that can support you when you are breastfeeding, during the precious first few years of your child's life. It will also help you meet the demands every parent of young children must face. A well-nourished person is better able to cope with stress than one who is inadequately nourished.

In my work with a pregnant woman, from the earliest prenatal visit, I place a great emphasis on nutrition. The reason is simple: there is overwhelming evidence that excellent maternal nutrition almost always results in healthy mothers and babies, while a poorly nourished mother is likely to experience complications during the pregnancy and birth, and her baby is also likely to have problems. This evidence ranges from scientific studies of many types to the personal experience of mothers and midwives who time and time again see the effects of excellent and poor nutrition.

But what is excellent nutrition? So many of us, raised on sugared cereals, canned vegetables, pizza, and TV dinners, have no clue as to what constitutes good nutrition beyond what we see and hear on television or in popular magazines or newspapers. Some shoppers may be familiar with the labels on packaged foods which tell us what the recommended daily allowance (RDA) of certain nutrients are. However, do we question where these standards come from, or how they relate to us? Do we even know what the nutrients are, what they do in our bodies, why we need them, and where we can get them? Many people remember the four basic food groups from elementary school or are familiar with the more recent food pyramid. However, we really have no idea what whole foods are or what variety of foods we should eat to ensure optimal nutrition. We can prepare our food in more wholesome ways, we can eliminate junk foods, and we can eat more fresh fruits and vegetables. I can recall my own first pregnancy when I put ketchup on my freshly picked organic kale and collard greens which my mate had lovingly harvested for me, in order to make them palatable. Before pregnancy I'd never eaten these highly nutritious greens which he, as a Southerner, had known since childhood. Now I devour these vegetables daily, as do my children, frequently with no more garnish than a dash of tamari.

In a culture that equates thinness with success, beauty, and health, women are afraid to eat for fear of becoming overweight. So we have a substantial population of women in our society with eating disorders (an estimated 1 in 5 women), many of whom are of childbearing age. Many women are so out of touch with their bodies that they don't even know when they are hungry, a result of suppressing their instinctual, life-preserving urge to eat. What often happens is that women try to get by on as little food as possible, living in a state of hypoglycemia, frequently overloading on sugar and carbohydrates to restore their low blood sugar level to a semblance of normality. This, combined with the fact that the few foods women permit themselves to eat are junk foods, it is no wonder that our country has a high rate of premature, underweight babies, and a high rate of pregnancies fraught with discomforts and problems. When you add to these issues the poor women whose access to healthy foods is difficult, and the omnipresent factor of stress which adds to our caloric and nutrient needs, we have a prenatal nutritional mess.

Yet all women can learn to eat well and to be informed about their unique nutritional needs. We can learn to be wise shoppers and to recognize that we pay more for packaged foods than for fresh foods, that buying junk food instead of nutritious food is throwing away our nutrition, money, and health, and that preparing our own foods, to whatever extent we can, is less expensive than eating out. Even women who are in high-risk categories for pregnancy complications due to the problems associated with poverty can bear healthy children when their diet is improved. Poor women of color have significantly higher mortality, morbidity, and congenital problems than white

women. It is essential that individual communities find ways to support those women who are at greater risk, such as providing free prenatal classes, promoting social services that provide prenatal care, and starting community gardens to provide seasonal fresh vegetables to pregnant women.

COMMITTING YOURSELF TO EATING WELL

The first step that a pregnant woman can take toward becoming well-nourished is to make the commitment to do so, knowing that she and her baby deserve it. Ideally the father or partner should also make the commitment to support the pregnant mother in shopping, cooking, etc. There will be days when a pregnant woman just doesn't feel like cooking but still really needs to eat well. Without some form of support, meals are likely to be missed or skimped, and mother and baby may go without adequate nourishment.

In order to be able to nourish yourself, you must reconnect with your instinctual sense of hunger, which is inherent in human beings. You will have to learn to eat when you are hungry, not for reasons such as frustration, anger, depression, or boredom. Likewise, you will have to learn not to skip meals due to emotional upset or stress. You must learn to love and appreciate your growing body, and eat without worrying about your weight (see "Weight Gain"). And you must learn what foods are necessary for optimal health first by studying, then by recognizing how different foods cause you to feel, and what you intuit you and your baby need. (See Chapter 3 for more information on using inner guidance during pregnancy.)

EVERY WOMAN IS UNIQUE

Every pregnant woman is going to have a unique appetite. She will come from a different ethic background, and seek different comfort foods. The best place to start to plan your diet is to list what you eat presently. From there, you can add foods that may provide you with the extra nutrients that pregnancy requires, and perhaps you'll be open to acquiring a few new tastes. The most effective way to begin is to write down what midwives refer to as a "diet diary." This is a record of all that passes your lips (i.e., food, pills, cigarettes). Five to seven days will give the broadest, clearest picture of your eating habits. A three-day diary is the absolute minimum. See the accompanying diet diary form that I give a pregnant mother, which outlines the ideal of three meals and three snacks daily. You can use any notebook to write in.

By glancing at this chart you can see that a pregnant woman will ideally be eating quite often. This does not mean that you need to gorge each time you eat. It does mean that you eat something nutritious every few hours. Ideally, every time you eat you should be meeting your daily needs. By eating a wide variety of foods from the Essential Nutrients section below, you will be doing just this.

Another excellent idea, taught to me by midwife Sarahn Henderson, is to create the ideal pregnancy diet diary. Using the same form, create a diet diary of what you would be eating for five days if you had an ideal prenatal diet. You can use nutritional guidelines from this book and others (see "Further Reading"). You will learn a great deal from this exercise, and might even come up with a few new ideas and recipes in the process.

DIET DIARIES

When I have a woman write down a diet diary, I have her keep a record of the intake of all substances over the course of five to seven days. The following samples represent a day from the diet diaries of several different women. All of the women are in mid- to late-pregnancy, as diet diaries done during the first trimester may reflect inability to eat optimally due to prenatal nausea (of course, it is still important to eat well when you are nauseous, and in fact, a healthy diet can often reduce nausea). Diet diaries are brought to an initial prenatal visit, and are reviewed as a part of the medical and personal history. The women in these samples began prenatal care with a midwife at the weeks gestation noted near the mother's name (all names are falsified for the purpose of confidentiality).

Diet diaries are assessed on the basis of general food groups as discussed later in this section, with the idea that a woman should ideally be eating a certain number of servings from each group. It would be impractical for a woman to record her food intake on the basis of grams, milligrams, international units, etc., and impossible for a midwife to evaluate her diet in this way, without knowing the exact sizes of individual servings, and specific nutrient contents of various brands of foods that might be used. For example, did the woman drink 6 ounces of soymilk or 10 ounces, and how much protein per ounce does that soymilk brand claim to have.

It is important to remember that there might be days that you don't eat optimally, but that the goal is to try to eat optimally as often as possible.

DIET DIARY

From_____ to_____

	Day 1	Day 2	Day 3	Day 4	Day 5
BREAKFAST					
SNACK					
LUNCH					
SNACK					
DINNER					
SNACK					
DRINKS *(specify)*					
SUPPLEMENTS					
OTHER					

Stephanie's Diet Diary

23 weeks pregnant with her third baby.

BREAKFAST
   2 scrambled eggs
   1/2 bagel
   water
   peppermint tea with milk and sugar

LUNCH
   manicotti with cheese and sauce
   green salad with alfalfa sprouts
   water
   milk

SNACK
   water
   apple

DINNER
   Potato omelette
   Rice and peas and beans
   broccoli, green beans, and carrots
   orange
   milk

EVENING
   water

Overall, this mother ate a very healthy diet this day. If you compare it to the recommended amounts, she received many of the servings needed for optimal wellness. Improvements might be in getting her complex carbohydrates from a whole-grain source such as brown rice and a whole wheat bagel, rather than the white flour variety. Her overall food choices reflect a wide variety of foods, and no reliance on sweets, empty calories, or junk foods.

Jenny's Diet Diary

27 weeks pregnant with her first baby.

BREAKFAST
   cheerios with blueberries and
     soymilk
   1 piece whole-wheat toast with
     strawberry jam
   prenatal vitamin

LUNCH
   3 1/4 ounce tuna
   wheat thins
   water
   raisins

SNACK
   apple juice
   iron supplement
   vitamin C

DINNER
   spaghetti with tomato sauce
   mozzarella cheese
   2 pieces whole-wheat garlic toast
   cucumber
   mineral water
   chocolate nonfat frozen yogurt

Jenny's diet contains few fresh vegetables, little protein, few calcium sources, and very little fluids. She shows a reliance on sweets for energy, which she probably craves due to the lack of whole grains and protein. She often had sugar in her urine, which would disappear after several days of moderating her sugar intake. She could add a salad to her lunch, a leafy green to her dinner, and a serving of squash, steamed carrots, or a slice of cantaloupe to one of her meals. To her spaghetti sauce she might add texturized vegetable protein, ground tofu, or ground beef for protein. At breakfast she might replace the cheerios with a whole-grain cereal. She could have a more substantial grain with her lunch, and perhaps some cottage cheese with the apple for her snack. She should increase her fluid intake.

Nita's Diet Diary

32 weeks pregnant with her second baby.

BREAKFAST
  2 whole-wheat waffles
  1 fried egg
  grapefruit juice

SNACK
  milk with ovaltine

LUNCH
  peanut butter and banana
  noodles and cheese
  green beans and red pepper

SNACK
  banana

DINNER
  artichoke with mayonnaise sauce
  large green salad with carrots, gar-
    banzo beans, and sunflower seeds,
    oil and vinegar dressing

OTHER
  2 1/2 quarts of water
  prenatal vitamins
  fresh carrot-apple juice

Nita has an excellent diet in general, and is conscientious in eating protein, vegetables, and fresh, wholesome foods. I might suggest a more natural alternative to ovaltine, as it contains a fair amount of sugar. Also, Nita might incorporate whole grains into her supper meal, or as part of her snacks.

Michelle's Diet Diary

25 weeks pregnant with her first baby, working full time as a health care provider in a busy practice.

BREAKFAST
  1 cup of decaffeinated coffee
  banana

SNACK
  crackers

LUNCH
  turkey with cheese sandwich

SNACK
  5 pieces of chocolate

DINNER
  tuna with pasta and cream sauce

OTHER
  2 quarts of water
  2 prenatal vitamins

Michelle's diet, even to the untrained eye, is obviously devoid of almost all nutritional value, short of 2 protein servings and plenty of fluids. In fact, she has far fewer nutrients than she requires and is actually further depleting her nutrients by drinking coffee and eating chocolate which rob minerals from the body. Michelle improved her diet somewhat by learning about foods that she could carry along with her to work, having prepared them in advance. Even still, her baby weighed only just over five pounds at birth, compared with all of the other babies in these samples which weighed at least 7.5 pounds, and she had a very difficult time establishing breastfeeding. Michelle needed a full education in nutrition for pregnancy health.

Amina's Diet Diary

33 weeks pregnant with her second baby.

BREAKFAST
　　prune/bran drink
　　2 pieces of whole-wheat bread with
　　　　peanut butter

LUNCH
　　carrot and celery sticks
　　cottage cheese
　　raisins
　　apple
　　crackers with cheese

DINNER
　　roast beef
　　potatoes
　　green beans
　　corn

EVENING
　　prune/bran drink

OTHER
　　1/2 gallon water
　　floradix (2x)
　　spirulina (2 tablets, 3x daily)

Amina has a good basic diet, but might add a calcium rich snack and a calcium serving to one of her meals. In addition, she rarely eats leafy green vegetables, and consequently, suffers from constipation. Leafy greens are also rich in calcium. A bed of lettuce for her cottage cheese and a serving of collard green with dinner might round out her diet nicely.

Diane's Diet Diary

30 weeks pregnant with her second baby.

BREAKFAST
　　orange juice
　　oatmeal with raisins

LUNCH
　　salad
　　cheese toast
　　cookie

SNACK
　　bagel with cream cheese

DINNER
　　potato
　　broccoli

OTHER
　　prenatal vitamins
　　calcium supplement
　　1000 mg vitamin C

Diane's diet diary is severely lacking in essential nutrients. Throughout her pregnancy she had recurrent bladder infections, sugar in her urine, and depression. She bled heavily at birth and was depressed after as well. Her diet is lacking in protein and calcium, contains no yellow or orange vegetables, and is heavy in sweets. She needs to add foods from all of the mentioned groups at each meal and snack, and try to find foods that are filling and non-sweet. In fact, when she tried this approach, the sugar did not show up in her urine samples.

The diet diaries in these samples come from women ranging from eighteen years old to their mid-thirties. These women have professions that include stay-at-home mothers, artists, musicians, school teachers, chiropractors, and medical doctors (not in that order).

To understand the evaluation of these diet diaries you will need to refer to the following information on specific nutrients so that you will know which foods provide which nutrients in these groups.

ESSENTIAL NUTRIENTS

Because it is ideal to get your nutrients from foods rather than relying on supplements, I am including a wide variety of food sources from which various nutrients are available. The best way to ensure that you are eating well is to include a wide variety of healthy, natural foods. Your best bets are foods that are as close to a natural state as possible—minimally processed with no additives or preservatives. The core of a healthy diet will be made up of whole grains, beans, fresh vegetables, fresh fruits, nuts, seeds, and smaller amounts of dairy products, and complementary amounts of meats, particularly fish and poultry. If you are unaccustomed to natural foods, try to find a few interesting cookbooks and begin to add healthy foods slowly to your diet. If you already are eating a very healthy diet, then make sure you are eating adequate amounts, needed by your growing body and baby.

Let your intuition guide you in your food choices. Suspend your conscious mind for a few minutes each day to allow messages to arise from your right brain or intuitive mode of thinking. If your intuition tells you to eat a piece of salmon, though you are an

RECOMMENDED DIETARY ALLOWANCES OF NUTRIENTS FOR PREGNANT AND NURSING WOMEN

Nutrient	Pregnancy	Nursing
Protein	74 g	64 g
Calories	2300	2500
Vitamin A	5000 iu	6000 iu
Vitamin D	400 iu	400 iu
Vitamin C	80 mg	100 mg
Vitamin E	15 iu	16 iu
B1	1.4 mg	1.5 mg
B2	1.5 mg	1.7 mg
Niacin	15 mg	18 mg
B6	2.6 mg	2.5 mg
Folacin	800 mcg	500 mcg
B12	4 mcg	4 mcg
Calcium	1200 mg	1200 mg
Phosphorus	1200 mg	1200 mg
Magnesium	450 mg	450 mg
Iron	30–60 mg	30–60 mg
Zinc	20 mg	25 mg
Iodine	175 mcg	200 mcg

(from the Food and Nutrition Board of the National Academy of Sciences, 1980)

DAILY RECOMMENDED PORTIONS OF SELECTED FOOD GROUPS

Protein	4 servings
Whole grains and complex carbohydrates	4-6 serving
Vitamin C foods	2 servings
Calcium foods	4 servings
Dark green leafy vegetables	2 servings
Yellow/orange vegetables or fruits	1 serving
Other vegetables or fruits	2 servings
Iron-rich foods	some daily
High fat foods	2 servings
Fluids	6-8 glasses

ardent vegetarian, you may choose your intuited needs over your ideals. Similarly, if you dislike collard greens but your body says "greens" you may have to develop a taste for collards and find a few delicious recipes! To develop this intuition, allow yourself to be very still and quiet for a few minutes, and then simply ask yourself or the baby what you need. Make a note of what you imagine the answer to be. Try this each day for a week and follow through on the messages that you receive.

Eat for nutrition and pleasure and you will meet your needs—enjoyment of food is one of the most important keys to good digestion, which must also occur if you are going to absorb and utilize the foods you do eat.

A general guideline of the food servings you need to eat *daily* is as follows:

- Calories: eat plentifully of healthy foods to ensure adequate calories daily—pregnancy is not a time to try to minimize calories.

- Protein: 4 servings

- Vitamin C foods: 2 servings

- Calcium foods: 4 servings

- Green leafy vegetables and yellow fruits and vegetables: 3 servings

- Other veggies and fruits: 1–2 servings

- Whole grains and other complex carbohydrates: 4–6 servings

- Iron rich foods: some daily

- High-fat foods: 2 daily

- Salt: daily in moderation to taste

- Fluids: at least 6–8 glasses a day

- Supplements: nutritious herbs, highly concentrated food supplements such as spirulina, and when necessary a vitamin/mineral supplement.

These daily serving amounts are known as "the daily dozen" in *What to Eat When You're Expecting* (Eisenberg, Murkoff, and Hathaway). They will provide you with a good framework to which you can add the healthy foods of your own choosing. Note that all of these requirements increase when you are carrying two or more babies. Remember, this is an ideal that you should try to achieve as closely as possible. Every woman will have better days and skimpier days, depending on how you feel and what is going on in your life. I also suggest that you pay attention to how you feel when you eat or miss a meal, or when you eat a healthy meal compared to a sweet snack. In time your body will come to crave the healthy meals over the empty foods.

The National Academy of Sciences has published recommended dietary allowances of nutrients for pregnant and nursing women (see chart). These numbers reflect the actual amounts of nutrients that pregnant and nursing women need in order to maintain a healthy pregnancy. When referring to this chart it is important to keep a few things in mind:

- We are all unique…so are our needs.

- The numbers in this chart reflect dietary needs to the best of present scientific knowledge. As knowledge changes and grows, so do charts such as this one.

- Following a chart of nutrients is less important than eating amply of a wide variety of whole, natural foods daily.

- A healthy diet comes from an open mind and a commitment to paying attention to your personal needs.

Following are descriptions of the common essential nutrients, along with their functions and the sources from which you can obtain them.

We are all unique and so are our needs.

—*A. J. R.*

— *Protein* —

Protein is one of the most abundant substances in the body, second only to water. It provides the structural framework upon which all body tissues depend for healthy growth. Bones, muscles, skin, blood, hair, nails, organs, and connective tissue are all made from proteins. The baby's formation of hormones, growth, metabolism, and sexual development are made possible with protein. Protein is necessary for basic chemical reactions, including the maintenance of fluid and pH balance. Protein encourages and contributes to the formation of antibodies necessary for fighting infection. If we have an adequate protein and carbohydrate ratio, our blood sugar level remains stable and we are provided with energy as we need it.

Protein provides the raw material for making the baby, placenta, and a strong uterus. It contributes to the formation of breast milk and is essential for healthy blood clotting. There are about 22 amino acids— the structural components of protein and the end products of protein digestion— needed by the body. All but eight of these can be produced in the body or converted into another kind should a shortage of any occur. The eight that must be obtained dietarily are called the "essential amino acids." These eight amino acids are available in many foods in varying proportions. However, for the protein to be used optimally by the body, they need to be present in specific amounts. Foods in which the amino acids are always present in these specific quantities are known as "complete proteins" and include such foods as meats, dairy products, and soybean products. Foods such as grains, seeds, nuts, and legumes are known as "incomplete proteins" as they are either missing or low in specific amino acids.

Vegetables also contain usable proteins, but in smaller amounts than the foods already mentioned. When eaten in various combinations they form complete proteins which are highly nutritious and assimilable by the body. See below for a discussion of protein combining.

Although protein may be converted into fat and stored in the liver it will not serve the same function as the original protein. Protein is not otherwise stored in the body and a continuing supply is necessary for the healthy functioning of all of our cells.

Protein deficiency may manifest itself as follows: abnormal growth and development, loss of muscle tone, lack of vigor and stamina, mental depression, increased susceptibility to infection, poor wound healing, and slow recovery from illness. Protein loss occurs through stresses such as injury and illness. During such times extra protein is required to replace or repair tissues. Childbearing, due to the increased size and amount of the mother's tissues, the baby's needs, labor, birth, postpartum healing, and lactation, requires a great increase in protein consumption. While protein requirements are influenced by a woman's size, nutritional status, and activity levels, it is generally thought that 75–100 grams of protein daily will fulfill the protein requirement for pregnancy. Eating at least four servings of protein rich foods as meals, with complementary high protein snacks (such as yogurt, cheese and crackers, hummus dip) daily will provide you with adequate protein. I personally have found that the lower end of this range is optimal, the upper end producing very large babies and difficult digestion. Inadequate protein intake during pregnancy is associated with toxemia.

An exhaustive list of protein quantities in different foods is beyond the scope of this

THE NATURAL PREGNANCY BOOK

book, but I direct you to *What to Eat When You're Expecting*, and all books by Gail and Tom Brewer (see "Further Reading"). *Holistic Midwifery*, written for health care professionals, also offers many pages of food servings and their nutrient quantities. It is clear enough so that you don't have to be a midwife to understand and make use of the information. By learning to recognize what foods are rich in different nutrients you will be able to construct a good diet for yourself.

— Carbohydrates —

Carbohydrates are the main sources of energy for all body functions including digestion and assimilation of food and all muscular activity. Carbohydrates provide immediately available energy for producing heat in the body. Broken down into glucose, carbohydrates provide fuel for the brain, nervous system, and muscle tissues; in the form of glycogen, carbohydrates can be stored by the liver and muscles. Carbohydrates, when available in excess, can also be stored throughout the body in the form of fat and used as reserve energy when needed. (The utilization of fat results in weight loss.)

Carbohydrates are needed in the largest quantity of all the nutrients required by the body. They make up the bulk of our diet. They are available in three main forms: simple sugars, starches (complex carbohydrates), and cellulose (the indigestible parts of fruits and vegetables that provide us with the fiber needed for healthy bowel functioning).

Simple sugars can be found in both refined foods (sugar, candy, soft drinks, chocolate, etc.) and unrefined foods (honey, maple syrup, and other natural sweeteners as well as in fruits). In these forms they are almost immediately digested, quickly raising blood sugar levels, and eliminating feelings of hunger. It is important to realize that the feeling of hunger, although triggered somewhat by falling blood sugar levels, is more than a signal to put more sugar in the body. It is also a call for vital nutrients. Both refined and unrefined sugars have the ability to satisfy hunger with quick fuel. This can lead us to forego eating nutritious foods that will provide us with longer lasting energy. This is true for fruits as well, though they do provide essential vitamins and minerals. Since excess carbohydrates are stored in the body as fat, you can actually become overweight at the same time you are becoming malnourished. Simple sugars are short-lived in the bloodstream, leaving us with sudden feelings of fatigue, depression, irritability, headache, and the need for another boost of energy. Persistent overconsumption of simple sugars can also lead to an overly large baby and maternal diabetes (with complications for both the mom and baby).

Starches are complex chains of sugar units. When carbohydrates are eaten in this form, the sugar units are separated and digested slowly, thus taking longer to reach the bloodstream and satiate hunger. This slow digestion allows the body adequate time to absorb the range of nutrients in these unprocessed starchy foods. With complex carbohydrates, blood sugar levels remain steady for a longer time than with simple sugars, so hunger is sated for a considerably greater length of time.

If carbohydrate intake is insufficient, the body will use protein and fat for energy. This leads to a harmful chemical residue in the body known as ketones, which if present consistently or in high amounts can be dangerous for both the mother and the baby. It is therefore essential that pregnant mothers base their diets around complex carbohydrates as their source of carbohydrates (4–6 servings daily), getting these from whole grains (brown rice, whole wheat, millet, oats, rye, barley, amaranth, etc.), seeds, and a variety of starchy vegetables such as potatoes (both white and sweet), squashes, and beets.

— Fats —

Fats, or lipids, are the most concentrated form of energy in the diet, providing twice as many calories per gram as carbohydrates and protein. Fats act as carriers of the fat soluble vitamins, A, D, E, and K. By aiding in the absorption of vitamin D, fats make calcium available to body tissues. Also, fats are important in converting carotene to vitamin A. Fat deposits surround, hold in place, and protect major organs. A layer of body fat helps the body deal with temperature changes in a room or outdoors and preserves body heat. There are three essential fatty acids (substances which give fats their different properties such as melting point, flavor, and texture). They are synthesized by the body if one of them, linoleic acid, is present in the diet. These unsaturated fatty acids are necessary for healthy blood, arteries, nerves, skin, and other tissues. They aid in the digestion of cholesterol.

Cholesterol is a fat-related substance and is needed to form sex and adrenal hormones, vitamin D, healthy blood, skin and nervous system, brain and liver tissue, and the bile which is necessary for the digestion of fats.

Although rare, a deficiency of fats will lead to a deficiency of fat soluble vitamins and related disorders. Excessive intake of fats could also lead to digestive and other health problems. It is accepted that one tablespoon of fat daily in the form of a pure vegetable oil (unrefined, cold-pressed oil), as well as foods rich in this nutrient, is plenty. Significant sources of fats are nuts, seeds,

vegetable oils, butter, margarine, dairy products, and fats in meat. Salmon, mackerel, and herring are excellent sources of essential fatty acids and can be eaten a couple of times a week. Essential fatty acids are also found in the oils derived from evening primrose, walnuts, black currants, flax seeds, and borage. Raw walnut oil or flaxseed oil can be added to salads and other dishes after cooking, or a supplement of 500 mg of any of these oils, with the exception of the walnut oil (do not exceed this dosage unless there is a specific reason for doing so), can be taken daily throughout pregnancy to ensure the adequate intake.

— Vitamins —

Vitamin A

Vitamin A is most noted for its role in preventing and fighting infections. It promotes healthy skin and mucous membranes, strong bones, rich blood, and keen eyesight. Proper digestion of proteins requires the presence of vitamin A. Requirements may vary greatly from person to person, and both deficiency and excess of this vitamin can be harmful. Therefore it is important to eat foods rich in vitamin A, but to avoid supplementation of this individual vitamin during pregnancy (other than what is in your prenatal vitamin if you are taking one).

Acute vitamin A poisoning can be recognized by nausea, vomiting, dry skin, diarrhea, hair loss, sore lips, and flaky, itchy skin. This usually only occurs as a result of excessive supplementation, and unless caused by chronic excess, will disappear soon after the vitamin supplement is withdrawn. In early pregnancy, however, excessive supplementation can result in permanent fetal malformations.

Symptoms of vitamin A deficiency include frequent colds and respiratory problems, sinus trouble, rough skin, acne, dandruff, and night-blindness.

Vitamin A is destroyed by light, staleness, drying of foods, and chemical fertilizers. It is leached out of the body by ingesting mineral oil. The body accepts vitamin A more easily in foods that are cooked, mashed, or puréed.

Rich sources of this vitamin include yellow and orange fruits, yellow vegetables, dark green vegetables, orange vegetables such as carrots and sweet potatoes, dairy products, eggs (especially the yolk), and liver.

Herbal sources include alfalfa, watercress, nettle, red raspberry leaves, dandelion, comfrey, nori, yellow dock, and lamb's quarters.

VITAMIN B-COMPLEX

The B-complex vitamins are grouped because they have similar functions and tend to occur together in nature. Similarly, a deficiency of a single B vitamin is less likely than a general B vitamin deficiency. They are essential for a healthy nervous system, as well as for the metabolism of carbohydrates, fats, and proteins. They also help maintain muscle tone in the gastrointestinal tract, and health of the skin, hair, eyes, mouth, and liver. Since they are water soluble vitamins, they are not stored in the body and must be ingested through the diet on a regular basis. Some of the B vitamins are produced naturally in healthy intestines.

There are quite a few B-complex vitamins. The following are considered especially important for health during pregnancy:

B1 (thiamin) is necessary for children's consistent growth, a healthy nervous system, and good muscle tone in the stomach, intestines, and heart. B1 aids in the conversion of glucose into energy and helps stabilize the appetite and blood sugar by the assimilation of starches and sugars. Signs of deficiency include constipation, loss of appetite, digestive problems, fatigue, apathy, uncertainty of memory, and nervousness. B1 is stored in the body only in very small amounts so daily intake is necessary. Found in the outer layers of grains, it is usually lost in the refining process. It is destroyed by heat, oxidation, and alkaline substances such as baking soda. Sources include whole grains (especially wheat germ), nuts and seeds, legumes, potatoes, peas, nutritional yeast, bananas, and avocados.

Herbal sources include dandelion, alfalfa, red clover, red raspberry leaves, nori, kelp, catnip, and watercress.

B2 (riboflavin) is necessary for the assimilation and digestion of carbohydrates, fats, and proteins. It aids in cell respiration. Maintenance of healthy skin, nails, hair, and good vision depends on vitamin B2.

This nutrient is found in nutritional yeast, whole grains (especially wheat), dried beans and peas, seeds (especially sunflower), leafy green vegetables, cottage cheese, milk, and organ meats.

Signs of deficiency in B2 include digestive troubles, skin and eye problems, cracking at the corners of the mouth, hair loss, poor lactation, sluggishness, retarded growth, dizziness, trembling, urinary difficulty, vaginal itching, and bloating of the body.

Herbal sources include rose hips, dandelion, dulse, kelp, and fenugreek.

B6 (pyridoxine) is required for a healthy nervous system and utilization of carbohydrates, fats, and proteins. It must be present for the production of antibodies and red blood cells. It helps regulate body fluids and aids in healthy muscle formation and functioning. It is associated with hormonal balance, and because of its importance in digestion and healthy muscles, deficiency is often associated with nausea and leg cramps in pregnancy. Depression may also be caused by a B6 deficiency.

B6 is destroyed by heat and ultraviolet light. Rich food sources include brown rice, wheat bran and germ, blackstrap molasses, nutritional yeast, bananas, salmon, and organ meats.

B12 is needed for healthy nerve tissue, fetal brain development, the production of genetic material, proper cell division, and the metabolism of many nutrients.

Because plants do not require B12 for their growth, plant foods, unless they have been fermented (encouraging the growth of bacteria which contain and help our bodies to synthesize B12) or fortified rarely contain this vitamin. Therefore, those on strictly vegan diets, containing absolutely no animal products, should consider using vitamin B12. Foods that do contain B12 include dairy products (with the exception of butter) and meats. Vegetarian sources include tempeh, miso, and B12-fortified nutritional yeast. However, the tempeh and miso contain variable and, according to some, unreliable amounts of B12. Because our bodies need only small amounts of B12 the addition of a small daily amount of dairy or other animal products to the diet will supply enough, as will a prenatal vitamin. Maintaining healthy intestinal flora with yogurt will also help with intrinsic B12 production.

The fact that our bodies store B12 for years is in some ways an advantage, but could also prevent deficiency signs from showing up for five or six years. Signs of B12 deficiency include a glossy, sore tongue, indigestion, abdominal pains, and diarrhea or constipation. Left untreated, serious mental and nervous problems may develop and eventually death may occur. Megaloblastic and pernicious anemia are terms used to describe deficiencies associated with vitamin B12.

Folic acid is a water soluble member of the B-complex group. It is essential for the formation of red blood cells and antibodies that prevent infection. A lack of folic acid can result in severe anemia in the mother and neural tube defects (such as anencephaly, a congenital absence of the forebrain, and spina bifida, an opening along the spine) in the baby. It is used in the breakdown and utilization of protein and is essential for healthy brain development. Digestive, mental, and emotional health are all related to folic acid intake. Folic acid is needed in much greater amounts during pregnancy, acting as a safeguard against anemia, miscarriage, premature birth, and birth defects. It is available in green leafy vegetables, wheat germ, nutritional yeast, eggs, whole grains, lentils, nuts, milk, and liver. As it is lost in the cooking process, care must be taken to eat raw leafy green vegetables daily and to regularly include several of these other sources in your diet.

VITAMIN C (ASCORBIC ACID)

Vitamin C is essential for the production of collagen, a protein needed for forming connective tissue in bones, ligaments, and skin, as well as in the healing of wounds and burns. It is needed to produce a healthy placenta, capillaries, and cell walls, and helps to prevent varicosities and hemorrhage. Vitamin C greatly aids in the assimilation of other nutrients such as folic acid, iron, vitamins A and E, and certain amino acids. It is very helpful in preventing and healing infections, and is quickly used up during stressful times. During pregnancy the daily dosage should not exceed 2000 mg, as it can lead to miscarriage in early pregnancy, and can cause a vitamin C dependency in the baby which can lead to scurvy in the newborn.

Found in most fresh fruits and vegetables, vitamin C is destroyed by heat, air, and light, and is also lost in cooking water. At least two servings of vitamin C-rich foods should be eaten each day. Excellent sources include green leafy vegetables such as raw or lightly cooked kale and collard greens, strawberries, peppers, citrus fruits, cantaloupe, alfalfa sprouts, and tomatoes.

Herbal sources include rose hips, watercress, dandelion greens, red clover, burdock, nettle, and alfalfa.

VITAMIN D

Vitamin D is a fat soluble vitamin, mainly available through exposure to sunlight and ingestion of fatty fish and fish liver oils, with smaller amounts to be found in butter, milk from grazed cows, and egg yolks. Fortified commercial milk is rich in a synthetic form of vitamin D.

Vitamin D aids in the absorption of calcium from the intestines and the breakdown and assimilation of phosphorous, both necessary for bone formation. It helps maintain a healthy nervous system, normal heart functioning, and normal clotting responses by helping the body absorb calcium. Deficiencies of this nutrient can lead to bone deformities and excesses of it can lead to dizziness, nausea, and weakness, similar to what is experienced from overexposure to the sun.

Herbal sources include alfalfa and nettle.

VITAMIN E

This is another fat soluble vitamin. The most common form is alpha-tocopherol which literally means "the substance required to bring forth normal births."

Vitamin E prevents the destruction of cells and vital nutrients, and it enables body tissue to function with less oxygen thereby increasing endurance and stamina. It is essential to certain types of metabolism, aids in cell division, and promotes health and healing of body tissue. Vitamin E helps prevent abnormal blood clotting and is said to increase the pain threshold.

It is abundant in whole grains, nuts, oils, eggs, wheat germ, legumes, and green leafy vegetables. Caution should be taken with any vitamin E supplementation during pregnancy as excesses may cause abnormal adherence of the placenta. Vitamin E can also be dangerous for those with heart or blood pressure problems, so any supplementation should be done carefully and intelligently.

— Minerals —

CALCIUM

The most abundant mineral in the body, calcium is needed in the formation of a baby's bones and teeth, and in maintaining the health of the mother's bones, teeth, and connective tissue. It is essential in controlling the coagulation of blood. Muscles cannot contract and release without it. Calcium helps maintain healthy nerves, normal metabolism, mineral balance throughout the body, and regular heartbeat. It is said to increase the pain threshold, and its effectiveness in promoting nerve and muscular relaxation prevents and reduces insomnia. Signs of calcium deficiency include irritability, insomnia, and leg cramps. Sources of calcium are milk, hard cheeses, and yogurt, leafy green vegetables, almonds, sea vegetables, salmon, and blackstrap molasses. It is important to maintain a balance of calcium and phosphorus in the diet as excess

We tend to think that a baby in utero is entirely cut off from the world that lies just beyond a thin layer of skin. We seldom consider the child within as a conscious being, capable of responding to sounds and the inner environment the mother creates through her sense of well-being or lack of it.

—Joy Gardner

of either will cause losses of both. Also, calcium and magnesium work together, and when you supplement calcium, take a supplement that contains both of these minerals. Be sure to eat four servings of calcium-rich foods each day.

Herbal sources include alfalfa, red clover, red raspberry leaves, nettle, chamomile, dandelion, kelp, and dulse.

IRON

Iron is present in every living cell. Its major function is to combine with other nutrients to create hemoglobin which brings oxygen to all the tissues of the body. Iron helps to build the blood, increases resistance to stress and disease, and allows for proper muscle contraction. It aids in protein metabolism, helps to improve respiration, and prevents hemorrhage.

Sources of iron include dark leafy green vegetables, dried fruits (raisins, apricots, black mission figs, prunes, currants, and cherries), blackstrap molasses, sea vegetables, dried beans and legumes, whole grains, eggs, red meat, and liver. You will need to eat several iron-rich foods daily.

Herbal sources include nettle, dandelion, yellow dock, kelp, alfalfa, watercress, and fennel.

IODINE

Iodine is needed for the healthy function of the thyroid gland, which is responsible for the rate of metabolism, growth and development, and mental balance. Deficiency may be signaled by frequent infections, weakness, nervous system problems, and low activity levels.

Iodine is found in sea food—fish and sea vegetables (kelp or kombu, dulse, alaria or wakame, hijiki, and nori)—and in iodized salt and sea salt. A few vegetables contain small amounts of iodine.

Herbal sources include watercress, kelp, dulse, and Irish moss.

PHOSPHORUS

Usually found in abundance in most diets, phosphorus is important for bone development, healthy teeth, and the healthy growth of fetal cells.

Herbal sources include alfalfa, red raspberry leaves, dandelion, watercress, caraway seeds, and comfrey.

ZINC

Zinc is essential for normal immune system functioning, healthy hormone production, organ development, healthy reproduction, and release of vitamin A from the liver. It also protects the bones and joints, as well as the prostate gland and sexual fluids in males.

Sources include oysters, other shellfish, herring, nuts, seeds, beef, eggs, chicken, turkey, fruits, and vegetables.

Herbal sources include watercress.

SODIUM

Sodium is an essential mineral for maintaining health during pregnancy. A deficiency of sodium is associated with swelling and toxemia in pregnancy. It is necessary for maintaining both fluid and electrolyte balance, as well as preventing muscular irritability. It is available in common salt, sea salt, and many foods. Pregnant women should reduce their consumption of junk foods which are heavily salted, but should salt their other foods to taste using a natural form of salt such as sea salt.

OTHER MINERALS

Other minerals, such as potassium which is needed for strong muscle contraction, and many trace minerals should all be available to you in your diet if you eating the quantity and variety of foods already mentioned.

VEGETARIAN AND OTHER NATURAL FOODS DIETS

There are four common variations on the basic vegetarian diet: the vegetarian who occasionally eats fish or chicken, but relies primarily on nonmeat sources for nutrients; the lacto-ovo vegetarian who eats no meats but does eat dairy products and eggs; the lacto vegetarian who eats dairy but no meats or eggs; and the vegan who includes absolutely no animal products in the diet whatsoever and frequently excludes honey as well.

A person on a macrobiotic diet eats whole grains, beans, vegetables, occasional fruits in season, sea vegetables, seeds, and nuts, with the occasional inclusion of fish. Such a person relies on the concept of yin and yang to create balanced menus to meet individual health needs and create harmony in the body, mind, and spirit.

A person on a raw-food diet believes that humans, like animals, should eat foods in a raw state. Emphasis is placed on fruits, vegetables, fresh juices, sprouts, nuts, and seeds (preferably sprouted). The idea is that cooked foods cause impurities in the body.

It is possible to meet your nutritional needs on any of these diets during pregnancy, if you give close attention to meeting these needs. Vegetarian diets that include a variety of foods are likely to include much less fat as well as fewer, if any, chemical additives and fewer overprocessed foods. Be open to your needs and don't get stuck on a preconceived idea. Respect your intuition whether you are a vegetarian wanting a piece of chicken, a vegan wanting a cheese sandwich, or a macrobiotic wanting a grapefruit in the middle of winter in Boston. The danger lies in becoming an extremist (admittedly, I consider a raw-foods diet extreme) and in excluding foods that might be just what your body needs. Of course there are many vegetarian ways to meet your needs if you choose to be strictly vegetarian—you must be willing to educate yourself about your nutritional needs.

Many natural foods diets are based on the idea that the body is dirty and needs cleansing through fasting. This is untrue and potentially very dangerous for pregnant women. Our bodies are capable of digesting meat, dairy products (unless a specific intolerance exists), and other foods often considered taboo. The key is moderation and balance. Also, foods serve different purposes. For example, fruits and raw foods cool us down and promote elimination while heavy carbohydrates and proteins warm us and help us to build our bodies. We must recognize what is appropriate for different seasons of the year and of our lives. Pregnancy is a time of building and nourishing, with elimination being an essential function for health, but not our primary goal.

Pregnant women need to eat with great care. They should avoid exposure to harmful additives as well as to residues from pesticides, and to antibiotics and hormones in animal products (dairy included). All pregnant women would do well to eat foods that are grown organically and are processed minimally if at all, with no additives or preservatives. Foods raised, grown, and prepared this way are not only safer to eat, but also retain more of their nutrient value than processed foods. While such good food may seem more expensive, it is actually worth the money as

Growing a baby is a big job requiring you to have good materials, enough to meet your needs and your baby's.
—*A. J. R.*

your body will be happy, and your medical expenses will be reduced. Chemical additives in food are associated with health problems ranging from acne to cancer. During pregnancy additives are particularly dangerous in the first trimester as they may impact on the development of the fetus. Hormones found in dairy products may imbalance a woman's own hormones, as well as cause her baby to grow overly big (even without these hormones, milk encourages babies to grow large).

Women who eat a healthy, well-balanced vegetarian diet may in fact enjoy a healthier pregnancy than women who rely heavily on the standard American diet which is laden with sugar and fat and excludes fresh vegetables, whole grains, legumes, nuts, and seeds. The primary concern for vegetarian women is that they get ample protein; if dairy is not eaten, foods containing calcium should be plentiful in the diet. There are many foods that can provide these nutrients, and in fact, in China where almost no dairy is used and a lot of dark green vegetables are consumed, the women have the lowest osteoporosis rates in the world. See the section on Calcium just above, and refer to books in the nutrition section of "Further Reading" for more information on calcium substitutes. I encourage women not to drink milk during pregnancy and to rely instead on nondairy calcium sources, as well as hard cheeses and active culture yogurt.

In order to obtain adequate protein from a vegetarian diet, these women must learn to combine their protein sources to create complete proteins, as described earlier in this section. The following shows the various ways this can be done:

1. Grains (rice, corn, wheat, millet, oats, rye, barley, etc.) can be combined with a slightly smaller amount of beans or legumes (lentils, peanuts, garbanzo beans, kidney beans, pinto beans, black beans, aduki beans, navy beans, soybeans, etc.).

2. Grains can be combined with dairy products.

3. Nuts and seeds can be combined with beans or legumes.

A few examples of complete proteins include rice and beans, macaroni and cheese, rice and tahini (sesame seed paste), pasta with peanut sauce, granola that contains oats, peanuts, and sunflower seeds, whole-wheat bread with peanut butter, tofu on toast. You don't need to eat complete proteins every time you have a protein food, but you should get 4–5 servings of complete proteins each day. I have enjoyed three completely vegetarian pregnancies, and one mostly vegetarian (in my last pregnancy I was inclined to eat fish and chicken and so I occasionally added these foods (organic poultry only) to my diet. The main advantage for me in including dairy as a regular part of my diet was the fact that it is easy to prepare and is a filling source of energy. One can eat rice, beans, and cheese, for example, and feel more filled than by eating rice and beans alone. Yogurt, or cheese and crackers, makes a great, filling, quick snack. Also, dairy foods are complete proteins, so I didn't have to be as concerned about combining foods as I would on a vegan diet. It takes a larger quantity of vegetarian foods to satisfy the appetite, than say a small piece of steak, but vegetarian food is also easier to digest, and not likely to result in problems such as constipation or weight gain due to the high fiber, low-fat nature of the foods.

I recommend that pregnant women do not drink milk because babies of mothers who drink a lot of milk tend to grow very big. I feel that this is a disadvantage in birthing. Milk molecules are also hard to digest, milk is high in fat, and it also contains hormones, both naturally occurring in cows, and sometimes added with cattle feed. These hormones are not beneficial to human health and may possibly be harmful.

If you are pregnant and vegetarian I can't overemphasize how important it is to eat a wide variety of foods in order to obtain all of the nutrients you now require. I've met many well-educated vegetarians whose diets were limited to just a few foods. Some rely on packaged foods. Processing is processing—it robs foods of nutrients. Also, many vegetarian women eat a lot of fruit and drink a lot of fruit juices, filling up on empty calories. Just being a vegetarian does not ensure that you are eating a healthy diet—it may mean merely that you are not eating unhealthy foods! If you plan to raise your child as a vegetarian, now is the time to do the research and feed yourself and your baby well.

SUPPLEMENTS

Recommending vitamin and mineral supplements to pregnant women is standard practice for most obstetricians and midwives. I vary my approach with pregnant women. For example, I check to see whether a woman is anemic or deficient in a specific vitamin or mineral, I look at her lifestyle (Is she under a great deal of stress? Is she already nursing a toddler or older baby? Or has she had close-spaced pregnancies in the last few years?), her commitment to eating well, and her tolerance of supplements. I for one got extremely nauseated and even vomited after taking supplements. I therefore did not take prenatal vitamins. When I was nursing my fourth baby and was busy with my older children and my work, I found myself wanting a supplement, and found no problem digesting it.

When a woman is pregnant and shows some stress or fatigue, or has a poor diet, a daily supplement can improve her well-being. When a woman is eating well (evidenced by her diet diary and an ongoing discussion of her eating patterns) and doesn't want to take a supplement, the addition of herbal infusions and syrups (see Chapter 5, "Herbs and Pregnancy Health") as well as concentrated food sources such as blackstrap molasses and spirulina (a blue-green algae) is generally sufficient supplementation. The former is an excellent source of calcium, iron, and B vitamins, while the latter is a source of high quality protein and many other vitamins and minerals. One to two tablespoons daily of each is an excellent addition to the diet. Molasses can be taken in hot water, added to a smoothie with yogurt, bananas, honey, and vanilla, eaten off the spoon, or in an iron tonic (see "Anemia" in Chapter 14 for the recipe). Spirulina can be taken in tablets, or can also be added to a smoothie. If iron deficiency is a problem, refer to "Anemia."

However you choose to enhance your diet, it is essential that you do so, as growing a baby is a big job requiring you to have good materials, enough to meet your needs and the baby's. Remember, though, that no supplements will substitute for good food.

CRAVINGS

As long as you are meeting all of your daily needs with healthy food there is no reason that you should not enjoy an occasional ice-cream or piece of cake, cookies, or a chocolate brownie. The main problems arise when you follow your urge for cravings that are downright unhealthy, such as coffee, cigarettes, sodas, or alcohol, which can interfere with nutrient absorption or may cause harm to your baby. Also, problems may arise when you use your craving as a substitute for nutritious foods. For example, if you work outside the home while you are pregnant and find yourself craving a chocolate bar at 11:00 A.M. each day, your body is really telling you that you need food energy. If you eat the candy bar, you are basically sublimating your appetite and not getting anything nutritious. You could carry a healthy snack with you to work, such as a container of yogurt and some granola, apples and peanut butter, a cheese sandwich, or a small thermos of soup, and eat this when you feel the craving. If, at the end of the day you've met your daily food needs and still want a dessert, have one. But even these can be made with nutritious and wholesome ingredients. (The cookbooks in "Further Reading" offer great dessert recipes .)

Frequently cravings are specific clues about our nutritional needs. Deciphering them may take a bit of detective work. For example, a pregnant mother in my practice craved the proverbial pickles and ice cream. She was busy tending to her two older children, both under three years of age, and didn't bother to eat. She then became ravenous for the pickles and ice cream. It struck me that her body perhaps needed more protein and calcium (the ice cream). As for the pickles, vinegary foods encourage our bodies to release calcium into the bloodstream. When I suggested she begin to improve her intake of protein and calcium, she reported that she had no more of those cravings. Frequently a craving for sweets is a physical need for more protein in the diet. Cravings for chips or pretzels can be a sign that you need more salt or even fats in your diet. Try to replace junk foods with wholesome choices and see how this affects your cravings. If you're eating well, and still want some ice cream, bon appetit!

WEIGHT GAIN

Because weight is such a big mental and emotional concern for most women (thin women don't want to gain it, fat women want to lose it, and most women compromise their eating because of it) I don't place any emphasis on weight gain in my work. The fact is, a woman can gain weight even on an inadequate diet. Therefore, I focus on what and how much a woman is eating, not how much she is gaining. I did the same for myself, weighing myself at the beginning and end of my pregnancies for curiosity's sake. When I begin to work with a woman, I will ask her if she knows her weight, and I will enter this in her chart. Then at subsequent visits I will ask her if she knows her weight, and if she does not, I will ask her if she wants to know her weight. If she says no, we don't check her weight. What is really important is whether the baby is growing and whether she feels and looks healthy. If so, there is no need, in my opinion, to be concerned about weight.

According to typical midwifery and medical standards, an ideal weight gain for a pregnant woman is about 25 to 35 pounds. Some women will gain more, some less, especially depending upon their pre-pregnant weight (very slim women may gain as much as 50 pounds while larger women may gain less). Women will also gain weight in unique spurts, not in neat little increments per month. Many women will gain moderately in the first months of pregnancy, only to make a big weight gain in the middle months of the pregnancy. Many women will slow down again toward the end of pregnancy, despite the fact that the baby may appear to grow rapidly during the last weeks of the pregnancy. Again, quality is more important than quantity in the area of weight gain. If knowing that you are gaining is going to make you sabotage yourself by consciously or unconsciously cutting back your food intake, then weighing should be abandoned. Similarly, if you go for a few weeks without gaining much weight, yet your baby is growing and your health is fine, it is wise to ascertain whether you are eating enough food, particularly if you exercise heavily. Each woman has a unique weight gain pattern.

CHAPTER 6

Herbs and Pregnancy Health

Herbs are used to promote health, spice up our lives, and restore health when we feel ill or out of sorts. There are literally thousands of herbs used around the world by different peoples for different conditions. Traditionally, herbs have been added to foods to improve the taste, promote healthy digestion, and prevent parasites and other infectious organisms from taking hold in our bodies. Herbs can be used to improve the quantity and quality of nutrients in the diet due to their high vitamin and mineral content. Many herbs are both safe and highly effective as remedies for both common health complaints and more serious conditions.

It is not hard to learn to incorporate herbs into your daily life, particularly when you choose from those that are known to be free of toxic effects. Herbs needn't be relied upon only when you are ill or uncomfortable. The best way to benefit from herbs is to use them daily as a source of nourish-ment. There are many herbs that can be used safely during pregnancy that not only provide additional vitamins and minerals to your diet, but also strengthen the womb, liver, digestive system, and urogenital tract. Herbs derive nutrients from the soil that many of our common foods may lack. Herbs used in moderation don't usually leave women feeling nauseated or constipated, as do many vitamin and mineral supplements, and the nutrients are more easily assimilated. Herbs are relatively inexpensive, particularly if you buy them in bulk. Tea drinking is a daily ritual in many parts of the world and can provide a nourishing ritual during your pregnancy.

The herbs mentioned in this book can be considered safe in pregnancy as indicated by generations of safe usage, as well as in clinical studies. Any exceptions are clearly noted. However, there are a few potential problems that should always be kept in mind.

First of all, no two people are exactly alike and therefore you cannot know in advance the exact effect an herb will have in your body (or your baby). It is best to rely on tried and true herbs during pregnancy and to begin with small amounts, gradually increasing dosage as appropriate and necessary. For example, chamomile is an herb considered completely safe and free from any toxic side effects according to extensive German research, yet because of its membership in the *Compositae* family, along with herbs such as ragweed, a rare individual may have an allergic reaction to it. Also chamomile does have emmenagogic properties, that is, it potentially promotes menstruation. However, in moderate doses this is extremely unlikely to be of consequence. With all herbs it is wise to proceed slowly and carefully.

If you are harvesting plants from the wild, make sure that you are identifying them correctly. Confusing the desired herb with a poisonous plant can be a fatal mistake. But even when purchasing a bulk herb, be certain that both the common names and the Latin names of the plants are what you are looking for (see Appendix II). (Plants have many different common names, but their Latin names are internationally accepted as a standard.) Also be certain to take herbal tinctures, pills, and capsules from carefully labeled jars so that no mistakes are made. Again this is especially important during pregnancy and with young children.

It is also important to follow general dosage guidelines for each herb. The idea that more is better is dangerous when applied to any medication, including herbs. Although most herbs are very gentle, their effects should not be underestimated. In Appendix I, Herbal Preparations, you will find general dosage guidelines.

When you are pregnant, further considerations arise. Herbs that you take during pregnancy will usually affect your baby as well as you. Herbs contain potent chemical substances, many of which have demonstrable effects on the body. Certain herbs, for example, contain volatile oils or alkaloids which can affect the functioning of the central nervous system, and when taken during the first trimester of pregnancy can interfere with the development of the baby's nervous system. Other herbs have what are known as emmenagogic properties—that is, they stimulate pelvic circulation. While this may be desirable when a woman is close to the time of birth, the result earlier might be the stimulation of contractions, perhaps even premature labor. Pregnancy is a natural process, and unless you are ill, it is unnecessary to use herbs other than as gentle toners and nourishers. If you are ill and wish to use herbs remedially, it is essential that you avoid herbs that are contraindicated during pregnancy, particularly during the first trimester. You should use herbs only according to recommended times and dosages. You should consult an experienced herbalist when you are unsure about the safety of using a particular herb during pregnancy.

HERBS TO AVOID DURING PREGNANCY

The table that accompanies this section lists those herbs most commonly contraindicated for internal use during pregnancy. However, there are some herbs on this list that may be used in small quantities for certain conditions, where the risks of using the herb are outweighed by the benefits. An example of this would be the use of very small amounts of goldenseal for severe diarrhea during mid-pregnancy, when diarrhea was causing the

A woman is the full circle, within her is the power— to create, nurture, and transform.

—Diane Mariechild

HERBS CONTRAINDICATED
FOR USE IN PREGNANCY

Alder buckthorn, *Rhamnus frangula*

Aloes, *Aloe vera*

Angelica, *Angelica archangelica*

Arnica, *Arnica montana*

Autumn crocus, *Colchicum autumnale*

Barberry, *Berberis vulgaris*

Bethroot, *Trillium spp.*

Black cohosh, *Cimicifuga racemosa*

Blessed thistle, *Carbenia benedicta*

Blood root, *Sanguinaria canadensis*

Blue cohosh, *Caulophyllum thalyctroides*

Broom, *Sarpthamnus scoparius*

Butternut, *Juglans canadensis*

Calamus, *Acorus calamus*

Calendula, *Calendula officinalis*

Cascara sagrada, *Rhamnus purshiana*

Coltsfoot, *Tussilago farfara*

Comfrey, *Symphytum officinale*

Cotton root, *Gossypium herbaceum*

Cowslip, *Primula veris*

Damiana, *Turnera aphrodisiaca*

Dong Quai, *Angelica sinensis*

Ephedra (Ma Huang), *Ephedra vulgaris*

Feverfew, *Tanacetum parthenium*

Ginseng, *Panax quinquefolium*

Goldenseal, *Hydrastis canadensis*

Gotu kola, *Hydrocotyle asiatica*

Goat's rue, *Galega officinalis*

Ipecac, *Ipecac ipechachuana*

Juniper berries, *Juniperis communis*

Licorice, *Glycyrrhiza glabra*

Lily of the valley, *Convallaria magalis*

Lobelia, *Lobelia inflata*

Male fern, *Dryopteris felix-mas*

Mandrake, *Podophyllum peltatum*

Mistletoe, *Viscum album*

Mugwort, *Artemesia vulgare*

Nutmeg (small amounts fine), *Myristica officinalis*

Osha, *Ligusticum porten*

Parsley (small amounts fine), *Carum petroselinum*

Pennyroyal, *Mentha pulegium*

Periwinkle, *Vinca spp.*

Peruvian bark, *Cinchona spp.*

Pleurisy root, *Aesclepius tuberosa*

Poke root, *Phytolacca decondra*

Rue, *Ruta graveolens*

Rhubarb, *Rheum palmatum*

Sage, *Salvia officinalis*

Sarsaparilla, *Smilax officinale*

Senna, *Cassia senna*

Shepherd's purse, *Capsella bursa-pastoris*

Stillingia, *Stillingia sylvatica*

Tansy, *Tanacetum vulgare*

Thuja, *Thuja occidentalis*

Wormwood, *Artemesia absinthum*

Yarrow, *Achillea millefolium*

mother to lose weight and become dehydrated. However, large doses of goldenseal during early pregnancy may damage the embryo. Also, certain herbs that are contraindicated by Western herbalists and Western scientific research for use during pregnancy are regularly used in other countries, such as dong quai prescribed as a blood tonic for pregnant women in China. It is wise to use such herbs cautiously, if at all during pregnancy, if you do not have prior herbal knowledge or the assistance of an herbalist. Pregnancy is not a good time to experiment with generally contraindicated herbs.

One group of herbs that has come under scrutiny are those containing pyrrolizidine alkaloids (PAs). These are suspected of causing liver damage in both adults and babies in the womb. Comfrey, coltsfoot, and borage are the main suspects, containing varying amounts of these PAs. It is therefore the most prudent to avoid the internal use of these herbs other than very occasionally and only after the first trimester of pregnancy. External use of comfrey is perfectly safe as PAs are not known to enter the body through the skin.

Herbs that contain other strong alkaloids (including those products which contain caffeine) and herbs that are considered to be strong bitters and which strongly promote digestive functions and metabolism are best avoided during pregnancy. Milder choices can be used in their stead. Herbs that strongly promote bowel peristalsis can also promote uterine contractions as well as bowel evacuation so it is best to avoid them. Other methods of promoting bowel functioning should be used, such as dietary changes, exercise, and nutritive laxatives. Most herbs with strong hormonal properties and those known to promote menstruation (known as emmenagogues) are to be avoided completely. Strong herbs used specifically to destroy intestinal worms are contraindicated as are the internal use of all essential oils.

Certain herbs in the accompanying table are considered safe for use only during the last few weeks of pregnancy, serving as "partus preparators." See the section "Herbs for Late-Pregnancy Health and Birth Preparation" in Chapter 11. Some of the late-pregnancy tonic herbs can also be used during labor, with the guidance of an experienced midwife or physician.

HERBS TO PROMOTE AND MAINTAIN PREGNANCY HEALTH

Using herbs helps us to connect with the natural world. What better or more primal time is there to do this than when we are pregnant? The optimal time to begin to use herbs is at the beginning of pregnancy, being careful to choose ones that are safe during the first trimester when the baby is still forming. But it is never too late to start. Herbs may be used singly or in combinations. If you begin to use herbs early in pregnancy, one cup a day will be enough, taken to the end of pregnancy. However, many of these herbs can be taken in larger quantities (as indicated). If you begin during your last trimester, you might want to increase the daily quantity of some of the nutritive herbs. This will also be indicated along with the description of the herb, preparation, and dosage.

Late-pregnancy tonics are not included in this list. Many of the herbs that can be safely used in late pregnancy are not safe earlier when the baby is in the formative months of the first trimester and they also can cause uterine contractions which could potentially lead to miscarriage. Herbs for late-pregnancy tonics can be found in Chapter 11, "The Month Before Birth."

It is simple and enjoyable to use herbs which provide us with a harvest of color, scent, and flavor in addition to their many beneficial qualities. Appendix I, "Herbal Preparations," will assist you in making infusions, oils, syrups, and other preparations, as well as in purchasing the herbs. Preparing your own tinctures, salves, and syrups is not only cost effective, it is an empowering way to create your own supplements and medicines.

As herbs are living beings harvested for our consumption, the respect and gratitude we give to our herbal preparations will also influence their healing potential. By allowing ourselves to be receptive not only to the pharmacological constituents, but to the vital essence that remains within the plants, we are opening ourselves to forces of healing that are beyond the quantifiable or reducible, that is, to the life forces which created the plants and ourselves. By growing plants or identifying them in the wild (even just some simple weeds common to backyards) you will gain a deeper appreciation for the subtle energies that invigorate herbs, and which you too will absorb when you partake of the healing plants.

The following herbs are some of my favorites for promoting and maintaining pregnancy health. I hope you will find a few favorites among these. They appear in alphabetical order, not by preference.

ALFALFA (*MEDICAGO SATIVA*)

This herb, a very mild mannered, common plant used as an agricultural cover crop, doesn't have dramatic healing properties, great beauty, or other outstanding features. What is remarkable about alfalfa is its high content of protein, vitamins A, D, E, B6, and K, calcium, iron, magnesium, phosphorus, trace minerals, and digestive enzymes. It is the most common source of chlorophyll and is also high in carotenes. The highly nutritive nature of alfalfa makes it an excellent addition to Nourishment Tea (see the box on page 70). It is a formula to be taken regularly throughout pregnancy to prevent anemia and other mineral and vitamin deficiencies, to prevent hemorrhage during childbirth, and to strengthen the many systems of the body.

BURDOCK ROOT (*ARCTIUM LAPPA*)

Burdock's tap root grows deep down into the ground, sometimes as far as two feet, making it both mineral rich and very grounding in its energy. Burdock is a prime liver strengthener and offers gentle support for the urinary organs. It also helps to balance the blood sugar because it stimulates the digestion and pancreas, it acts as a gentle laxative, reduces skin complaints such as itching, and in its role as a blood purifier prevents outbreaks of herpes infections. It is purported to have been used for centuries as an herb to promote strength and uterine tone before and after birth. It has a sweet, slightly bitter taste.

Burdock may be taken in a variety of ways. You can take it as an infusion with other herbs, using up to 1/2 ounce of the dried root or 1 ounce of the fresh to 1 quart of boiling water, drinking up to 2 cups daily (it is excellent combined with dandelion root); in tincture form, about 20 drops twice a day for purely preventative use, more for remedial purposes; and as a vegetable (known as "gobo" in Japanese). In order to derive maximum nutritive benefits, use burdock regularly as an infusion and as a vegetable. Macrobiotic cookbooks will provide you with numerous recipes for the preparation of burdock root; here is a simple one that I love:

Burdock Root Sauté

Heat one tablespoon of oil in a skillet and add half an onion, sliced. Sauté for a minute

---

or two. Add an eight-inch piece of burdock root and one large carrot, both sliced into matchsticks, and sauté for a couple of minutes more. Add 1/4 cup of water and one tablespoon of tamari (soy sauce), cover, and simmer for twenty minutes. Add a few cups of chopped kale and simmer ten more minutes. Add more tamari to taste, and enjoy while hot. When you develop a taste for burdock you can add a four-inch slice of kombu (kelp) cut into small squares at the beginning of cooking, along with a few tablespoons of extra water.

CHAMOMILE
(ANTHEMIS NOBILIS; MATRIARCA CHAMOMILLA)

This is one of my two favorite herbs (nettle being the other) when I am pregnant. Chamomile eases digestion and quells nausea, relieves heartburn, reduces insomnia, promotes gentle relaxation, relieves mental tension and headaches, reduces cramps, provides calcium, prevents constipation, prevents urinary tract infections, and improves the appetite. Chamomile, when steeped for 10 minutes in a covered vessel (1 tablespoon of the herb to 1 cup of boiling water) and then very slightly sweetened with honey, has an exquisite taste. It can be sipped each evening before bed to induce peaceful sleep, or sipped during the day as a general tonic. Baths of chamomile infusion can also be taken to promote peace and relaxation. For this purpose I love to combine chamomile and lavender in an infusion and add this to the tub.

CAUTION: *For women with a history of miscarriage or who have been spotting and are within the first four months of pregnancy, do not exceed one cup a day, as chamomile can promote menstruation.*

Though this is rare, persons who are allergic to ragweed may also have a reaction to chamomile, which comes from the same family, so try a small amount and let it sit in your mouth. If you notice any itching or any other side effects, do not use this herb. Again, this is very rare but the possibility should not be ignored.

DANDELION ROOT AND LEAVES (TARAXACUM OFFICINALE)

Not only is dandelion highly nutritious, but when you eat the leaves as greens or drink the root in infusion, it is a digestive tonic, liver strengthener, and kidney and bladder ally. It also helps to regulate both blood sugar and blood pressure. By promoting liver functioning, dandelion aids in making iron available in the body, much of which is usually stored in the liver. In early pregnancy dandelion tincture helps to alleviate nausea and relieve a sour feeling in the stomach, and throughout the remaining pregnancy dandelion root relieves itching of the skin and helps to prevent such problems as gallstones, indigestion, fatigue, and even toxemia. To use, add chopped fresh dandelion greens to salad or sauté them with garlic and add a dash of lemon and tamari. They are slightly bitter but delicious. The root can be taken as an infusion similar to burdock root, or combined with burdock for improved taste. Tincture of the root and leaf can also be taken for medicinal benefits, though the nutritional value will not be as great this way.

FALSE UNICORN (CHAMAELIRIUM LUTEUM)

While this wild herb with its long flowering spike is not a nutritive tonic, it has long been used to strengthen uterine tone before, during, and after pregnancy. It is particularly suitable for women with a history of miscarriage as well as for women with a history of uterine prolapse. Other benefits include its general ability to regulate hormones and to benefit liver and digestive functioning. It is fantastically bitter and is therefore better taken in tincture form, up to 20 drops three times a day in early pregnancy, and then periodically throughout the rest of pregnancy as needed. As it is an endangered plant it should be used sparingly.

GINGER ROOT (*ZINGIBER OFFICINALE*)

Ginger root has long been employed as a digestive stimulant and gas expeller. While it is contraindicated in large amounts during pregnancy due to its strong ability to stimulate circulation in the pelvis and bring on the menses, it is an excellent herb for sluggish circulation, nausea, chills, and diarrhea. It can also be taken for colds. It is perfectly safe to sip cupfuls of the warm tea once or twice day. To prepare the tea:

Ginger Tea

Steep 1 teaspoon of the freshly grated root in a cup of boiling water for 10–20 minutes, keeping the cup covered while steeping to retain the precious volatile oils. Sweeten with honey and enjoy.

Ginger tea can also be made stronger and used as an invigorating foot bath for aching feet at the end of the day.

KELP (*LAMINARIA SPP.*)

A sea vegetable, kelp is an ideal nutritive supplement for pregnancy, being rich in a variety of minerals and vitamins in abundant quantities. Kelp also helps to reduce growths (such as fibroids), nourishes the thyroid and endocrine glands, and supports pregnancy health. Kelp may be cooked as a vegetable (often sold under the name kombu—see above under burdock root). Or you can add a 4–8 inch piece of the whole "leaf" to soups, stews, and grain dishes. Powdered kelp can

also be used, especially by those who don't particularly relish the taste. (I love the taste now, but it took me a few tries to get used to it.) You can purchase kelp capsules or make your own by filling "00" capsules with powdered kelp. Two capsules, up to four times a day, is a good dosage.

LAVENDER (*LAVENDULA OFFICINALIS*)

Lavender is a lovely purple flower with a strong floral fragrance. Use it as a relaxing tea and as a soothing addition to your bath. It will promote sleep, reduce anxiety, lift depression, and calm heart palpitations. It also relieves gas and indigestion and stimulates the appetite. I generally use it by adding a pinch of lavender to my chamomile tea, or I add a few drops of lavender oil to my bath, especially if I am

stressed, or before bed. Lavender also makes a calming addition to massage oil.

LEMON BALM (*MELISSA OFFICINALIS*)

Another herbal nervine, lemon balm calms the spirit, reduces tension, and promotes excellent digestion. Lemon balm has a delightful flavor that reflects its uplifting qualities. It can be added to chamomile and lavender teas, or prepared alone. Cover when steeping to retain its essences, using about a tablespoon of dried herb or two tablespoons of fresh leaves to one cup of boiling water. Let it sit for fifteen minutes. Lemon balm can be added to other infusions and teas to improve their flavor. (See the Appendix for definitions of infusions and teas.)

MOTHERWORT (*LEONURUS CARDIACA*)

In some women motherwort may promote contractions and bring on the menstrual cycle in early pregnancy. It has useful properties: it reduces anxiety and thus helps with stress; it is especially helpful for women prone to hypertension. The common name of this herb implies its use as a healing herb for mothers, and its botanical name, *Leonurus cardiaca*, reveals its reputed ability to strengthen the heart and promote courage. Take this when under stress or if you have hypertension or heart palpitations. Do not exceed more than 10 drops at a time, up to three times in a day, and not for more than five days in a row until the last few weeks of pregnancy when the dosage may be increased.

It can be taken safely in tea form. The alkaloids that are emmenagogic are not extracted in water, only in alcohol. It is therefore the tinctures you should be particularly careful with.

NETTLE (*URTICA DIOICA*)

Second to none, nettle is a pregnancy herb par excellence, supplying appreciable quantities of highly usable vitamins and minerals, promoting healthy kidney function, strengthening the blood vessels, reducing varicosities, and decreasing the likelihood of hemorrhaging at the time of birth. Nettle should be a regular addition to the diet of pregnant women, as it is very effective in nourishing the blood and preventing anemia (see the recipe for Nourishment Tea on page 70). For optimal health take infusions daily, up to one quart. To prepare, steep one handful of dried

nettle in a quart of boiling water for one hour. Fresh nettle, the richest form of this herb for its nutrients, may also be prepared as a vegetable, similarly to dandelion greens (handle carefully as the leaves pack a sting which is painful to some), or taken freeze-dried in capsules. Nettle tincture is useful for remedial purposes but nettle in the form of infusion, juiced leaves, fresh, or freeze-dried preparations are most effective for nourishment.

OATSTRAW (*AVENA SATIVA*)

This herb, which comes from the same plant as oats that we eat as a grain, is an excellent gentle nervine that is rich in calcium and magnesium. It is a component of Nourishment Tea (see the box on page 70) which I encourage mothers to drink regularly throughout pregnancy. Drink oatstraw tea to promote relaxed nerves and healthy muscle functioning, also to increase your calcium intake, and to prevent insomnia, cramps, and other related pregnancy discomforts.

PARTRIDGE BERRY (*MITCHELLA REPENS*)

Partridge berry is considered one of the best uterine tonics for pregnancy. It is also a mild nervous system tonic.

It can be taken as a tea or mixed with other herbs of your choice, or added to Nourishment Tea using a tablespoon of this herb per quart of water, a few times a week. It can also be used as a late-pregnancy tonic as described in Chapter 11.

RED RASPBERRY LEAVES (*RUBUS IDAEUS*)

Perhaps no other herb has such a highly proclaimed folk reputation for use during pregnancy as the leaves of the red raspberry plant. Rich in vitamins and minerals as well as a substance known as fragarine, which tones uterine muscles, this herb is said to nourish the muscles, tonify the uterus, and prevent hemorrhage due to both its high iron content and astringent qualities. It is

Nourishment Tea

This is my favorite beverage in pregnancy. It is a nutrient supplement (iron, calcium, and many vitamins and trace minerals), and is an overall "partus preparator" or birth preparation brew. The dried herbs can be mixed in a large batch to have on hand. The tea is delicious both hot or cold and it can be enjoyed by your whole family. You can vary the quantities of the ingredients, or add and omit herbs from time to time. It is safe to drink this brew throughout pregnancy, during labor, and is beneficial for the postpartum as well, as it helps with milk production.

2 parts red raspberry leaf
2 parts nettle
1 part oatstraw
1/2 part alfalfa
1/2 part rose hips
1/4 part red clover
1/4 part spearmint leaf

Mix all of the dried herbs together and store in an airtight container away from heat and light. To prepare your infusion, take 4 tablespoons of the mix and place in a quart-size jar. Add boiling water to fill the jar, cover, and let steep for a minimum of thirty minutes, a maximum of 2 hours. Strain, sweeten, and drink 1–4 cups daily.

one of the main ingredients in Nourishment Tea (see the box at left), and can be taken as a tea (2 tablespoons of the dried herb per cup of boiling water; steep 20 minutes) regularly throughout pregnancy.

ROSE HIPS (ROSA CANINA)
High in vitamin C, a nutrient essential to both health of the circulatory and immune systems, rose hips make both a nutritious and delicious addition to Nourishment Tea, and may be used regularly throughout pregnancy as a beverage. I particularly love rose hips and peppermint prepared as a sun tea as a summer beverage. I sometimes add lemon balm and fennel seeds to this mix as well, then sweeten it with honey for a wonderful tasting, nutritious brew.

ST. JOHN'S WORT (HYPERICUM PERFORATUM)
Though this herb is not to be used regularly as an internal remedy during pregnancy, I include this plant (also known as St. Joan's wort) because it is a fantastic external remedy when used as an oil, for treating aching muscles, a sore back, sore ligaments, and sciatica. Simply put a small amount of the reddish oil into your hand and rub into the affected area. Internally, St. John's Wort may be used homeopathically for these same indications, taking a 30x dosage as needed.

WILD YAM (DIOSCOREA VILLOSA)
This herb has a remarkable ability to prevent miscarriage, reduce severe prenatal nausea, and is a valuable liver strengthener. It also helps to reduce cramping, muscular tension, and intestinal gas. I prefer to use it as a tincture, in a general dose of 15 drops 2–3 times day for general purposes, and up to 30 drops every 4 hours or more for more serious complaints such as threatened miscarriage or hyperemesis.

YELLOW DOCK (*RUMEX CRISPUS*)

Yellow dock is an excellent liver support and supplies appreciable quantities of iron and other minerals. It also prevents and remedies constipation, making it a beneficial herb for many pregnant women. It can be taken as an infusion or syrup (see Iron Tonic Syrup in Part II, under "Anemia") for its overall beneficial properties as well as mineral content, or as a tincture, which will not provide many of the nutrients but will still support digestion, hormonal balance, health of the skin, and reduction of anemia by stimulating the liver to make iron more available throughout the body. Dosage is 1–2 tablespoons of syrup daily, 1–2 cups of infusion daily, or 15–30 drops of tincture 2–3 times a day.

Exercise and Posture

EXERCISE

Exercise is vitally important for health in pregnancy. It increases circulation, which promotes well-being and prevents depression; it helps oxygenate the blood, reducing fatigue; it prevents the build-up of tension in the muscles; it reduces pelvic congestion and thus cramping, low backache, ligament pain, and constipation; it prevents congestion of blood in the lower extremities, reducing leg cramps and tension as well as varicosities. Exercise promotes tone in the muscles, making the body ready for birth, aids recovery of organ tone and placement after birth, and also prevents prolapse of the pelvic organs There are also many specific exercises and yoga postures that can be used to relieve common pregnancy discomforts.

More important, exercise will help you become comfortable in and enjoy your body. Exercise will relax you as it tones your body. Many women resist exercising because they associate it with our cultural emphasis on a thin, tightly toned body. Feeling that this cultural ideal is too hard to achieve (in fact it is not our goal here at all), many women give up before they even try. Many women have also had discouraging experiences in school physical education classes or locker rooms which have prompted a negative association. And many women are so accustomed to being sedentary that they must muster up the will to get moving. Even 15 minutes a few times a week can be beneficial.

One excellent way to help you overcome resistance to exercise is to refer to it as *movement*. In what ways do you enjoy moving your body? What feels good to you—dancing, walking, yoga, Tai Chi, horseback riding, swimming, tennis, aerobics? Choosing a gentle form of movement that is safe for pregnancy is the most advisable way to begin. If you've not ridden horses before on a regular basis, this is definitely not the time to start! Similarly, some forms of movement such as swimming (although highly beneficial for both toning and relaxing) might be difficult if you don't have access to a swimming pool or reasonably warm lake.

I can recall hiking trips I took, prior to my first pregnancy, with a heavy backpack, sweating, crying, and becoming exhausted from the weight of the load. Though I have always been physically flexible and have enjoyed bicycle riding, swimming, walking, and dancing, I had never been an athlete, muscularly developed, or particularly engaged in sports. During my pregnancies I chose yoga as a gentle form of toning my muscles, learning how to identify those muscles and to relax them. I learned to enjoy the sensations of my body moving and the feelings of warmth, improved circulation, improved digestion, better sleep, and mental wellness that rewarded my efforts. In addition, I loved to feel my baby moving as I moved with and around my growing child. For more vigorous exercise I took brisk walks and often turned on music with a great beat (my preference being reggae and African drumming) and let loose, dancing. The latter I did in privacy, with my kids or with my husband. Dancing freely is my favorite form of movement even now, and it is something my entire family enjoys. We put on music and dance through our housecleaning! Belly dancing, originally developed as a form of abdominal and pelvic toning for pregnant women, is also an excellent way to exercise prenatally.

In these years of having babies and making movement an enjoyable part of my life, I have really learned to appreciate and enjoy my body, and my strength and endurance have improved dramatically. How you choose to move your body while you are pregnant is less important than that you do so. Dance,

play, get lively, and learn to enjoy your body, whatever size, shape, or tone you are in!

Exercise, when taken to the extreme every day, can have deleterious effects during pregnancy. First of all, childbirth requires as much the ability to release our muscles as it does muscle firmness. In fact, women with backgrounds in professional dance or athletics may have a more difficult time giving birth than those women whose muscles are looser and less toned. If conscious awareness of relaxation is not included as part of exercising, then exercise may actually be self-defeating. Intense exercise also uses up precious calories and nutrients, and if these are not replaced, then exercise can actually contribute to undernourishment. Finally, for many women, heavy exercise, particularly aerobics and similar workouts, reflect control issues and a lot of inner tension. Women may be trying to control their shape, stamina, or to prove their strength without taking the time to feel good about who they are.

The ability to give birth requires an ability to yield and to let go. While this does not mean giving up the control associated with autonomy, it does mean that you must give up a sense that you can make your body do whatever you want it to do. For example, while exercise is energizing, it cannot provide you with the rejuvenation that you derive from a nap—if you need to rest, don't

Poor posture

Good posture

push your body with a workout, and don't resent your body for its physical needs. You can't exercise away your stress—you have to reduce stress in your life at its source.

Many of us experience our bodies as what we inhabit rather than what we are. Often we don't like our bodies, comparing ourselves to fashion models, whom few of us resemble. Not liking our bodies translates to not liking ourselves. Exercising in an attempt to look like somebody else is psychologically unhealthy; it disturbs your ability to appreciate yourself for your uniqueness. As your breasts, hips, and waist grow during pregnancy, you may judge yourself harshly rather than seeing yourself as a gorgeous, well-nourished pregnant mama—an image of a creation goddess. If you are not feeling positive about yourself, you are less likely to take excellent care of yourself, so do something about that attitude! It will save you a lot of pregnancy and birth problems.

Be certain to balance exertion with periods of relaxation. Swim a couple of laps, then float on your back for ten minutes, then repeat this sequence; ride your stationary bicycle or do your step aerobics, but intersperse this with a few minutes of deep relaxation. Or end your sessions with five to ten minutes of guided visualization (read on for details) or deep relaxation in a tub. The activity followed by the rest will help you to identify areas of tension in your body which you can then deliberately and progressively release. This is perfect physical preparation for birth. As you move and relax, pay attention to the sensations of the baby moving or being still within you, and notice how this changes as you relax. All of this will better enable you to allow your baby to move easily through your pelvis and into your arms. As you both move and relax, communicate your enjoyment and love to your baby.

Remember, it is possible to hurt yourself, even with gentle forms of movement such as yoga. As your belly grows, your center of balance will change somewhat, and you may find various positions or activities more challenging. There is no need to prove anything to anyone, or to show that pregnancy doesn't slow you down. To some extent, it should! Pregnancy is a time to listen to and honor your body's messages, not ignore them.

POSTURE

Posture is rarely discussed as an important component of prenatal health, and this is unfortunate because proper posture can prevent many pregnancy discomforts such as low back pain, shortness of breath, and indigestion. I also believe that proper posture can reduce the incidence of urinary tract infections due to stasis of urine in the ureters, as these are less likely to be compressed.

Aside from the fact that many Americans already have poor posture with a tendency to hunch their shoulders forward, pregnant women have the added tendency, as pregnancy advances, to allow the lower back be pulled forward by the weight of the growing belly. This produces the typical sway-back of late pregnancy, also known as lordosis, and accentuates the waddling gait of late pregnancy, as the legs are displaced from the hip bones being pulled forward.

While it is natural for pregnancy to affect your posture to some extent, you can learn to maintain excellent posture throughout pregnancy simply by practicing. Good posture, when standing, is as follows. Your head is held high, shoulders are held back but not stiffly, lower back does not curve forward but remains relatively straight, your tailbone is tucked under so that the tops of your hip bones are not pulled forward, and your feet should be slightly apart. When you are walking you can practice maintaining excellent posture by keeping your tailbone tucked. To keep your pelvis in a position of good posture use your abdominal muscles to pull it up in the front and use the muscles of your buttocks to pull your tailbone down.

When you hold yourself up properly, you are lifting your diaphragm and stomach off your belly, allowing more room for breathing and for food in your stomach. You can feel the difference simply by sitting in a chair in a slouched position, and then switching to an upright, erect posture. Or if you sit down and either feel out of breath or full in your stomach, try sitting up straight. If you find yourself slouching when you sit, practice sitting taller by pushing your lower back toward the back of the chair (so that you minimize the curve in your back) and let your feet rest squarely on the floor, with your legs dropped slightly apart. If needed, you can put a small pillow behind your lower back and another behind your head and neck. This is especially good if you plan to relax in the chair. Similarly, when you are sitting up and reading in bed, sit upright, using pillows for support to prevent you from slouching.

Whenever possible, sit tailor-style on the floor. This will improve the strength of your back muscles, and you receive the added benefit of exercising your muscles as you get up and down.

When you lie down, use pillows to ensure comfort. For example, if you lie on your side, rest your bent leg on a pillow to prevent the weight of your belly from pulling on your lower back. You can also tuck a small, soft pillow under your belly to lift your belly slightly off the bed. Many women like to place a pillow between their knees when lying on their sides, rather than the pillow under their legs. Either way, it is helpful to have plenty of pillows on your bed as pregnancy advances, so that you can try a variety of positions. Comfort while you sleep will prevent you from the feelings of irritability, indigestion, and muscle aches that so often accompany a fitful sleep.

ESSENTIAL MOVEMENTS FOR PREGNANT WOMEN

There are many excellent books on prenatal exercise and yoga (see "Further Reading"), so here I will provide you with only ten prenatal exercises. These are the ten movements and poses that I have found to be beneficial to the circulation, pelvis, and digestion. They will help you identify, stretch, tone, and relax the muscles that will be called upon when you give birth. These exercises can be done individually, or as a set. The order given is a logical progression, but not from the easiest to the most difficult. You can decrease the number of repetitions if you are not accustomed to exercising, or increase them for a more vigorous workout. Use the descriptions and pictures together to best understand the movements. Begin slowly, and rest for at least five full minutes when you have completed the movements. You can follow an exercise session with a relaxation technique (see Relaxation Techniques in the next chapter).

I enjoy visualizing my baby surrounded with light as I do each exercise. Soothing music in the background also facilitates relaxation and concentration. I find it helpful to begin each session with a few minutes of relaxation, neck rolls, and deep breathing. Always exercise on a firm, but soft surface.

The Standing Twist

1. Stand upright with your feet about 12 inches apart. Extend your arms out to each side.
2. Exhaling, bend forward at the waist so that your upper body is parallel to the floor.
3. Now inhale as you resume the standing position, legs still apart and arms extended. Gently twist to your right, pivoting your right foot slightly.
4. As you exhale, bend forward over your leg, so that your upper body is again parallel to the floor.
5. Inhale and resume the standing position.
6. Repeat steps 1 and 2, again bending to the front.
7. Follow steps 3 and 4, but this time bending to your left.
8. As you inhale, return to center, and repeat step 1.

Repeat positions 1 through 8 up to 10 times.

1.

2.

3.

4.

The Yogic Squat

1. Stand upright, feet about 12 inches apart, knees slightly bent, and raise your arms over your head, with your hands joined and pointed toward the ceiling. Inhale deeply.
2. On the exhale, begin to lower your head toward the ground, one vertebra at a time, until your hands touch the floor.
3. Let your buttocks down toward the ground and as you inhale, slowly allow your body to assume a squatting position.
4. Hold this squat for as long as you can. If you are unaccustomed to squatting, begin by holding the position for a count of 10 seconds. Eventually you will able to increase this to several minutes.
5. If you wish to repeat this exercise more than once, you can reverse the steps until you are again in a standing position with upraised arms, and begin again with step 1.

The Butterfly Pose

1. Sit upright on the floor, flat on your buttocks.
2. With your legs bent at the knees and open to the sides, bring the soles of your feet together.
3. Holding onto your feet with your hands, draw your heels as close to your crotch as possible.
4. Gently "flutter" your knees up and down, gradually bringing your knees closer to the floor.
5. Accompany this exercise with gentle inhalations and exhalations.
6. Maintain this pose for a greater length of time at each session. Draw your feet in further and bring your knees closer to the ground for increasing difficulty.
7. *Optional*: You can try to touch your head to your feet for an added stretch to your inner thighs. Do not try to flutter your legs while you do this.

The Forward Bend with Variation

1. Sitting upright on the floor, extend your legs to the side, keeping them straight. Inhale deeply.
2. As you exhale, slowly lean forward, bringing your belly and chest as close to the floor in front of you as possible.
3. On your inhale, sit straight, maintaining the leg position.
4. Repeat up to 10 times, getting closer to the floor the more you practice, and holding the forward bend longer.
5. *Optional*: You can also alternate bending forward over each individual leg.

The Centaur (Created by Jeannine Parvati Baker)

1. Bend one leg under you and stretch the other straight behind you, as in the picture.
2. Your hands are in front of you as if your palms are pressing flat against an imaginary wall.
3. Hold this position for up to 2 minutes, then switch legs.
4. *Optional*: Maintaining the leg positions, twist your torso slowly toward the side of the extended leg, and lean back toward your foot. Switch legs and repeat on the other side.

The Bridge

1. Lie flat on your back with your knees raised and your heels flat on the floor.
2. As you breathe in a relaxed rhythm, grasp your ankles with your hands.
3. Continue with the relaxed breathing, and slowly lift your buttocks off the floor as if an invisible string were drawing your belly button toward the ceiling.
4. Hold this position for up to 30 seconds, then lower your buttocks to the floor.
5. Repeat up to four times in a row.

Pelvic Rock

1. Get into a hands and knees position with your back parallel to the floor.
2. As you exhale, let your belly drop toward the floor.
3. Now inhale, arching your back like a cat.
4. Repeat this sequence up to 20 times, following a gentle breathing rhythm.

Leg Extensions

1. In a hands and knees position, gently lift your left leg backward and upward, letting your foot reach toward the ceiling.
2. Return your knee to the floor.
3. Repeat up to 20 times, then repeat with the right leg.

Leg Lifts

1. Lie on your left side.
2. Raise your right leg to the ceiling and make gentle circles in the air with your foot.
3. Lower your leg.
4. Repeat up to twenty times, then roll onto your right side and repeat with the opposite leg.

The Lumbar Stretch

1. Lie flat on your back, legs extended and arms stretched out to the sides.
2. Slide your right foot up and bring your knee toward your chest.
3. Keeping your shoulders flat on the floor, twist your hips until your right knee touches the floor near your left hand.
4. Breathing gently, hold this position for up to 30 seconds.
5. Return to position 1, and repeat on the opposite side.
6. This can be repeated up to three times on each side.

From this last posture you can easily go into a relaxation position, using pillows as necessary to support your legs, belly, and head and neck.

PELVIC HEALTH

Most women lack an understanding of their pelvic organs and muscles—where they are, what is normal and healthy, even how they look and feel. Yet this awareness can help you prepare yourself for the birth experience, as well as enable you to maintain lifelong pelvic health. Few women realize how much birth can be facilitated by the ability to consciously relax the vaginal muscles. In addition, pelvic tone will prevent a host of female problems in later life such as uterine prolapse and urinary incontinence. Sex will be improved, digestion will be healthier, and you are less likely to experience problems such as hemorrhoids. *The New Our Bodies, Ourselves* is perhaps the best resource for understanding your anatomy, and I encourage you to include this book in your personal library as a reference manual.

I will, however, provide a basic idea of the structure of the pelvic bones, the yoni, and the pelvic floor muscles. Refer to the accompanying diagrams for visual assistance. The pelvis is a large, bony cradle or bowl that is open at the top and bottom, with various openings within the bony structure allowing for muscles and blood vessels to pass through and attach to the bones. There are the following bones: the ileum, the two hip bones which form crests just below your waist on either side of your abdomen, the ischium, which form the central portion of the hip bones and form the bones commonly referred to as your "sit bones," and the pubic bones which meet at the center of your pelvis near your pubic hair line. In the back of the pelvis are the sacrum and the coccyx, also called the tailbone. Your pelvis contains the birth canal, urethra, rectum, bladder, uterus, fallopian tubes, and ovaries. There are ligaments which connect the uterus to the front, back, and sides of the pelvis, and muscles which form a sling beneath the uterus, making up the birth canal, supporting and surrounding this and the other structures. It is these muscles which can be identified and strengthened so that you can work effectively during birth to open your bottom and also prevent some of the health problems I've already mentioned.

In order for you to identify these muscles, collectively referred to as the pelvic floor, you must learn to feel comfortable with your sexual organs. Look at anatomy drawings to help you understand what is what, and if you wish (I highly recommend

PERINEUM AND PELVIC FLOOR

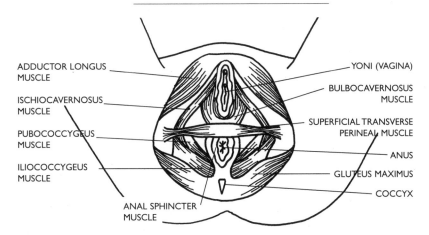

ADDUCTOR LONGUS MUSCLE

ISCHIOCAVERNOSUS MUSCLE

PUBOCOCCYGEUS MUSCLE

ILIOCOCCYGEUS MUSCLE

ANAL SPHINCTER MUSCLE

YONI (VAGINA)

BULBOCAVERNOSUS MUSCLE

SUPERFICIAL TRANSVERSE PERINEAL MUSCLE

ANUS

GLUTEUS MAXIMUS

COCCYX

One mother I worked with referred to orgasms as "assisted Kegels."

this) look at yourself in a mirror. You can visually observe yourself tightening and releasing the muscles that surround your external genitals, the same muscles which you would tighten and release to urinate.

— The Kegel Exercise —

Learning to stop and start your urine flow while you sit on the toilet is an excellent way to identify your pelvic muscles (always be certain to release all of the urine before you finish). Then once you are familiar with this sensation, you can do it whenever you wish. It is known as the Kegel exercise in honor of the physician who developed it as a treatment and for prevention of urinary incontinence. For those of you in a sexual relationship, making love provides a great opportunity for practicing this tightening and releasing, with your partner confirming how tight you can squeeze your muscles during your sexual experience. (Orgasms are natural tighteners of these muscles. They also promote pelvic blood circulation. One mother I worked with referred to orgasms as "assisted Kegels.") Kegel exercises can be done up to 100 times a day (double that if you've already had problems with incontinence or prolapse).

However, tightening and releasing these muscles is not enough. Women must also learn to tighten the muscles way up in the birth canal in order to gain optimal benefit. This requires some practice, and it can be difficult and even tiring at first. Your midwife can help you to identify these muscles by showing you where they are in your vagina. Or you can feel for yourself. Look in books, or ask your mate to let you know when you are squeezing his fingers or penis. Try to imagine yourself tightening your muscles way up inside behind your pubic bone, not using your thigh or abdominal muscles while you squeeze.

— The Elevator Exercise —

Another pelvic exercise is often called the "elevator" by midwives and childbirth educators. The basic imagery is that your yoni is an elevator shaft and you are raising an imaginary elevator from the ground floor (your vaginal opening) to the fourth floor (high inside) using just your muscles. You do this slowly floor by floor, then release slowly, floor by floor. You can also release your muscles to the basement by letting them get super relaxed, an excellent practice for totally releasing your muscles to birth your baby when she or he is crowning (the head is showing and about to be born). The elevator can be done ten times each day in addition to the above exercises.

— Happy Birthday Exercise —

A final pelvic exercise, one of my favorites, I gleaned from renowned childbirth educator Sheila Kitzinger. This is one in which you imagine that your vaginal walls are a piece of paper onto which you are imaginarily writing "Happy Birthday" using your muscles with which to write. Beginning at the vaginal opening you "write" the "h" and continue upward tightening and moving your muscles to form all of the letters in these words. You can write any way you want to, but always cross your "t" and dot your "i." Do this ten times each day along with 100 Kegels for optimal pelvic health.

Note: In order to remember to do the above exercises, choose certain times each day to do them routinely, for example after each time you urinate, when you wake up, go to sleep, and before each meal or snack, or every time you stop at a red light in your car or are at a checkout counter in the grocery store.

— Squatting —

Squatting is another way to tone your pelvic muscles and is a great position for practicing the exercises described above. Women in traditional cultures worldwide squat daily in order to cook over fires, wash laundry in the river, etc., naturally promoting pelvic health. The majority of women in traditional cultures are also reported to have had smooth and easy births. Try to squat for ten minutes (or more) each day, building up to it slowly if you've never squatted before. You can squat while you watch TV, play with a toddler, or read a book. Any time that you think of it, squat. Putting a book under each of your heels can help if this position hurts the back of your legs initially. By the end of your pregnancy you'll be able to squat much more easily, and much to your benefit!

MASSAGE—PASSIVE EXERCISE

Traditionally, pregnant women were given extensive massage often by the midwife, this being the central component of prenatal care. The pregnant woman might have been massaged weekly or more often throughout pregnancy, with a thorough massage of the belly, hips, and legs. This allowed the mother to be aware of and relaxed in her pelvis, and allowed the midwife to identify the baby's position and massage the baby into the right place if need be. I feel that this physical contact is essential for pregnant women who want to be touched soothingly, especially for women who have a low interest in sex, but still want a lot of physical contact. In addition, I am convinced that the babies love to be massaged even while in the womb, much as children love it all throughout childhood (what adult would turn down a massage?).

— Benefits of Prenatal Massage —

This healing modality is nearly absent from the care of pregnant women in our culture. And this is a great loss. Prenatal massage has numerous benefits. Being a form of passive exercise it promotes circulation which in turn oxygenates the mother's (and baby's) entire body, reducing sluggishness, nausea, fatigue, and depression. It also promotes the release of nutrients stored or stagnant in various parts of the body, and helps to relieve congestion of blood which can result in varicosities and aches. (*Warning*: varicosities should never be directly massaged as this may release a blood clot which can result in a dangerous embolism.) Massage gently tones the muscles and helps the mother relax deeply. It can be an excellent sleep promoter for women having sleeping difficulties. It encourages good posture which in turn prevents both backache and overstretching of the anterior uterine ligaments. But most important, massage helps a woman get in touch with her body. It is an inwardly focused experience which allows her to feel comfortable physically and provides a time and place for identifying and relaxing muscular tension. This is a very important preparation for birth.

Ideally, the father of the baby will massage his partner regularly throughout her pregnancy, even if it is simply a nightly belly rub or foot massage (the latter being my favorite way to fall asleep late in pregnancy). One needn't be a professional masseuse in order to rub someone firmly and strongly or softly and tenderly, depending upon individual preferences. One only has to be receptive, willing, and sensitive to areas of tension. Massage provides a wonderful opportunity for partners to show their wives how much they appreciate them and is also a ripe time for the dad to feel and talk to the baby. If there is no partner in the picture, another friend can give you a massage periodically—as a gift or as a trade. (Nonpregnant friends would probably appreciate a back rub or foot massage, and this is nice way for pregnant women to give loving energy, too.) Or you can treat yourself to an occasional professional massage.

Midwives can learn to incorporate massage, taking time at least in a couple of prenatal visits to rub a mom out. This can help to develop the feeling of trust and relaxation between you. It also provides an opportunity for you to teach the pregnant woman's partner how to give her a massage, and allows you to identify areas where she may be holding tension, helping her to identify and release these. It may provide the mother with much needed touch, especially if she is single or is the mother of young children and is putting out energy all day but has little time to replenish herself.

General Tips on
— Giving a Massage —

Giving an effective massage is really quite simple. The first thing to do is to create a relaxing atmosphere. You will need a dimly lit room that is warm, with a quiet and comfortable spot in which a pregnant woman can relax—plenty of pillows on hand will enable even women in late stages of pregnancy to find a workable position. Soothing music such as the sound of rain or another natural element can help induce a relaxed state.

If the woman will be removing her clothing then you will need to provide a sheet with which she can cover herself. You will need to expose only small areas at a time, such as an arm, leg, or her back. This will reduce her feeling of vulnerability and provide her with some warmth.

While it beyond the limits of this book to offer thorough instructions for massage, I will provide you with a general idea of how to proceed with a full body massage. Always remember that for a general relaxing massage (in contrast to a specifically remedial massage) your sensitivity, gentleness, and willingness to listen to the mother's needs are all it takes.

Before you begin, remind the mother to use the bathroom, otherwise you can be sure she'll have to get up at some point to pee, or she'll be holding onto her muscles, preventing complete relaxation. Then help her to find a comfortable position—lying on her side with one leg over a pillow works well. Now, using a small amount of massage oil, begin by rubbing her feet gently. If the mother wants a firmer and deeper massage you can then press more deeply, but in each area begin gently to allow the muscles to respond and relax to your touch. Work your way up the legs, then proceed to massaging the neck and shoulders. Next position the mother on her side, if she isn't already, so that you can rub her back. Gently work down her back and over her buttocks. Afterward, you can gently massage the mother's belly, rubbing your hands over it to help her relax her abdominal muscles. If at any time the woman falls asleep, let her rest.

If you wish to massage just one area, such as her feet, simply massage that area more minutely. When massaging the belly, always remember the baby, speak to the baby, and massage her or him, too!

The Need for Rest

My partner's grandmother, when she was in her late eighties, would always comment whenever she saw one of my babies napping, "Oh he (or she) is going to grow another inch." She believed that sleeping helps babies grow. There may be scientific evidence that supports this idea, as our metabolism and hormonal levels do differ between waking and sleeping states. Nevertheless, when we rest, we are taking the energy that we would normally use outwardly to be productive in the world, and turning it inward so that this same energy may be used for rejuvenation, repair, rebuilding, and regrouping. This is true on many levels, whether rebuilding cells or healing from illness or injury, to taking time out or making space for our thoughts and feelings.

At no time is this need for rest greater in your life than when you are pregnant. Your body is doing an incredible amount of work growing a baby. Your physical output is great, your hormonal levels are extremely high, and you also tend to be losing sleep. If you have young children, you are already even more likely to be exhausted. You must be careful to rest when the older kids nap, or when dad or a friend or relative takes the kids for a while. (This is the responsibility of fathers and other members of your community. Anyone who has the right to brag about the kids should also help take responsibility for them.) I cannot overstate the importance of allowing yourself to rest each day of your pregnancy. If you don't allow yourself to rest you will be more likely to experience fatigue, nausea, indigestion, constipation, lethargy, irritability, emotional swings, and depression. Exhaustion also makes birth and postpartum infinitely more challenging.

RELAXATION TECHNIQUES

Taking time to rest does not necessarily mean taking time to relax. Relaxation specifically means letting go of mental stress and physical tensions, at least during the time you are relaxing. You can't make economic difficulties or a leaking roof disappear by relaxing, but you can call a twenty-minute moratorium on worrying, long enough to tune into who you really are. Since most of us store our anxieties in our muscular, nervous, and skeletal systems, learning to release your worries will help to unlock areas of physical tension as well.

In addition, learning to relax is an essential skill for moving through the birth experience and into parenting with grace and joy. Learning to relax will allow your birth canal to be the path of least resistance. The following exercises are a small sampling of ways to learn to relax. For deeper stresses and anxieties refer to Part II, and whenever necessary seek out supportive listeners or professional counselors.

- Find a comfortable, quiet place where you'll be uninterrupted. (Remember to turn the ringer off on your telephone.)
- Put on quiet, peaceful music to help create a relaxed mood.
- If you have insomnia or find it difficult to relax try these techniques: First take a warm bath and drink a cup of your favorite relaxing herb tea (a chamomile and lavender combination is excellent).
- If you are a restless type, do yoga or even take a brisk walk. This can help relieve your body of excess energy. Exercise is also a great way to relieve muscular tension,

and relaxation is a perfect follow-up to any exercise.
- Empty your bladder before you begin so you're not interrupted by the need to urinate for at least thirty minutes.
- Be certain to prop yourself adequately with pillows so that you don't become uncomfortable lying on your back. These exercises can also be done in a chair or lying on your side.

— Deep Breathing —

Close your eyes and imagine your baby floating or snuggled happily in your pelvis, surrounded by a golden-pink glow. Now take a deep breath in through your nose and imagine that breath traveling down through your body to your womb. Let the breath encircle the baby, washing gently over her or him, then let it rise slowly back up through your chest, through your throat, and back out of your nose or your mouth. Repeat this eight or ten times, feeling yourself with each breath being washed over with your baby's love. You can continue to repeat this until you feel deeply rested or until you fall asleep. You can also follow this up with another relaxation practice.

— Progressive Relaxation —

Close your eyes and take a few deep breaths, strongly blowing the air out of your mouth after each breath. Continue to take deep, gentle breaths, allowing a slow and gentle exhale after each inhale, as if your breaths are coming and going as waves gently lapping against the seashore.

Now, beginning at your toes, let a warm, tingly, and comfortable feeling spread over each toe. Wiggle your toes slightly, one at a time or all together. Now let that warm feeling spread s-l-o-w-l-y over your feet. Feel all tension and fatigue leaving with your next exhale….

Work your way over your entire body, continuing from your feet up to your head. Relax each area of your body slowly, deliberately releasing your muscles as you go along. Imagine your breath as fingers that are massaging away tension in specific spots. (You can also begin at your head and work your way down to your feet.) Pay extra attention to releasing the muscles in your pelvis, abdomen, and buttocks, areas where women tend to hold tension. Many times you'll find that you've fallen asleep before you get all the way from your feet to your head or vice versa. This is fine and good.

— Creative Visualization —

This process emphasizes the qualities of using your imagination as above. Creative visualization, however, focuses on using imagery to induce inner processes for facing and resolving dilemmas or for imagining yourself how you would like yourself to be. There are many audio tapes now available that have visualizations with lovely music in the background. You can also have someone read a guided visualization to you or tape record your own. Some excellent visualizations can be found in the books *Transformation Through Birth*, *Silent Knife*, *Pregnancy as Healing*, and *Motherwit*.

The accompanying box provides an example of a visualization you can do for letting go of anxieties. I was inspired to create this after reading *Motherwit* (by Diane Mariechild). To begin, follow the general relaxation instructions and a brief version of the progressive relaxation to bring you into a more deeply receptive state.

Releasing Anxiety: A Creative Visualization

Imagine yourself in a place that is your idea of absolute beauty, security, comfort, and safety. It can be any setting you like—the beach, the mountains, or a cozy chair in a favorite room. This is a place you can return to in your mind whenever you wish to do so.

Here in this space you can safely allow your worries to surface, knowing that they cannot harm you. Now take each image, worry, fear, or anxiety, and one at a time, watch it grow smaller and smaller. Help it to dissolve before your eyes, let it be washed away by rain or waves, or let the wind whisk it far away. The images are dissolving until they no longer exist. These fears can no longer harm you, they are released from your heart. Feel yourself lighter, relieved of carrying unnecessary burdens.

And now imagine your most cherished ideal for yourself and your family. Whatever it is that you consider nourishing and important, conjure up this vision. Let this vision grow larger and larger. Let yourself be filled with the joy of this image (pause for a few minutes until you feel filled with this sensation).

These positive feelings will grow and develop as you nourish them each day. They are a part of you now and always.

When you are ready you can return to your regular awareness filled with the joy of nourishing yourself and your baby. Slowly open your eyes, and take a few minutes to breathe deeply before you get up.

SPENDING TIME
OUT OF DOORS

Pregnant women are a living metaphor for the Earth, which carries and sustains us from Her very body. In a sense a pregnant woman becomes a microcosmic representation of the Earth.

Natural pregnancy health is facilitated by spending time in fresh air. Walk barefoot, feel the sun on your face and the wind in your hair. Sit on the Earth feeling the pull of gravity drawing you close to her, work in a garden, stroll along the beach, take a walk in a cool, quiet woods. There is no greater recipe for pregnancy health—for confidence in your body and clarity of mind—than recognizing your relationship with the forces of nature.

Too often women become accustomed to a sedentary daily routine, lived mostly in the confines of houses, offices, cars, stores, etc., going out primarily when it is necessary to go from one place to the next. This type of lifestyle can cause you to become mentally and emotionally contracted, dwelling on fears, anxieties, stresses, and the mundane details of housework, etc. While I acknowledge that not all of you who are reading this book will have access to pristine natural settings in which to expand your awareness of the world around you, most women can take a walk in a park, along a river, or near a pond. I myself grew up in an inner city and know that some connection with nature is always possible— even if it's just admiring a tree or the clouds in the sky, or enjoying the purifying sensation of rain on our faces. Being close to nature is a reminder that you, too, are a beautiful part of the miracle of life.

CHAPTER 9

Physical Changes During Pregnancy

While every woman is unique in her pregnancy, there are certain physiological changes that occur regardless of body type, size of the baby, or other factors. The degree to which these changes become uncomfortable, however, can be influenced by nutritional habits, exercise, heredity, available support, and personal outlook. Understanding the changes you are experiencing can help you relate to your body with acceptance and approval, knowing that it is adjusting just as it should. Of course you should feel free to discuss all questions you have about your body with your midwife or other health care practitioner.

YOUR BREASTS

The increasing hormones in your bloodstream can cause breast sensitivity and even extreme tingling or tenderness soon after you conceive and even before you miss your first period. These sensations usually quickly abate, though you may experience heightened sensitivity in your nipples throughout pregnancy and breastfeeding.

As pregnancy advances, women will notice small raised bumps around the areola (the dark area surrounding the nipple). Called Montgomery's tubercles, these are small oil-secreting glands that keep the nipple lubricated. The nipple and areola will also become darker. As pregnancy progresses some women notice a yellowish or cream-colored discharge coming from their nipples, a wet spot on their bed sheets near their breasts, or a bit of crusted matter in their nipples. This is colostrum, the first "milk" that is in the breasts, and which will last for the first few days after birth until your real milk comes in. During pregnancy you will want to look at your nipples to see if they are erect, flat, or inverted. If they become erect in cool air or when you feel sexually aroused, then you are ready for breastfeeding; if they are flat or actually dimple inward even when squeezed or stimulated then speak with your midwife or a La Leche

League leader to learn how to prepare your nipples for nursing. There are simple things that you can do that will enable your baby to latch onto your nipples with greater ease, but which should be done before the birth for an optimal transition to breastfeeding your baby. Flat and inverted nipples need not prevent you from nursing your baby.

Your breast size may increase substantially during pregnancy which can lead to discomfort, especially if you already had large breasts. If this is the case, a supportive bra in the appropriate size can be helpful, even if you haven't worn one before. You may notice that the veins on your breasts and on your chest are more visible, appearing like the blue lines on a map that mark the location of rivers. As your breasts increase in size and weight you may notice silvery lines: these are stretch marks.

It is also normal for the breasts to feel slightly lumpy due to enlargement of the alveoli (the milk glands). However, it is sensible to feel any lumps carefully to be certain that they are part of normal breast changes. Learning to massage your breasts can be part of a regular practice of loving your breasts, and will help you to recognize cyclical changes as you become more familiar with your body. In this way you are likely to notice any problems should they arise without the anxiety that a formal breast exam conjures up. Of course, any suspicious lumps should be further palpated by your midwife or other health care practitioner, and, if necessary, further information should be sought to determine the nature of the lump, as pregnancy does not prevent breast cancer (though according to research studies, extended breastfeeding substantially decreases the risk of developing this disease). Remember, however, that most breast lumps are not cancer.

During pregnancy it is important that you be honest with yourself about how you regard your breasts. Many women harbor anxieties, measuring their breasts against cultural standards. If you are unhappy about your breasts this can hinder breastfeeding. For example, if you have always felt that your breasts are small and inadequate you may also worry whether you can produce enough milk (small breasts can produce as much milk as large breasts), or if you are embarrassed about your breasts you may hesitate to nurse your baby in public, and may feel uncomfortable and inhibited in general. Talking to your midwife or a La Leche League leader can be helpful.

YOUR YONI

Vaginal changes also occur early in pregnancy, with the birth canal becoming a purplish color and the amount of vaginal discharge increasing. The yoni and vulva become quite engorged during pregnancy due to increased blood flow to the area. This can greatly increase sexual sensitivity and pleasure. The increased amount of discharge can cause considerable wetness, to the point of it being completely normal to change your underwear during the day.

Increased wetness can also promote the growth of vaginal organisms such as yeast. This can lead to itching, burning, or irritation, increased need to urinate, discomfort during lovemaking and, depending upon the type of organism, can cause the discharge to become thicker with a creamy, yellowish or greenish color, with an odor ranging from a mild "bread-yeast" smell to a strongly unpleasant fishy odor. (See "Vaginal Infections" in Part II for treatment suggestions.)

In addition to the birth canal and vulva becoming engorged, so does the cervix. It also becomes softer and more likely to bleed if it is touched or scraped. Therefore it is not uncommon for pregnant women to notice a few spots of blood, or pink-tinged vaginal mucous, after sex.

DIGESTION CHANGES

Most pregnant women are familiar with the digestive changes that pregnancy brings—an increased sensitivity to smell, a change in food preferences, slower digestion, nausea, indigestion, lack of appetite, and bowel changes. Most of these changes are due to increases of progesterone and estrogen and to the increasing pressure of your growing baby and uterus on your digestive organs. There might be increased sponginess of the gums—hormonal changes cause them to bleed more easily. Pregnant women should take care to brush and floss regularly but gently, and to maintain an excellent diet rich in iron, vitamin C, and bioflavonoids.

To some extent some of the digestive changes of pregnancy are unavoidable and normal. However, with excellent nutrition and attention to rest and exercise, many prenatal digestive discomforts can be reduced or prevented.

URINARY TRACT

Due to increased blood volume, pressure from your growing womb, hormonal changes, and incorrect posture, pregnant women experience a marked increase in the need to urinate. This can be as frequently as every couple of hours during the first trimester and even more frequently during the last months. Most women will also need to urinate at least once during the night, but sometimes as often as two or three times in late pregnancy. You may also need to go

when you stand after having been sitting for a while, and as soon as you get in the car to go on a long journey! Most pregnant women will notice that they don't urinate quite as frequently during the second trimester. This is because the weight of the uterus has lifted somewhat off the bladder. If you are experiencing extreme urinary frequency, discomfort when you urinate, backache, frequent uterine contractions, or flu-like symptoms, see "Urinary Tract Infections" in Part II. It is beneficial to use herbs such as dandelion, nettle, and chamomile regularly as they promote kidney health, prevent urinary tract infections, and have general nutritive value.

Due to the pressure of the womb on your bladder, you may notice that you occasionally dribble a bit of urine when you sneeze or if you run or jump. This may also be due to weakness of the pelvic floor muscles. It is to your long-term advantage to begin now to strengthen your pelvic muscles to prevent later problems of incontinence or prolapse of your pelvic organs (see "Urinary Incontinence" in Part II).

UTERUS AND BELLY

The most obvious change your body goes through during pregnancy is uterine growth. This transformation is generally very exciting, though at times anxieties may arise. You may wonder how much more you can really stretch, or will you ever be able to see your toes without bending over. A pregnant woman's belly receives a great deal of public attention as well, some of it welcome, some unsolicited and unwelcome. Strangers and friends alike rarely fail to comment on how big or small a pregnant woman is, on whether she carries her baby like it's a boy or a girl, and so on. With all of this attention it is easy to overlook the

It is an honor to become a parent. A mother is the doorway through which we gain entrance into this world.

—Diane Mariechild

incredible miracle that your body is manifesting.

The uterus grows from the size of a small a pear to a large watermelon. Your womb increases in weight from a couple of ounces to about two pounds. It is an incredible structure capable of growing to such a size and then returning to its pre-pregnant size in a matter of weeks. In addition it serves the marvelous purpose of sending your baby forth from your body and into the world. The layers of the uterus also have built-in mechanisms for contraction that prevent excessive bleeding after the birth.

Your womb will grow steadily throughout pregnancy (see illustration), with the baby having occasional periods of more or less rapid growth. By about twelve weeks the top of the uterus, called the fundus, can be felt just above the pubic bone, and by twenty weeks the fundus is usually at about the level of your navel. At approximately thirty-six weeks your uterus will be pushing up against your diaphragm and you'll probably be wondering how much bigger you're going to grow. Then about two weeks before the baby is likely to be born, the baby will drop down slightly into the pelvis. While this gives you more breathing room and room for food, you'll likely be urinating a lot again. For some women who have already given birth, this shift, known as "lightening," may not occur until labor begins.

Of course all of this growing means that your body is doing a lot of stretching and growing around the middle (and everywhere else). Many woman are afraid of putting on weight, fearing that they'll never lose it again. It is true that pregnancy changes our bodies. In general we become just a little softer and certain changes such as stretch marks are permanent, though they do fade with time. If we can accept the beauty of our bodies for who we are, not comparing ourselves to a cultural ideal, and commending ourselves for our incredible ability to bear children, these changes will be accepted and needless tension will dissolve. In fact, if we could redefine the standards of beauty for women's bodies, our whole culture would be healthier and more sane. It is up to women to claim our pregnant bodies as beautiful and powerful. Only by each one of us changing our attitudes can society change its attitudes. We are not meant to be teenagers forever—we are meant to become women, with all of the aging and stretching that goes along with this transformation.

During pregnancy you may notice periodic and irregular tightenings or contractions of your uterus. This is not generally an uncomfortable sensation; you may merely notice that your belly feels very hard for a matter of seconds. These contractions may get more frequent or last longer as you get closer to the time of labor. They are more likely to be noticeable in your second or succeeding pregnancies. You are also likely to notice such contractions after orgasms. These contractions are in fact beneficial as they serve to tone your uterus and help to regulate pelvic blood flow. Only if they become regular, of stronger intensity, or progressively closer together more than three weeks before you are due will there be any need to contact your midwife or health practitioner to try to stop the contractions.

SKIN AND HAIR

For most women pregnancy brings enhanced hair and nail growth, with hair becoming lush and thick for the duration of the pregnancy. I've also heard stories of women's hair changing color during pregnancy, generally becoming darker, though I've never heard any scientific reason for this phenomenon, nor have I seen it. Many women will notice accelerated hair growth on their underarms and pubic hair as well. This usually stops after the birth, and in fact much of the new growth may fall out during the first year after birth.

Your skin can also go through a variety of changes during pregnancy, ranging from darkening of the nipples, development of the line of pregnancy that extends over your abdomen, and the mask of pregnancy, a brownish discoloration over the eyes and on the forehead, that resembles a mask (and is perhaps a sign of folic acid deficiency), or an increase or a decrease of pre-existing skin troubles such as acne or eczema. Itching may also be noticeable, particularly as pregnancy becomes advanced. Whether the problems clear up or are exacerbated depends upon your diet. The healthy functioning of your liver will help to process the hormones that can trigger skin troubles. Healthy bowel and kidney functioning will also help to reduce skin problems as the task of elimination will not rest so heavily on the skin if your other systems are performing their eliminatory functions optimally.

During pregnancy and through the first months after birth, women generally sweat much more than usual, with a stronger odor. This increase in sweat is both due to hormones stimulating the sweat glands and due to the extra heat of pregnancy from increased metabolism and subsequent sweating, a cooling mechanism. Again, a healthy diet with good elimination should reduce strong body odors, and a natural deodorant (one that contains no aluminum, is based on natural ingredients, and is not an antiperspirant) may also help. In her book *Holistic Midwifery* Anne Frye suggests taking 1 to 2 tablespoons daily of liquid chlorophyll to help reduce body odor and provide extra nutrients at the same time.

BONES AND MUSCLES

Contrary to popular assumptions, pregnant women do not suffer bone loss or tooth demineralization if they eat a well-balanced diet. In fact, pregnancy enhances calcium uptake, and though some bone loss may occur during lactation, this is replaced when your child stops nursing. Of course, a nourishing diet rich in minerals is essential.

Due to the influence of hormones, in late pregnancy you will notice that your joints, especially in your pelvis, feel looser. You may notice tenderness, or outright discomfort, or a feeling of mushiness. You may even notice clicking sounds in your pelvis as you walk or roll over in bed. It is this same loosening effect that allows the pelvic bones to separate slightly to accommodate the baby's head. You should pay attention to your posture, as the loosening of the joints and the slight relaxation of the abdominal muscles can lead you to sway your back and consequently develop low-back pain. All of these changes are more likely to register as complaints and discomforts if your muscle tone is already lax, particularly if you've had a number of children already. Regular exercise, both before and during pregnancy, and good posture are beneficial.

TOUCH, SOUND, AND SMELL

Sensitivity to touch and sound are generally enhanced (much to the chagrin of mothers with toddlers!) as is the sense of smell. It is very common for pregnant women to be irritated by noise and sensitive to touch.

The sense of smell is greatly exaggerated, though the nasal mucosa may become engorged, leading to a slightly stuffy nose. Taste may be either enhanced or decreased, depending upon the woman, but either way it is usually noticeably altered. Spatial awareness is also frequently altered—for example, it is not uncommon for a pregnant woman to miss the last step going down a flight of stairs, when her belly prevents her from seeing the step. Her sense of balance may also be affected. Some pregnant women notice that they drop things more easily or that their short-term memory seems fuzzy at times. These are all temporary changes, may not occur at all or only rarely, and may have to do with nutritional needs—for example, anemia may affect mental clarity as less oxygen may be delivered to the brain than is optimal.

Emotional Changes by Trimester

Just as pregnancy changes us physically, it changes us emotionally. Such change is a normal and healthy part of becoming a mother. Because a woman is emotionally sensitive, she can reflect on her fears, anxieties, concerns, and joys. The themes that infuse women's emotional and psychological issues are very similar, often reflecting the specific stage of pregnancy the woman is in at the time.

Your emotional state can affect your health and your baby's health either beneficially or detrimentally. Stress and joy can increase or reduce tension levels, reduce or enhance immunity, change heart and respiratory rates, and so on. Therefore your emotions deserve as much attention as your nutrition or exercise plan. Past experiences such as a miscarriage, difficult pregnancy or birth, or problems with a surviving child can all surface as anxieties, as can childhood traumas. Also, depending upon individual circumstances, women will have their own concerns, such as being a single mother, a mother who works outside the home, a mother carrying two or more babies, or a mother in a stressful partnership.

You may feel, as do many pregnant women, that you are the only one experiencing anxiety, ambivalence, fear of birth or motherhood, or sexual tensions with your partner. You may assume that your problems are overwhelming. Internalized stress is no small matter. It can lead to insomnia, poor eating habits, high blood pressure, rapid pulse, poor weight gain, and many other symptoms. Not addressing these symptoms can lead to complications in your pregnancy or in giving birth. It is vitally important that you work up the courage to talk with your midwife so that you can resolve the problem and feel good about yourself. This section is intended to let you know that most women have many anxieties during pregnancy, and that you are definitely not alone or crazy!

FIRST TRIMESTER

The first trimester can be considered a time of integrating the fact that you are pregnant. For some women this will be a joyous realization, having wanted a child. For some women the news will be a surprise. Some women will be outright unhappy to be pregnant, having not planned or wanted a baby at the time.

Some ambivalence is usual in pregnancy and will not cause physical harm to the baby. If you are experiencing ambivalence or if you do not accept the fact that you are pregnant, you can discuss the matter with your midwife or health care provider. She can guide you in letting your baby know that it is nothing personal, that you have some issues to work through. It may take several months to integrate the pregnancy, particularly if it was unexpected. This ambivalence is generally increased by the nausea, exhaustion, and the other physical discomforts common to the first trimester. As these discomforts begin to subside it is very common for the ambivalence to subside as well. However, it is a good idea to discuss your feelings openly with your partner, midwife, or trusted friend so that you don't overload yourself with worry or guilt.

Feelings of nausea and other physical discomforts can also cause you to feel extremely incompetent and dependent, particularly if the nausea is severe or you have other responsibilities such as children or work that you don't feel capable of doing. This can lead you to feel very discouraged about your ability to cope with pregnancy and to wish it were all over. Being dependent on your mate for extra help can also lead to tension, especially if he does not understand how terrible you feel. If both of you discuss your situation with your support person(s) it can help resolve the tension and help you get the support you need without feeling guilty for needing it.

How a partner responds to the news of your pregnancy can also influence you. You may get angry at him, feel rejected and depressed, or worry whether you may have to bear the child as a single mom. Many women find that during pregnancy they feel an intense desire to be with their partner practically all of the time to develop a very intimate connection. Unfortunately, men who are feeling anxious about the responsibility of fatherhood or who are not accustomed to such bonding may feel boxed in. Open communication and learning to feel centered are essential skills for a healthy relationship. While it is perfectly reasonable to want the baby's dad to be excited about having a child, many men experience a wide range of complex emotions, and may not have the grace to show excitement so that you can feel secure in the situation. Hopefully you will both come to a place where you can joyously support each other in welcoming your child into the world. Nevertheless, you must first learn to feel secure in yourself.

The hormonal changes of pregnancy can cause strong emotional fluctuations and a heightened sensitivity that can lead to unexpected, new emotional outbursts, such as weeping, anger, taking things personally or feeling rejected (particularly with your mate), and sentimentality (such as crying over a children's story or a song on the radio that would never otherwise make you gush). Nausea, fatigue, and hunger can exacerbate some of the more unpleasant outbursts. On the brighter side you are also likely to experience new levels of elation, sexual union, and joy, and a deep connection to living beings.

The first trimester is often accompanied by a sense of disbelief that you really are pregnant. I can recall that with each of my four pregnancies I would expect to see menstrual blood each time I wiped after urinating. Many women will wait with baited breath for any physical indications of pregnancy, and with each increase or decrease in breast tenderness or nausea will think, "Oh, I really must be pregnant," or "I guess I'm not pregnant after all." Even with a positive pregnancy test, women will wonder if it was a false reading.

If you have a history of miscarriage, you may anxiously wait until you are past the point where the miscarriage occurred in the previous pregnancy. This can be a very stressful time in which you don't allow yourself to become attached to this new little person, afraid that this baby too could be lost to you. However, the actual process of working to connect with your baby, as painful as this may seem, can help you to maintain your pregnancy. Even if the baby is not going to stay with you, a strong spiritual bond can exist for you, and you can help that being on its way. Similarly, a woman may put off bonding with her baby prenatally until she receives the results of prenatal testing (i.e., amnio, alpha-fetoprotein), which confirms her baby's wellness, rather than loving the child regardless. If you are planning to keep your baby even in the presence of a potential abnormality, there is no reason to avoid developing an emotional bond with your baby prenatally, and for as long as you are gifted to enjoy his or her presence.

SECOND TRIMESTER

During mid-pregnancy most women will feel at the peak of health and energy. At this point your belly has become more obvious and your baby begins to move, giving you a very tangible sense of her/his presence. This movement will make the experience finally real for the father as well, enhancing your connection together. People, even strangers, may notice that you are pregnant and you may find it fun to receive the extra attention.

The second trimester, however, is not without its own emotional nuances. General concerns such as finances or other problems may still worry you, and if you are looking after other children, particularly toddlers, you may still feel more tired than you do usually. The middle trimester is often a time of reflecting on your own childhood and on your relationship with your mother. It is perfectly natural for you to need your mother's support during pregnancy, yet at the same time to evaluate what your mom did that you would or would not want to do with your own child. In this generation, many women who want to have natural pregnancies and follow natural birthing and parenting styles may find it difficult to call upon their mothers, as most women in previous generations did not have such experiences and do not know how to talk to us about nutrition, birthing consciously, or breastfeeding our babies. This can lead to you rejecting your mother, and prompt tension in a relationship which you want to be nourishing. You also may want your mom to treat you as an adult woman. But because she may give advice or treat you as a child, you may feel unacknowledged in your own transformation into motherhood. All of these feelings may be confusing, but in the long run, can often bring you closer to your mom. For women who come from seriously abusive families, the complexity of issues may be greater and may have an impact on your pregnancy and parenting experience. It can be helpful to seek the support of an experienced counselor and to discuss such matters with your midwife.

Another common concern that women express during this time is a deep fear that something horrible will happen to their mate, leaving them alone with the baby. In fact, many women have such fears about birthing the baby without the dad that it will bring them to tears. This anxiety can cause these women to worry when their partner is late in arriving home and can also cause them to get angry if he didn't call to let them know he'd be late. If you are economically dependent on your partner, you may worry about how you would support yourself if a tragedy occurred. To reduce your anxiety, you can ask your partner to give you general notice if he won't be at an expected place at an expected time. Clear communication from you can let your partner know how important an issue this is to you.

The second trimester is also a time when women tend to become obsessive about dreams (which may be exceptionally vivid during pregnancy) and about comments people make (which are not always considerate). For example, it is not uncommon for a woman to have a dream that her baby has a deformity, nor is it uncommon for someone to tell a pregnant woman a pregnancy or birth horror story. You may find yourself wondering over and over if a worrisome dream is true or if a person's horror story is some kind of message that this is going to happen to you. While these ruminations are

perfectly normal, they don't help you feel positive about your baby or pregnancy; so the only purpose they serve is to help you to find your confidence and courage. Trust that you are doing your best by consciously caring for yourself and your baby.

THIRD TRIMESTER

By late pregnancy you may be feeling more physically tired again, needing to rest in the afternoon or go to sleep earlier. If you already have kids you may find yourself falling asleep while you put them to bed. You probably have to urinate a couple of times at night, and you may find it hard to eat much before you feel full. In general, all of these sensations may propel you to feeling ready to give birth. At the same time, you may feel overwhelmed by preparing your supplies or getting your home ready for the baby. Many women become obsessive about having a clean house, scrubbing areas that are usually overlooked such as the corners of cabinets, the baseboards, or spots on the walls. This seems to be a normal, almost instinctive need at this time. However, it is important that you are able to let go of being compulsive, trusting that you will be ready when the time is right, and that as long as your home is generally clean, the baby doesn't really care how the cabinets or baseboards look.

You may not feel obsessively worried about your mate any longer, but may now worry that you yourself may die giving birth. This seems to be a particularly worrisome thought for women who already have children. You may also worry that if you and the baby are okay, something may happen to one of your older children. Such anxieties are perfectly common and reflect how important your family is to you. They may also help you see how much you value your life and your commitment to your baby. We are too often trained to expect the worst or to feel as if we can't have it all, causing us to mistrust the future. This is, again, a time to call upon your trust in yourself that if you've done all you can (and likely you have) to be healthy, then you are healthy. It is very rare for women to die in childbirth in affluent countries such as this.

You may also feel depressed about the size of your body, uncomfortable in all of your clothes, and awkward as you engage in physical activities. Physical fatigue may cause those of you who already have children to worry how you will cope with the baby. Remember that you will have hard days and smooth days, and that the better you eat, rest, and refresh yourself emotionally, the better you will cope in the future. Sex may also feel awkward at this stage. You and your mate may need to try different positions so that you feel comfortable. If you honor the beauty of your pregnant body (and take care to exercise regularly to maintain your limberness), you will feel more comfortable in late pregnancy and have a more positive body image.

Toward the end of pregnancy many women find themselves more "spaced out" than usual. You may find yourself daydreaming about your birth or baby, or preoccupied with other details that you feel the need to attend to before your baby is born. While you are no less capable of dealing with concrete tasks, you may prefer to bask in a warm bath, take a long walk, or write in a journal. It is normal and actually beneficial to take the time to tune in to your more intuited needs at this time. A natural birth is best facilitated when you are able to enter into a relaxed, reflective, and intuitive state.

The Month Before Birth

During the last four to six weeks of pregnancy you may, like many women, feel eager to prepare yourself for birth and to meet your baby. This anticipation is welcome. You may also face new discomfort now that you have become so ripe with child, such as the need to urinate frequently, difficulty in eating due to less physical space in your stomach, more fatigue if you are caring for older children or working outside the home (or both), difficulty finding a comfortable sleeping position, heartburn, indigestion, and so on. Hopefully you have read earlier sections of this book and have been able to bypass most of these complaints, or at least have found natural approaches for addressing these discomforts and so have greatly reduced them.

Late pregnancy is a transitional time in which you may feel ready to move beyond pregnancy and hold your baby in your arms. This is a healthy and natural readiness that helps to prepare you mentally to welcome birth. It is also a time when utmost patience is required, particularly as you approach your due date. Each baby comes in his or her own unique time. During these last weeks of your pregnancy you may have many questions for your midwife or other care provider, especially about birth and caring for babies. There are no silly questions, and since you will be seeing your care provider more regularly, you can use the time to become better informed.

As the end of your pregnancy approaches, you may also begin to wonder whether you can really do it, or feel that you just aren't ready yet. This is a common anxiety, a reckoning with the forces of birth that you are about to face, and an awareness of the great responsibility of parenting. There may also be other anxieties or feelings of ambivalence. The best way to resolve these is to discuss them openly. By admitting worries and asking for help you are more likely to facilitate your birth. By holding back you may actually hold the birth back, as your hormones and muscles mirror your emotions. Midwives are usually prepared, willing to listen to your concerns and help you face and work through these feelings. By acknowledging and addressing your doubts, and arriving at a place of confidence before you enter labor, you will be in a stronger state of mind for birth.

How well you care for yourself during late pregnancy can strongly set the tone for your birth experience. This chapter is devoted to helping you continue caring for yourself optimally during these last weeks of pregnancy so that the tone you set is positive. It explores ways that you can prepare your body and nourish your spirit so that when the time comes for your baby to be born, you will be ready, willing, strong, and healthy.

NUTRITION AND REST DURING LATE PREGNANCY

A mother who enters labor tired and poorly nourished stands a very great chance of not being able to cope with the intensity of the process, of having a dysfunctional labor in which her uterus does not contract effectively, and of eventually requiring interventions that enable her body to birth or be delivered. Sleep and nutritional deficits are easy to prevent and even cure during pregnancy for most middle-class American women. It is therefore of tremendous importance that you pay close attention to your body's needs during this time.

— Sleep and Relaxation —

When you are tired, stress seems magnified and pain is less tolerable. When you are fatigued, emotions seem to take on a life of their own and your body will function less effectively. It is standard for you to tire more easily during late pregnancy than at other times in your life; you are working constantly, even when at rest, to grow your baby. When you ignore your body's need for rest problems begin to arise. The simple solution is to rest regularly, napping in the afternoon whenever possible and getting to bed early (I generally recommend that women try to get to bed by 10 P.M. during the last weeks of pregnancy). These habits will ensure that you will be well rested so that if you begin labor at two in the morning, for example, you will have had some sleep.

If you are unable to take a regular afternoon nap, a short period of deep relaxation can substitute. Chapter 8 provides several suggestions and techniques for deep relaxation. It can be done before you go to sleep at night, enhancing your sleep. It can't be overstated that you must be well rested during late pregnancy. Birthing can take a long time and you will be able to meet this challenge only if you meet your body's needs beforehand. It should be clear that fatigue can actually prolong labor.

— Nutrition —

For most women, late pregnancy brings fluctuations in appetite ranging from being ravenous to not having much appetite at all. Your increased appetite will be in proportion to growth spurts that your baby has in the last weeks of pregnancy. A loss of appetite often occurs at this time because you have a sense of fullness as your growing baby presses against your stomach, leaving much less room for food than you had earlier in the pregnancy. It is important to maintain excellent nutrition throughout your pregnancy, since this will keep you in top preparation for birth, which requires an enormous expenditure of energy. If you find that you are tired of the same-old-same-old, treat yourself to a new recipe book or ask your friends or your midwife for recipe suggestions. Sometimes just having a change of foods can spark your appetite.

As your baby grows and you find it difficult to eat a quantity of food at one sitting, you may want to eat small but frequent meals throughout the day and into the evening, avoiding foods that might contribute to heartburn (tomatoes and peppers are common culprits). It is very important to eat sufficient complex carbohydrates, proteins, and iron foods at the end of pregnancy. The complex carbohydrates will help maintain stable blood sugar levels, keeping your energy levels steady as well. The increased protein and iron are essential, the protein for the rapid development of the baby's brain, and the iron for storing in the baby's body for the first six months of life. If you have a consistently poor appetite, anemia may be an underlying cause, and should be treated using the recommendations found in Part II, under "Anemia."

HERBS FOR LATE PREGNANCY AND BIRTH PREPARATION

In addition to the herbs you are taking for nutritional purposes (see Chapter 6) there are several herbs that can be used to relieve late-pregnancy discomfort and that tone and relax your uterine muscles, preparing your body for birth. Many of the herbs in this latter category were taught to us by Native American women who have long used herbs in late pregnancy for the purpose of easing birth. Many of these herbs are inappropriate for use prior to the last three weeks of pregnancy due to their ability to stimulate labor; therefore use them only after 36 weeks of

pregnancy, and only as recommended with the guidance of an experienced herbalist. Following is a list of herbs and how they can benefit you, as well as four recipes for late-pregnancy tonics. You should feel free to create your own formulas as well. Refer to Part II for herbs that address specific complaints, such as leg cramps or high blood pressure, which may also occur during late pregnancy.

Black cohosh, which is not botanically related to blue cohosh (but is commonly used along with this herb), helps to relax the cervix and uterine muscles, relieve irregular uterine contractions and promote more regular ones, and also to reduce blood pressure by dilating peripheral blood vessels. This herb is also commonly included in late-pregnancy tonics, and should be used with the same precaution (see below) as blue cohosh, as it can also cause side effects such as headaches, dizziness, and nausea.

Blue cohosh has developed a notable reputation for its effectiveness as a late-pregnancy uterine tonic, preparing the uterine muscles for birth. It should be taken only in the last three weeks and may be especially beneficial for women with a history of going far overdue or of having been induced in past pregnancies. Women who have not been having Braxton Hicks contractions may specifically want to take a late-pregnancy tonic with blue cohosh to stimulate labor. Begin in small doses and increase them as the due time approaches, or just after. Some women find that using this herb causes nausea and light-headedness. If you experience any of these side effects, discontinue usage and the symptoms will abate. Do not use before 37 weeks gestation as a birth preparator as it may stimulate contractions, and do not exceed more than 20 drops of the tincture, four times daily, without the guidance of an experienced herbalist or midwife.

Chamomile is nutrient rich and can be taken daily as a lightly steeped tea to reduce both muscular and nervous tension, bringing a definite sense of calmness, reduced aching, and reduced anxiety that might contribute to elevated blood pressure. I frequently went to sleep in late pregnancy after a warm cup of chamomile tea, which induces enough relaxation to promote a gentle sleep. However, this herb can be used freely during the day without slowing your reflexes or making you sleepy. I also enjoy the beneficial effects of chamomile tea during labor. As it is sometimes considered a gentle emmenagogue, it is best to avoid if you have had late-pregnancy bleeding.

Cramp bark has properties that you might expect based on its name. While it tones the uterine muscles in preparation for birth, it generally serves to promote muscular relaxation, relieving uterine cramping and spasms, leg cramps, low back pain, as well as pressure in the groin. It can be used during pregnancy, and makes an excellent addition to a late-pregnancy tonic as shown on page 104, either in infusion or tincture. Black haw, which may be slightly stronger, can be used interchangeably with cramp bark. These herbs can help to reduce arterial blood pressure, relieve anxieties, and prevent irregular uterine contractions. As it is a hypotensive, women may feel slightly dizzy if they stand up too quickly.

False unicorn root also makes an overall excellent uterine and hormonal tonic and can be a beneficial addition to a late-pregnancy routine. It is quite bitter, making a tincture a good choice if you are going to take this herb regularly.

Partridge Berry is a highly esteemed partus preparator—that is, an herb that prepares your body for birth. It tones the uterine muscles while promoting gentle relaxation. It helps to reduce backaches, leg cramps, anxiety, and tension, and also tones the urinary tract and the bowels, making it an all-around ally for women in late pregnancy. It can be taken in infusion or tincture form, and you will find it in the formulas listed below. While it can be used throughout pregnancy, it is most beneficial in the last four to six weeks.

Motherwort, already mentioned several times throughout this book for its wonderful ability to promote relaxation and reduce emotional anxiety, as well as to strengthen the heart and prevent hypertension, can be used during late pregnancy for all of these same purposes. Before 36 weeks it should be used sparingly, or in infusion rather than in tincture form, as it contains substances that can stimulate the uterus, but it can be used in slightly larger amounts in late pregnancy. As it is very bitter, tincture is the most palatable form for using this herb. Take up to 20 drops at a time for anxiety or high blood pressure, not to exceed four doses daily, five days a week.

Nettle throughout pregnancy continues to maintain kidney health, prevents late-pregnancy urinary tract infections, prevents excessive fluid retention, and helps to regulate the blood sugar. Using nettle infusion regularly throughout late pregnancy may also prevent anemia and heavy bleeding at birth. Up to a quart a day can be taken.

Wild yam is an excellent hormonal regulator, and I therefore like to include it in a late-pregnancy tonic. It is also useful for reducing irritable cramping during late pregnancy, for stress, and as a urinary tract antiseptic.

As for remedies, yes, the herbs are powerful healers in and of themselves, but healing is deeper and more than the plant. Healing is will and intention—the strong desire for life.

—A. J. R.

Late-Pregnancy Tonic Recipes

Late-pregnancy tonic recipes should include herbs that both tone and relax your uterine muscles as well as your nerves, helping you to stay relaxed and well rested while preparing your body to give birth. Here are four recommended formulas:

Combine 1 part each of red raspberry leaf, partridge berry, false unicorn root, and cramp bark, and add 1/4 part of wild yam and motherwort. Steep 4–6 tablespoons of these herbs in one quart of boiling water for 30 minutes. Strain and drink 1 to 2 cups daily.

Combine equal parts of false unicorn root, partridge berry, blue cohosh, and cramp bark. Prepare 4–6 tablespoons of this mixture as above. Dosage is the same.

Take 10 drops each of the following tinctures 3 to 4 times daily during the last month of pregnancy, increasing the dosage to 20 drops each 3 to 4 times daily during the last week before you are due: false unicorn root, Mitchella, blue cohosh, and cramp bark.

Take the following formula according to the dosage and amounts of the preceding formula: blue cohosh, black cohosh, wild yam, motherwort, and false unicorn root.

In addition to one of these formulas, take 500 mg of evening primrose oil or black currant oil daily for the last four weeks of your pregnancy. Do not increase the dosage unless you are overdue and your cervix is "unripe" (not yet soft) according to a vaginal exam. In this case you may double the amount, but do not take more than this. These oils contain substances that support prostaglandin production, a hormone in our bodies responsible for cervical ripening. Semen also contains prostaglandins, and regular intercourse in late pregnancy can help to prepare the cervix for birth.

PREPARING YOUR BODY FOR BIRTH

Your body, unhindered, knows exactly how to give birth and nourish a baby. There are several ways that you can promote and enhance these natural abilities, including vaginal muscle awareness, the use of herbs, and regular body movement, which should be emphasized in the last four to six weeks of your pregnancy.

Vaginal muscle awareness was touched upon in Chapter 7; refer to this chapter for a full discussion of the muscles involved in birth, as well as the importance of Kegel exercise. During late pregnancy you can increase this awareness by practicing vaginal muscle massage. This technique is commonly referred to as perineal massage; you or your partner massage and stretch the external vaginal muscles to enhance suppleness and to prepare you for the sensation of your baby causing you to stretch during the crowning of its head when it is about to be born. Unfortunately, emphasis has become placed on using this technique to prevent tears. Tears are best prevented when the woman has the ability to relax the yoni, not by having it stretched. I have offered this technique to help you to become comfortable with your vagina, identify areas where you may be holding pelvic tension, and learn to relax your muscles.

Your midwife can provide instruction for vaginal massage at a prenatal visit, particularly at a visit to your home if a home birth is planned or this is where you feel most relaxed. You can do vaginal massage on yourself by inserting your index and middle fingers into your birth canal either while you are in a bath or while standing with one leg on a chair. If you are quite supple you might be able to do it lying in bed, propped on pillows. Your mate can also help you by doing the massage. The idea is to feel for areas that feel tight both in the vaginal canal and along the perineum, and gently massage them while you deliberately try to identify and relax these muscles. This will enable you to do this during birth, allowing your baby to be born with minimal resistance.

Vaginal massage can be done a few times a week or even daily, using either plain vegetable oil, a mild massage oil, or an oil that is specifically for perineal massage, sometimes available through mail-order birthing supply companies. An excellent blend can be made at home following the instructions in Appendix I for making an oil. Comfrey leaf and root, calendula, St. John's wort, lavender, and calendula are some herbs that may be included in such an oil. Vitamin E oil also makes an excellent addition since it benefits the skin as well as helping to preserve the oil.

Love-making is also an excellent way to prepare your yoni for birth if this is something you enjoy during late pregnancy. You may have to be creative in finding positions in which you are comfortable, but the movements of your pelvis are excellent for toning your uterus and your vaginal muscles. Love-making can be creative in other ways, without intercourse, if intercourse is too uncomfortable for you.

As discussed in Chapter 7, regular movement during pregnancy in the form of dance, yoga, swimming, walking, or other gentle but strengthening activities helps you become closely attuned to your body. This is essential preparation for an active and positive birth in which you are able to work cooperatively with the birth energy. Late pregnancy may require you to slow down some or to modify your activities, but it is highly beneficial for women to remain physically active even until the last minutes of pregnancy. Physical activity will keep your heart and lungs prepared for the work of labor, and will help to keep your blood pressure steady, your circulation excellent, and your stamina and endurance up. However, physical activity is effective only if it continues to be in harmony with your physical needs and your baby's needs. Such exercise should help you get loose and relax your muscles as well as tone your muscles.

PREPARING FOR BREASTFEEDING

Breastfeeding provides your baby with both perfect nourishment as well as the continuity of closeness with which your baby is so familiar. Many women wonder whether they will be able to nurse their babies—whether they will have enough milk, whether they have the right nipples for nursing, and so on. These concerns arise more from internalized cultural messages than reality. Most well-nourished women will have a plentiful supply of milk for their babies and most women's nipples are just fine for breastfeeding. Occasionally a woman will have flat or inverted nipples, where the nipples do not become erect when stimulated such as by touch or cold, or they actually dimple inward. Women with flat nipples will usually be able to nurse without any prenatal preparation of their nipples other than massaging the area around the nipple (on the areola, the dark circle around the nipple) to break up any tissue adhesions that might prevent the nipple from protruding. Frequently women will have flat nipples before their first baby is breastfed, but will have erect nipples after having nursed their first child.

If you have truly inverted nipples you will want to consult with a La Leche League leader or a lactation consultant for information on how to prepare your breasts for nursing. Nipple shields, small plastic cups with a hole in the inner layer, which are worn over the nipples for a period of time each day, exert gentle traction on the nipples, encouraging them to come out before the baby is born. You may also need a bit of extra support with nursing after your baby is born, but even if you have fully inverted nipples you can nurse successfully—it may take a bit more determination.

There is no need to "toughen" your nipples by rubbing them vigorously with a towel or any such technique, but you may wish to go without a bra periodically if you are comfortable doing so, and let your shirt rub against your breasts. Also, if you are able to expose your nipples to a bit of sunshine now and then, even through a window (but preferably directly), this may be beneficial. Again, none of these steps are necessary for successful breastfeeding. Excessive nipple stimulation can actually cause contractions!

If milk production is a problem refer to my book *Natural Healing for Babies and Children* for a comprehensive discussion and suggestions that are highly effective.

WHAT YOU NEED AFTER THE BABY IS BORN

While this book is not about postpartum care, there are certain preparations for the immediate days after birth that you will need to have made during your pregnancy. Late pregnancy is the time to make sure that you have the supplies you will need for your baby, as well as the support you will need for caring for yourself, the baby, and the other members of your household while you are recuperating from the birth.

— Baby Supplies —

I've never been a big supporter of baby paraphernalia. There is very little equipment that you need for your baby during the first months of life. A car seat is essential, as there is substantial evidence that babies in car seats are the safest passengers in moving vehicles, but aside from that, all you really need are cloth diapers and diaper covers, appropriate clothing (you will need very few newborn-size things since most breastfed babies will outgrow these in the first week or so), a baby hat (babies lose a lot of heat when their heads are exposed), a diaper bag, a baby blanket, a few receiving blankets, and a handful of soft washcloths. A sling baby carrier is a useful addition to this list. Later on, a high chair or Sassy seat is helpful, and simple toys. A backpack for carrying a baby, in my opinion, is indispensable. Playpens, cribs, a host of plastic toys, bath tub inserts, pacifiers, bottles, and so on are really unnecessary if you are going to be with your baby and breastfeed. Baby stuff is big business, not necessities.

— Help After the Birth —

During pregnancy, I have my clients consider who of their friends or relatives might be able to come to their home a few hours after the birth to help prepare a nourishing meal for the couple or the family, to run linens that might have been used at the birth through the washer and dryer, and to look after the other children. This allows both the mother and father the freedom to rest and bask in the presence of their newborn without interruption, and ensures that everyone will be well cared for. While for most women, birth is not a traumatic event (in fact, you may feel very energetic immediately after the birth), it is important that you allow people to cater to you. This is a time for you to allow yourself to be nourished by those who care for you.

If you would prefer not to have company in the immediate hours after birth, you can still prearrange for a friend to leave a meal outside your front door, so that all your mate or midwife has to do is warm it and serve it to you. You can also have meals in the freezer that merely need to be defrosted and heated. You can prepare and freeze these in advance, or ask friends and relatives to gift you with meals that can be frozen. One of my clients was given a casserole shower by her friends. Guests brought a dish for the mother to freeze for both her late pregnancy when she might not have the energy for cooking, and also for after the birth. This was very liberating for the both the mother and her mate, as dinners did not have to be a concern for several weeks after the birth.

If you have older children, particularly if they are under seven years old, you will also want to have someone at home with you at least for the first week after the birth who can tend to their needs. This will help the children feel cared for, as well as prevent you from becoming exhausted.

If you are in a situation where you live far from relatives, or have just moved to a new town and don't know many people and can't easily arrange for support, you might want to hire a doula, a woman whose profession it is to provide postpartum care for mothers. A doula will come to your home for the number of hours that you agree upon and will do the housekeeping, grocery shopping, meal preparation, and laundry. Some will even pick children up from school and bring them home. Most doulas also have basic knowledge about newborn care,

breastfeeding, and the needs of new mothers, and can therefore provide valuable emotional support and answer some questions that may arise. To find a doula in your area ask local midwives, obstetricians, or La Leche League leaders. The address for Doulas of North America is listed in "Resources."

CELEBRATING PREGNANCY

Pregnancy provides a wonderful opportunity to celebrate not only the coming of your baby, but the transformation of your own life as well. In our country the traditional form of celebration is to give the mother a shower shortly before the baby is due, passing on to her positive stories of birth and motherhood, as well as giving her everything she needs (and sometimes doesn't need) for the baby. While this ritual has the potential to be a time to disseminate valuable information as well as to encourage and empower a woman about to cross through the doorway that is birth, it is often less relevant, though still a memorable occasion. In addition to this celebration, or in lieu of it, I'd like to share with you the tradition called the Blessingway. I also want to share an enjoyable activity—making a belly mask—that results in a terrific conversation piece as well as a long-lasting *objet d'art* that tangibly honors your pregnancy experience.

— *The Blessingway* —

The term Blessingway derives from the Dine (Navaho) culture and language, but such rituals are germane to peoples all over the world. This ritual, taught to me by my mentor, Jeannine Parvati Baker, has become popular among midwives across North America as we have sought to reclaim and

"As you do unto your unborn children, so they will do unto the world."

—*Thomas Verny, MD, from a workshop on prenatal psychology*

create meaningful rituals and beautiful celebrations for our life cycles.

The Blessingway is a ritual that can be done to honor, celebrate, direct, and emphasize any significant life changes that are occurring, such as a new job, a move, a marriage, a graduation, the onset of the first menses, menopause, a birthday, and so on. While it is a celebration it is not a party; it is a ritual, a time of focus and concentration on the subject(s) for whom the ritual is being created, and a time to give birth in an atmosphere that reflects the purpose of the ceremony.

The Blessingway has three basic parts: the opening of the ritual, the body of the ritual, and the completion of the ritual. While there are certain elements that are commonly included, they are not fixed. You can create your own ceremony using original ideas or those you glean from other sources. There are several useful books in the Appendix and many others to be found in bookstores. Singing is an important and uplifting aspect of the Blessingway. Look for tapes at women's bookstores. I highly recommend tapes by Lisa Thiel, Alicia Bonnet, and Libana. The songbook *Songs of the Earth* by Anna Kealoha (Celestial Arts Publishing, Berkeley, California) is a rich source of songs from many religious and spiritual traditions, both old and new, and has many songs appropriate for ceremonies such as this. Many of these songs are quite simple and have repetitions that make it easy to follow along in a large group, even if people haven't heard the songs before.

The Blessingway does not need to follow any specific denomination. You can infuse the ritual with your own religion, but if you are not part of any organized religion you can extract elements from a variety of cultures and religions or create a nature-centered ritual.

A Blessingway can be given by a close friend, relative, your midwife, or it can be done by yourself or with your mate and children. It is usually done in the weeks just prior to your due time. Blessingway guests should include only those people with whom you are very close and with whom you feel positive and comfortable. Blessingways can be women-only, women only except for your mate, or mixed. A small group is better with Blessingways, as it is easier to remain focused.

Supplies for a Blessingway are variable but the main ingredients are objects that symbolize pregnancy, life, babies, relationships, the powers of nature and Earth, etc., which can be used to create an altar or centerpiece for the gathering. Guests can bring gifts to decorate the altar. Additionally there should be lit candles, flowers, comfortable seating (lots of floor pillows and soft chairs), and a special area arranged for the guest of honor, the mother. To the Blessingway each guest should bring a small gift for the mother, preferably homemade, or of simple and natural materials if purchased. This gift can be a poem that is appropriate, a new hairbrush or hair clip so that she has something new and personal for herself after the baby is born, a gift for the baby, or even the promise of several meals or help with older children just before or after the new baby is born. Also each guest should bring a dish to contribute to a pot-luck meal or snack after the ritual. Ideally, one person will get a list from the mom as to whom she wants at her Blessingway, and this person will then call the guests and tell them what to bring. The Blessingway should not cause extra work for the pregnant woman, unless of course, you are planning the Blessingway yourself.

Before you begin the Blessingway, create an atmosphere in the area that invites peace, contemplation, and comfort. You are creating a sacred space. Let people know exactly when you will begin, as late-coming guests can disrupt the energy of the ritual once it gets going. I find that Blessingways done indoors are facilitated by semi-darkness and candlelight. Blessingways held outside are quite beautiful as well.

OPENING THE RITUAL

Opening the Blessingway involves several aspects or actions on the part of the person facilitating the ritual: welcoming everyone and explaining what the ritual is about and why you are doing it. You needn't be historically accurate; simply explain your intention to create a meaningful way of honoring and supporting—Blessing the Way—of your friend who is about to give birth. (If you are doing this ritual by yourself or with your mate you may wish to mention your intentions for this ritual rather than the explanation.) This explanation can also help anyone unfamiliar with the idea of ritual, who may associate it with something scary or horror-movieish. Let folks know that the Blessingway is a participatory event, that you are just helping to keep it focused on the purpose of blessing the mother.

Next comes a purification. I prefer the technique known as smudging. I use smoke to ritually remove any energy, thoughts, or feelings that may negatively be influencing any of the guests or the mother, and to welcome in positive and loving energy. To smudge, you light the herbs cedar and sage and allow the smoke to circulate around each person by holding the lit herbs near their body (use a bowl or a large shell to contain the sparks and ashes). You can blow on the herbs to direct the smoke around the person's body. A nice way to smudge is to have each person smudge the person to their left, going clockwise around a circle. To

order smudge sticks that are made for this purpose see "Resources." If you know other purification techniques you can substitute your own methods.

Finally, the invocation is spoken, that is, a prayer to invite and welcome all of those spiritual forces (use your own terms: angels of birth, spirit guides, your own higher powers, forces of nature, Great Mother, Heavenly Father, God, whatever your belief system holds for you) that will assist this mother on her path. The tone should be reverent, the room receptive to these spiritual allies, and the prayer slow and eloquent.

This invocation can be given by the person organizing the ritual or someone else in the group. During the smudging or purification, songs can be sung.

THE BODY OF THE RITUAL

This part of the ritual is focused on nurturing the mother, encouraging her sense of support and empowerment and creating a collective positive intention for her safe and joyous experience of birth. It is a time for each guest to share his or her love individually and as a group for the mother and baby. These are the steps that I usually follow when giving a Blessingway. They are open to your own creative input.

Note: After each step in the ritual it is pleasant to punctuate the celebration with singing. My friend Lisa Olko created handwritten lyrics sheets almost ten years ago that I continue to use at Blessingways. You

waters rising
moon filling me
this vessels holds firm
but is ready to
overflow at any time.
so ready for my baby
to be born

—A. J. R.

can write your own by jotting down the words to several songs that you might want to sing. Then photocopy enough pages to hand out to the guests so that each person can follow along. Hand drums, rattles, and other simple percussion instruments can help set the tempo for the music. These are easy to play and add richness to the singing. You can ask guests to bring instruments if they have any. In fact, when I plan a Blessingway I call each guest about a week before the gathering and let them know that they can contribute to the ritual by bringing items for the altar, flowers, a verse, poem, song, or thought to share.

1. Going around the circle clockwise, each guest introduces herself, and tells why she came and what she would like to contribute to this ritual. Each person should have the opportunity to place something special on the altar should she so desire.

2. The person facilitating the group can lead the guests on a guided visualization, perhaps of imagining giving birth as they would wish it to be. Begin the visualization with a deep relaxation exercise so that everyone has the opportunity to relax and benefit from the ritual. (*Motherwit* is an excellent book filled with relaxation and visualization exercises that can be adapted for rituals.)

3. Give everyone the chance to return to a sitting position in the circle and introduce the idea of grooming the mother. This involves massaging the mother's feet in a foot bath, brushing her hair, and generally doting on her. Utmost sensitivity to the mother's needs and sense of personal space is essential. For the foot bath use a rectangular bucket wide enough for her feet and with enough water to reach her ankles. Add

herbal oils to scent the water and float a handful of herbal potpourri in the bucket, or prepare a strong herbal infusion and let her soak her feet in this. Lavender, rose petals, calendula, mint, lemon balm, and other aromatic herbs are wonderful. While her feet are soaking and massaged by two of the guests, a third person, perhaps the mother's closest friend, sister, or mother, will brush the pregnant woman's hair (sprinkle a few drops of lavender or rose oil on the brush for added effect) and then style it using hair clips, ribbons, etc. This is symbolic of preparing her "head-space" to be ready for birth and mothering. A flower garland, which is easily homemade with a bouquet of flowers and wire, makes a perfect crown after her hair is completely groomed. I also have a special Blessingway gown that was a gift to me, that each mother dons at the beginning of the grooming part of the ritual. After each Blessingway it is washed and put away until the next Blessingway.

After the hair is done and the feet massaged, the two women at her feet rub cornmeal over the woman's feet, rather than drying them with a towel. This gives the feet a nice glow, wishing luck, protection, and prosperity for the mother as she walks along her path.

4. When the grooming is complete and all of the grooming supplies set aside, the next step is the Give-away, when each guest has the opportunity to address the mother. I like to go around the circle clockwise once more and have each guest say something special and positive that they remember from her own experience of giving birth. If she has never given birth, she can relate some other special experience. Each person will then present her gift, either reading a poem she may have brought, or explaining the gift. This is often a teary experience, so give plenty of time for each person to speak. However, if anyone starts getting negative or goes on and on, you may have to graciously move the energy along.

Another lovely thing to do, taught to me by midwife Diane Bartlett (Whapio), is to give each person a slip of paper, a pen, and have some strips of ribbon available. Have each person write a prayer, wish, or blessing for the mother and baby on their paper, then pass around a small basket. All wishes should be for the highest good of the mother and baby. Tell each guest to read their wish aloud in turn, and as they do, put the paper in the basket and attach ribbons to the basket. When this is completed you will have a beautifully decorated wish basket that the mom can look at for inspiration whenever she desires, one that will be a beautiful keepsake for the baby. The actual gift giving can be done when the basket has been completed.

COMPLETING THE RITUAL

To complete the ritual the facilitator can ask if anyone has anything further to share. It is nice if all of the guests hold hands and sing. A very special song that was taught to me is as follows. I don't know who wrote it.

> *Dear ones, Dear ones*
> *Can I tell you how I feel*
> *You have given me such treasures*
> *I love you so.*

This is sung to the tune of "Soul Cakes," a familiar old folk song.

Once done, thank all of the participants, most especially all of the helping angels and other beneficent beings who have blessed the mother's way. Welcome everyone to join in a feast and celebration. You have completed the Blessingway ritual.

— *Making a Belly Mask* —

This simple, inexpensive project is the creation of an actual plaster cast of your belly, best done in late pregnancy for full effect. It is made with the same techniques and materials you use for making plaster face masks. Here's how to do it:

Purchase about three rolls of plaster gauze at a local craft store. This is plaster impregnated gauze used for making face masks. You will also need a small jar of Vaseline, an old plastic bucket, and a few rags.

Because it is a messy project, it is best done either out of doors where the rain or a garden hose can wash away the drips of plaster, or indoors on a drop cloth or inexpensive shower curtain liner. It is preferable to have someone help you with the process.

To begin, assemble all of your supplies and fill the bucket with warm water. Take your clothes off (you can leave a bra or short tank top on) and stand on the plastic or drop cloth. Measuring horizontally across the areas to be covered, cut strips of the gauze in pieces long enough to cover your belly (and torso if your want to include your breasts), and additional gauze to add two to three layers of thickness.

Now smear a thin layer of Vaseline onto the areas that you will be plastering. This will prevent the materials from sticking to you or hurting when you pull them off. You don't need to smear Vaseline onto your pubic hair—the plaster doesn't stick well in hair. Then, following the directions on the package of gauze, dip the strips into the warm water and begin applying them to your belly. The general idea is to make overlapping horizontal layers leaving no places uncovered, and continuing until you achieve the shape of the belly that you want. When you are finished applying the strips, allow the cast to dry for about five minutes, then remove it from your belly, smooth out the edges by folding them back a bit, and put in a dry, protected spot to harden completely. It will take about 24 hours to be dry enough to paint.

Paint with acrylic paints, and have someone spray or paint it with a lacquer or glaze for extra protection. If you must spray it yourself, do so only in a well-ventilated area, preferably outdoors.

Pregnancy as a
Time for Transformation

PREGNANCY AS A RITE OF PASSAGE

In many cultures, including our own as evidenced by communions, bar mitzvah and bat mitzvahs, graduations, weddings, baby showers, and other celebrations, it is important to mark life transitions in tangible ways as rites of passage. The ceremony is a marker indicating that a person has learned what is necessary or has grown to a stage of development that gives him or her the privilege of entering a new stage. In traditional cultures, rites of passage are used to mark the transition from youth to adult responsibility in a tribe, village, or community. During this time the initiate must demonstrate her or his ability to withstand or endure certain challenges and will also receive knowledge imparted by elders about the new stage to come.

In our society little recognition is given to the major transformative nature of pregnancy, which, along with its culmination in the birth of a child, is a lengthy rite of passage into becoming a mother. One can call pregnancy a liminal stage, that is, "a phase of becoming." Women becoming mothers are neither given the special recognition as initiates, nor imparted the skills that teach and support them to be strong women and capable mothers through the teachings of elders. But we can change all this by acknowledging the important transformative qualities that pregnancy has in a woman's life.

By viewing pregnancy as a rite of passage you can take it upon yourself to make the most of the process, looking at the entire pregnancy experience not simply as a means to an end (the birth and the baby) but as a valuable process in and of itself. You can make a firm and courageous attempt to become a powerful woman, learning to trust your body, and your innate wisdom. By doing so, you will come to realize that the aura of strength and wellness with which you fill and surround yourself will infuse the baby with these qualities as well.

AN OPPORTUNITY FOR PERSONAL GROWTH

Pregnancy can be viewed as an opportunity to resolve conflicts from the past that may hinder your sense of empowerment. Pregnancy is a time of heightened emotional sensitivity, a perfect time to learn to work with your emotions. It is a time to develop the strength to deal with your issues with grace, confidence, and determination. These are the same attributes that will see you through birth.

It is perfectly natural and healthy to expect that as we walk through the doorway of pregnancy and birth we feel fears—we are, after all, facing the unknown. This is inevitably challenging as we grasp the enormous responsibility of motherhood, as well as recognizing the intensity of the birth experience. And there seems to be benefit in

what I refer to as "the work of worrying." I've noticed that women who do some healthy worrying during pregnancy and admit to having fears or anxieties are actually engaged in resolving conflicts. Women who deny—either consciously or uncon-

sciously—that they have fears about birth, the baby, motherhood, their marriage, etc. tend to have a more difficult experience of birth. If you can actively look at a particular concern, prepare or educate yourself about it, and then let it go, once you've done what you can to address, resolve, or at least contemplate it, then you are actively working out your fears. It is by addressing such fears or concerns that you can find the inner strength for creative problem solving. For example, if you already have toddlers and find yourself pregnant, you may feel anxiety about how you will handle all these responsibilities. Creative problem solving might include arranging support for a while after the birth, making menus or freezing foods during your pregnancy to have for after the birth, and affirming each day your ability to nurture yourself so that you maintain the energy to care for your family.

You might also choose to relieve bouts of anxiety by writing in a journal, nurturing yourself with tea and a bath by candlelight, crying on your mate's shoulder, or drawing a picture of yourself with images of abundant love being showered down upon you by an imagined loving mother. Such visualizing can help to increase your sense of greater energy and support.

SELF-EMPOWERMENT

Empowerment refers to the ability to know what one needs and to feel confident to meet those needs. However, for many women, trained since childhood to be accommodating and passive, this is no simple feat. For a pregnant woman to give herself and her child the best care possible, she must relinquish passivity and empower herself to make choices in her health care.

In the present health care system that denies individuality for the sake of efficiency, predictability, and cost-effectiveness, women must become empowered if we are to receive the care we want for ourselves and our families. To accept treatment that is not truly in our best interest is to allow ourselves to become victims. When one chooses something, this is empowerment; when one allows oneself to be manipulated, coerced, or frightened into accepting something, this is victimization. I always remind my clients that they are the ones in charge of their health care decisions, not the midwife, doctor, or anyone else. Short of an emergency situation, it is your voice and your needs that should determine the care you receive.

So how do you become empowered to make health care choices? Often it takes a difficult experience before a woman is empowered. But you don't have to have an initial experience in which you have felt victimized to bring about such revelation. Determination to trust your body and gradually learning to do so is an excellent place to start. Trusting your inner voice, your intellectual abilities, and your mental competence, and then speaking up for yourself or following your feelings are also ways to empowerment. Telling a doctor, for example, that you didn't like a negative comment he or she made about pregnancy, birth, or your body, or asking a neighbor not to tell you negative birthing stories is empowerment. Rather than meekly accepting a negative comment for the sake of being polite or for fear of offending someone, you must protect and care for yourself.

Listening to your body, an important aspect of empowerment, means taking the time to be body-centered each day. Because pregnancy brings so many new sensations,

this is a ripe time for becoming aware of your body. As you respond more readily to your body's cues, they will become more apparent. In the same way, you will increasingly trust your intuition and common sense. You have to trust that you know what is best for you. You can elicit information, advice, opinions, and support, but then you will have to decide how *you* feel about things.

Experience, too, is empowering. Many women have never had the opportunity to spend time with babies and young children, have never seen a woman breastfeed, and have never changed a diaper. Therefore many women enter motherhood feeling that they lack the skills necessary to care for their young. While much of mothering is highly intuitive, not all of it is. It does help to spend time around babies. The opportunity to assist another mom with the care of her baby, letting her know that you want to be familiar with the feel of a newborn and to feel comfortable with changing diapers, etc. can raise your level of confidence and your sense of empowerment. Reading books to educate yourself about the basic facts about pregnancy, birth, and parenting can be empowering. Learning infant massage, infant CPR, or other skills, and hearing about other women's positive birth experiences also can be empowering.

Empowerment is taking an active stand that acknowledges your intrinsic worth as a human being and honors your right to choose whether to say yes or no. It is choosing to replace self-doubt and undermining behaviors with self-loving actions, protective of both you and your family. It is only by each of us actively making self-empowering choices that we will create the attitude in our culture that pregnant women know best what they and their babies need for optimal well-being.

In my life the physical acts of birthing have been an incredible means for sourcing my power.
—Diane Mariechild

Affirmations for
— Nurturing Yourself —

Affirmations are a powerful tool for personal transformation. Repeating these messages to yourself is a way throughout your day to consciously and deliberately create an inner sense of well-being: the best times are when you wake, during the course of your day, and before you sleep. By repeating affirmations you slowly but surely remake your thought processes into those that foster wellness. Affirmations are not used to suppress or deny concerns, but rather to dispel nagging anxieties that do not benefit you. They are useful for dispelling the negative messages we have all internalized—for example, that our bodies are not trustworthy, that our intuitive awareness is inferior to science and technology, that we are unworthy of joy and success, and so on. The following list of affirmations are a sampling of what you might use:

- I am a strong and capable woman.
- My body knows exactly how to nourish my baby.
- I have enough love to share.
- I give myself the right to accept love and nourishment from others.
- My baby is healthy and beautiful.
- I love my pregnant body.
- I will let my labor and birth be its own unique experience.
- I embrace the concept of healthy pain.
- I trust my ability to give birth with strength and power.

If you find yourself countering an affirmation—for example, if you tell yourself, "I am a strong and healthy woman" but a little voice pops into your mind saying "no you're not, you're weak"—try to figure out whose voice you have internalized and how that happened. Even if you can't figure it out, you may gain an interesting insight. Don't let such negative messages undermine your efforts—as you persist in the affirmations, you will replace the old, self-defeating messages. Remember, language not only expresses your thoughts, it shapes both your thoughts and our culture. Merely by shifting your attention to the positive, without denying your concerns, you can nurture health and enthusiasm.

Because pregnancy is a time of great sensitivity and a portal into a new phase in life, it offers you the opportunity to recognize and release your fullest potential as a woman. This in turn will nurture your confidence as a mother, and as an advocate for other pregnant women and other mothers. By holding the intention to be healthy and joyous, and by admitting to and resolving doubts, old beliefs, and negative internal messages, you can grow joyously through this rite of pregnancy, becoming stronger and more powerful in the process.

For further suggestions on honoring pregnancy see "Celebrating Pregnancy" in the preceding chapter. For more on the healing and transformative powers of pregnancy, and releasing emotional and psychological blockages, I recommend the following books: *Transformation Through Birth*, *Pregnant Feelings*, *Birthing Normally*, *Silent Knife*, *Open Season*, and *Pregnancy as Healing, Volumes I and II*, all listed in "Further Reading." Also see the titles on women's spirituality listed in that section.

— Spirituality —

Each of us has her own spirituality. For some this might be the religious experience they have in a synagogue, church, mosque, or sweat lodge. For some, spirituality might be experienced during a walk through a sunlit wood, through hearing waves crash against the shore, or by listening to the sound of rain. The experience of spirit often connects us to something that includes but is somehow larger than our individual selves. Pregnancy offers you an opportunity to experience a heightened sense of your spirituality, because during the precious months of pregnancy you are an individual, yet you are also more than this. It is a period of time during which your connection with something beyond yourself is more apparent than in a nonpregnant state—it is at once physical and transcendental.

The awareness that you are participating in the process of creating life may also enhance your spiritual awareness, as you may find yourself connected to the realm that your baby is in, a realm that is at once physical and at the same time mysterious and unseen. Even ultrasound testing, which makes a baby visible during pregnancy, does not explain the mystery and miracle of the pregnancy process.

You may also experience a heightened awareness of spirituality if you find yourself dreaming about angelic realms, "hearing" your baby talking to you, or experiencing an unexplainable "knowing" of who your baby is and what your baby needs, or have other insights about your pregnancy, birth, or child. I find that during my own pregnancies I also have increased experiences of precognition, for example, thinking of an old friend minutes before she phones or receiving a letter from her in the mail. This section discusses ways in which you can develop the spiritual aspects of your life during your pregnancy, and how you might use your spirituality to bring you closer to your intuitive awareness, as well as closer to your strength as a woman.

— Nourishing Your "Womanplace" —

There is eminent value in taking time regularly throughout your pregnancy to create a sacred space where and when you take time to honor yourself, other women, family, babies, pregnancy, and birth, and affirm and nourish your great strength as a woman.

Within each of us resides what writer and midwife Nancy Cohen has referred to in *Open Season* as our "womanplace." This term refers to the part of us that innately knows how to be pregnant, nourish our babies, birth, and live our lives in a creative, empowered, and intuitive way. It is impossible to deny even by a scientific standard that we are capable of what can be termed intuition, or extrasensory perception (see sidebar). Pregnant women, as do all women, have access to this womanplace for information. But first, each of us must identify and then nourish this place. You may identify your womanplace as residing in a distinct area of your body depending upon the ways that you express yourself creatively—for example, an artist may identify with her hands, a gardener with her feet planted firmly on the ground, another woman with her heart or womb. To make your womanplace come alive for you, you must nourish and call forth this part of yourself.

You can make this place real within you by actively awakening it through ritual and creative expression. Ritual is simply a time set aside regularly for active attention to your womanplace and for creative expression. How do you like to be nourished with beauty and what kindles your soul? I enjoy putting on music that makes me dance, and after working up a sweat I like to feel that

A particular mother had developed a sacred time of connection with her baby and very late in her pregnancy (over a week past her due date) had the distinct feeling that her baby was going to be born in the caul, that is, with its water bag still intact around the baby. I told her that some cultures consider this an auspicious sign, and that it is certainly possible, though very rare. That night she began labor, and a few hours later she gave birth to her daughter—in the caul as she'd predicted!

—A. J. R.

creative place strong and alive within. I also like to sing and drum in a dark room with lit candles, or in my garden. I enjoy drawing. Do whatever nourishes your sense of strength and brings you closer to your true self, where you feel a sense of spirit beyond your mundane self and where you feel strongly attuned to your body. It could be a walk in the woods, planting flowers in a garden, making love, or having a water fight with your kids. Visualize your womanplace, even draw what it should look like. Set up a special place in your home, perhaps on the top of a bureau or night table, to remind you of your womanplace. Place objects there that reflect the strength of women, the power and beauty of nature, of pregnant women, and mothers. This will serve as a visual reminder of your strength and connectedness with other women and the forces of nature. Nourish that place of creativity and aliveness often and it will be alive for you when you birth and when your kids are little and you need to find your inner resources of energy and patience. By doing so, you also give your children the great gift of energy, as they see your vitality and are supported by you in developing their own place within.

Support of the Women's
— Spirituality Movement —

The women's spirituality movement can also help you to move closer to your womanplace. Through the writings of such women as Merlin Stone, Marija Gimbutas, Riane Eisler, Vicki Noble, Anne Kent Rush, Starhawk, Jeannine Parvati Baker, Elizabeth Davis, and many others, and through our own spiritual practices and social commitments, we re-awaken to the divinity and strength of women. Ancient traditions reveal that long before written history, female deities were recognized and revered as much as "God the Father" is now. To reclaim the self-respect we deserve for our varied roles and talents both as nurturers and women of social power is incredibly revitalizing. Similarly, awareness of women's great contributions to political and environmental change also gives us a sense of collective strength, pride, and power. We come to realize that spirituality, politics, and women's status are all intimately connected to the environment we create for pregnancy, birth, and motherhood, and that, in reclaiming our strength and wisdom, we can make this world a healthier place in which to live, birth, and raise children.

Your Changing Family

THE WOMAN'S POINT OF VIEW by Aviva Romm

Whether this is your first baby or your sixth, each pregnancy and baby brings changes to the family structure as you and your mate adjust to your changing needs and the needs of other family members. Older children may be delighted or they may groan, the youngest has to adjust to the idea of a sibling, and your family budget has to stretch just a little bit more. Approached with a healthy awareness of the stresses involved, the changes of pregnancy need not be overwhelming. Pregnancy can be a joyous time of celebration, anticipation, and integration of this new being into your life.

YOUR RELATIONSHIP WITH YOUR MATE

Regardless of how long a couple has been together, pregnancy and a baby change your roles, expectations, and needs. Women who have careers and who now choose to be home and women who have never had a job may begin to feel dependent upon their mates and lose their sense of competence and value, both so important in the transition to motherhood. These feelings may cause a woman to act more childlike or cling to her partner, or conversely, to withdraw. For men pregnancy will hopefully bring a sense of increased responsibility, but along with this may come the shadow of feeling burdened, overwhelmed, or scared. This may cause him to withdraw from his partner, seeing her as the object or cause of these feelings.

In school we are not taught "Communication Skills 101," or "Relationship Skills for Sophomores" (literally, "wise fools"), and we therefore all too often go bumbling through our relationships. Of course, not all marriages work out and it isn't always healthy for women and men to put up with intolerable or abusive situations for the sake of commitment. But many marriages began as loving relationships, and it is often merely a lack of relationship skills along with mundane pressures that cause marriages to fall apart.

— Common Sources of Tension —

Because pregnancy causes each parent to feel new concerns and pressures, as well as causing them to re-evaluate their needs and expectations for support, this can be a time of stress. In addition, parents may begin to discuss and disagree about how to raise the child—for example, parenting styles, religion, how and where to birth, and whom to choose as a care provider, and so on.

A common source of tension for pregnant couples is how the pregnant woman's physical and emotional needs should be met. For example, when a woman feels consumed by nausea in the first trimester she may feel too ill to keep up with the responsibilities she typically attends to, and may want her mate to help out more. He may respond with irritation, even accusing her of exaggerating her illness in order to shirk her responsibilities. She may then become angry at him in addition to blaming herself for feeling so horrible. Such tension can cause the relationship to suffer throughout the pregnancy.

As a pregnant woman's body grows and changes, she may feel insecure about her appearance and may look to her husband for reassurance. While it is important for a woman to like her own body regardless of another's opinion, her mate's attraction to her or rejection will influence her sense of self. If a woman perceives that her mate is rejecting her pregnant body, or if he actually is, this can be a very painful situation. It seems to me very sad that any man wouldn't find his pregnant mate beautiful; however, this issue often arises for couples. The man may be confused by finding himself attracted to a mother—a new way of seeing his sexual partner. Usually a frank discussion facilitated by a counselor or a midwife will clear the air and resolve misconceptions.

Sexual needs are also a common source of stress. A pregnant woman may not feel like having sex during the first couple of months, if she is extremely nauseated or fatigued, or very late in the pregnancy. If suddenly she isn't interested in intimacy, he may take this as rejection. Other pregnant women may feel like having sex more often than ever. If he is not a person who wants to make love frequently, she may take this as rejection. If either partner is afraid to hurt the baby or feels embarrassed making love "with the baby there," this can create sexual tension. A useful guidebook to love-making

during pregnancy is *Making Love During Pregnancy* by Elizabeth Bing and Libby Colman. For ideas on creative relationships as well as intimacy see *The Couple's Comfort Book* by Jennifer Louden.

— Healing Tensions —

If you are both committed to being together, there are skills you can learn that will enable you to integrate your differences and transcend the difficulties in order to create a vital, dynamic, committed loving relationship. The book mentioned above by Jennifer Louden has many creative ideas for improving communication, rejuvenating a relationship, and enhancing intimacy both sexually and in general. Another book that my husband and I have enjoyed over the years is *The Shared Heart* by Joyce and Barry Vissell. This book takes a look at the spiritual dimensions of a relationship, offering many exercises for nourishing a committed relationship.

The foundation of any marriage has to be two strong individuals who agree to be together because they love each other and enjoy each other's company. Each of you must work on your own ability to be loving, compassionate, strong, caring, and sensitive. Then you can give love because you want to, without your entire sense of self resting upon your partner's response. However, a healthy marriage must be mutually satisfying; if the responses you receive do not nurture you, this will not be a mutually happy situation.

A couple must be able to communicate their needs and expectations openly and truthfully. Both partners must feel free to express themselves and must be able to listen to the other with the heart. It is not fair to have expectations that are not expressed, then resent the other for not meeting these expectations. You cannot expect someone to read your mind, a common mistake that pregnant women make when they want their mates to anticipate their needs. It is fair, however, to expect your partner to see your needs as important, since you are carrying this child for both of you. How one expresses needs can also have an impact on whether they are heard. "Love, would you please rub my back" sounds vastly different than "Why don't you ever offer me a back-rub? You know I'm tired!" While an empathetic partner might respond lovingly to either message, the first is certainly more likely to elicit the desired response. Again, expressing messages clearly and from your loving heart is essential, especially if you want to be heard by a loving heart. The section later in this chapter, "A Man's Point of View," provides further insights on the importance of the father's (or mate's) role in the relationship during pregnancy, and should be read by both of you.

WHEN YOU ALREADY HAVE CHILDREN

Pregnancy the first time around is quite a different experience than when you have other children to care for. Most first-time moms do not have the same amount of household work and demands that a mother who already has children may face. If you already have children, particularly if they are young, you are apt to be more tired than when you were having your first baby. Yet so many women seem to forget this simple truth and berate themselves for falling asleep at eight o'clock when their four-year-old goes to bed, letting housework slide a bit more than usual, or eating peanut butter and jelly for lunch instead of a high-protein meal with a fresh green salad.

I am writing this section to simply remind you of the importance of taking good care of yourself. It is important to learn to ask for help and to be easy on yourself. Do let your toddler watch an afternoon movie so that you can take a nap. Let your husband help you prepare meals, and enlist older kids in getting household chores done. While

P.B. and J. sandwiches are okay once in a while, by all means don't skimp on your meals. Fatigue can be reduced by eating well and getting plenty of rest, but if you try to be a supermom you'll probably be exhausted no matter what you do, and your pregnancy and birth may be more difficult for you. Learn to set limits without feeling guilty, and trust that you are a good mom and deserve time to nourish yourself and the baby.

Involving Siblings
— in the Pregnancy —

I can barely describe the magic and wonder on a child's face when she or he sees a newborn sibling for the first time. As a midwife this is one of my favorite moments. Yet not all siblings react with keen interest when they meet a new brother or sister. Much resistance can be prevented and even melted

The baby moves around so much each day. It feels wonderful to have this reminder that we are welcoming this new little one into our family.

—A. J. R.

away, by integrating and welcoming children into the life of the baby before it is born.

As a baby's life begins at conception, the best time to tell older children that you are pregnant is soon after you find out. Should you miscarry, you can explain this to your children gently in a nonthreatening and age-appropriate way. By making your children insiders in the process and sharing the pregnancy as a family experience you will give them months to integrate the idea of a new family member. Nor will your children be confused by your mood changes or your changing body. You will not only be allowing your children to feel secure in the knowledge that they are important, respected members of the family, worthy of knowing such important news, but you will be providing essential education in the pregnancy process. Children who have a realistic perspective on pregnancy and parenting may be more thoughtful in preparing for their own families, and may choose to do so in a more responsible fashion than those who have never been involved in a pregnancy or the care of a young child.

When children are involved in the pregnancy from the beginning they tend to marvel with you at the changes in your belly, the kicks and rolls of the baby in your womb, and the sound of your baby's heartbeat. Children will usually, if not either pushed with the idea or protected from it, develop a healthy anticipation and eagerness to meet this little being inside you.

A lengthy discussion about having siblings present at the birth is beyond the scope of this book, but if you plan to have your child attend the birth, there is no finer preparation than being included in the prenatal care, becoming familiar with your birth attendants, and being exposed to your naked pregnant body. If you view pregnancy as a normal fact of life, so too will your children, and if you extend this view to the birth, your child will do the same.

It is empowering to young children to feel that they are capable people and important members of your household. You can ask your toddler to help you prepare a meal for you both and let him or her know that this feeds the baby as well. You can ask your older child to watch a toddler for an hour while you rest or stretch, or you can invite your children to stretch along with you. You can teach them with books and videos about how the baby lives in your belly. You can ask your midwife or physician to help the children feel the baby's head, feet, or bottom when she palpates your belly at prenatal visits. Of course, if your child is shy about this, she or he should not be forced to participate. If you have been open with your older children all along, they are likely to want to be involved, and most toddlers love to be in on the action.

When children attend prenatal visits with their parents I always invite them to feel and listen to the baby. I've even done a mock prenatal on little ones who insist that they are also pregnant. I've had little ones hug me when I've left their homes after a sibling has been born, and thank me without being prompted for helping their mommy with the birth. This always moves me to tears. And as I watch the closeness of these children with their younger siblings, I am reminded of the value of welcoming siblings into the process of pregnancy.

THE MAN'S POINT OF VIEW by Tracy Romm

A woman's experience of pregnancy can be enhanced by the participation of a loving support person, whether it be her mate or another close friend. This section was written by my partner and the father of our four children, Tracy Romm. This section offers ideas on how to support your pregnant partner, how to meet your own needs, and how to honor your changing role as you become a father.

While it takes both a man and a woman to conceive a child, that is the point when any biological necessity for male participation in this sacred act ends. The fact is that women can grow and birth a child independently of the father. Sadly, an increasing number of women in our modern societies are compelled to do exactly that.

Just because men do not bear or birth babies themselves, however, does not mean that we don't have a vital role to play in childbearing. When we help to conceive a child, when we become a father, we assume a host of life-long responsibilities to both mother and child. Although many men define this role primarily in material terms—being the breadwinner—it is clear that other men are searching for more.

Pregnancy and birth present men with a powerful opportunity to cultivate our nurturing qualities and to bond in deep and lasting ways with our mates and children. The benefits of fathers' active participation in childbearing for optimal maternal, child, and overall family health has been amply documented in the research litera-ture. Nowadays, childbirth educators routinely expect fathers to attend classes, and some childbirth systems assign to fathers a key role at birth. In sum, all signs point to a shift in the way men perceive their place in the childbearing cycle.

Yet how ill-prepared so many of us are. I remember all too well the dominant images of fathers in my formative years. One of the Desi Arnaz and Lucille Ball shows depicted an almost hysterical Desi trying desperately to cater to the every need of an almost equally hysterical Lucy—to the point of an all-hours search for the proverbial pickles and ice cream. Yet where did it get him? At the birth he became the stereotypical figure of the pacing father in a cramped waiting room, pockets full of cigars, grasping for any word from any white-clothed figure with authority.

There are reasons to wonder whether our current Hollywood models are any better prepared to show us the way. A recent movie, *Nine Months*, featured a successful psychologist who took almost the full term of his mate's pregnancy to willingly make a commitment to mother and child. In the end it required the video image of an ultrasound to win him over, convincing him that the fetus was a child worth loving and working for. In the end, however, he was reduced to a bumbling idiot as he rushed his wife to the hospital, culminating in an adrenaline-induced brawl with another expectant father in the delivery room at the very moment his wife gave birth. At least we men have made it to the birthing chamber!

This section acknowledges the unique and important role for fathers in pregnancy. When all is said and done, we are usually the single most significant other in the life of our mates. As they grow this baby, they look to us for many types of support—emotional and spiritual no less than material. Pregnancy is a dance, admittedly a new one for many of us, and it often takes a while to learn the steps. Take heart. To paraphrase an African proverb, if you can walk you can dance, if you can talk you can sing.

— Becoming a Father —

You become a father when you conceive a child. There should be no debate about this assertion. Whatever the conflicting medical and spiritual positions about when life begins, it is certain that at the moment of conception a man enters into a deeper and more intimate relationship with a woman. She now carries within herself a part of his biological essence merged with hers—and the whole is greater than the sum of its parts. The relationship now has a tangible nature that cannot be simply wished away or erased. (How many men who have experienced the loss of a child through abortion, for example, can really forget that event, even if they supported or encouraged the abortion in the first place?) This realization can be exhilarating or terrifying. For most of us it is both.

When Aviva and I confirmed the conception of our first child, I was truly exhilarated. I felt as if I were walking on air—literally. All of the pressing concerns of my life seemed to melt away in the rosy glow of those first days. Perhaps I was more fortunate than many because I knew that I wanted this child. For a man who feels ambivalence about assuming the responsibility of fatherhood or even about his commitment to the mother, it must be much more difficult. One point to keep in mind is that doubts are common and most men experience them.

Am I ready to be a father? Will this child interfere with my life? Can I afford this (another) child? Do I really want to be in a life-long relationship with this woman? Will the child be healthy? It is okay to let yourself ask these questions and others. In fact, it is probably healthier in the long run to begin to face your shadows at the outset rather than to deny them. Many men report that becoming a father unleashed emotions and thoughts that were not usually part of their waking consciousness. You might find yourself, for example, reflecting more deeply on your own childhood, and specifically on your father's place in your early years. Remember that pregnancy is a process that lasts nine months and that you have time to grow. At the same time don't get lost in your doubts; don't forget to enjoy the moment, for the glow can grow faint at times.

Pregnancy produces some of the most profound changes to a woman's body and psyche that I can imagine. These changes are often so gradual that at any one moment they are imperceptible. The result is that it is often easy to forget what is really going on. We get so caught up in the stresses of day-to-day living that we forget we are in the midst of this extraordinary experience that is like nothing we have ever faced before. There are no simple road maps; no one person, not even this book, can fully prepare you for what lies ahead. If you expect the familiar, particularly if you are a first-time father, forget it.

Supporting Your
— Pregnant Partner —

Pregnancy requires surrender. Unfortunately this word has negative connotations for most men in our culture. Surrender implies giving up to a stronger person or position; it implies defeat. This is decidedly not what I am trying to convey here.

To say that pregnancy requires surrender is to acknowledge and even honor the fact that the childbearing woman must—by biological necessity—accept that many aspects of her life are no longer under her control. It is a 24/7 task: twenty-four hours a day and seven days a week she is growing this baby inside of her belly. Everything about her life may be in a state of flux, of change. The predictable is fleeting, whether we are speaking of sleeping patterns, eating habits, emotions, clothing styles and sizes. Anyone who has experienced pregnancy with his partner remembers the restaurant where she ordered a delectable meal, only to turn it away after the first bite. Or the new urgency on finding access to a public bathroom and in packing snacks for excursions out of the home, particularly in late pregnancy. In my many years of marriage to a practicing midwife, I have noticed that the women who do not surrender to these pregnancy changes, these new needs and desires, frequently have the most difficult transitions into birth and motherhood.

What does this mean for the new father? A number of years ago I came across a slim volume entitled *Your Baby Is Your First Guru.* Translated literally, *guru* means "spiritual guide." The kernel of wisdom I gathered from this book is that learning to cheerfully accept the needs of your mate and baby and to make them a priority in your life develops your inner strength and your ability to face the ups and downs of life generally. We all know that life is not a straight line; we do not start and end, traveling along a predictable path as in a board game. There will be crossroads of decision and detours, as well as peaks and valleys. We will never have total control over all of the challenges life presents to us. We do have some measure of control over the attitude with which we face them. What better place to start than with our own mate and child!

At the same time, to surrender does not mean that fathers have to mimic the pregnancy experience itself. Although many men report sympathetic changes in their own biology during pregnancy—such as morning sickness, insomnia, weight gain—the ideal model of partnership during pregnancy focuses on supporting the childbearing mother. Rather than mimicking her symptoms, we would be wiser to envision ourselves as the willow tree. Willows are renowned for their flexibility when the winds are gusting, yet they are rarely uprooted. Our task is to bend to our mate's needs, yet not to lose our sense of rootedness. Our mates will be looking to us throughout pregnancy, as well as during birth, for steadiness and reassurance. How can we provide these to her if we are so caught up in our own changes?

The downside is the danger that *you* may begin to feel unsupported. If mother and baby become the center of your universe, who will fill *your* needs? In the process aren't you becoming hen-pecked, tied to your wife's apron strings, less of a man? Please know that the surfacing of resentments is a very common experience for expectant fathers. It would be surprising otherwise in a culture where male programming calls for men to be in control and to wear the pants in the family. Even those of you who are not

The path of the mother should be given its deserved value as a sacred and powerful spiritual path.
—Tsultrim Allione

bound by these stereotypes may feel resentful at times of the incredible amount of effort that pregnancy demands of your mate and thus of you. Being pregnant together, in the fullest sense of the word *together*, does not mean that you and your mate have to do everything alike and at exactly the same time. As you nurture your partner, do not forget to nurture yourself. While pregnancy

is not a time to go out to sow your oats in a last-chance fling at freedom, it is okay to continue to cultivate your interests and to meet your needs.

The key is to align yourself with your mate and baby in total love and understanding. Assume your full responsibilities as their protector. I know this notion may strike many as sex-role stereotyping, but my experience is otherwise. Becoming a father activates our protective instincts; most women want us to be protective at this time if for no other reason than they are incredibly preoccupied by the internal demands of pregnancy, including being fiercely protective of the child growing within them. But being protective does not mean that we have to dwell in the land of fight or flight. Perhaps advocate imparts a truer sense of our role than protector.

As an advocate you are acting in the service of your pregnant mate to ensure that her best interests are always the priority. This requires your willingness to listen and to respond to her expressed needs. Even though male programming may tell you that

you know better, you must maintain an open mind, affirm your mate's best intentions, and be fully prepared to yield to her requests. And, if necessary, you must offer your mate a gentle reminder when pregnancy calls on her to grow or change in ways she may resist or does not see. The fruits of this attentiveness and caring are a healthier mother and pregnancy, as well as improved communication and a deeper trust that will continue to nurture your relationship through the demands of raising a family together.

Becoming a Part
— of the Pregnancy —

Serving as an advocate allows fathers to assume an active and full involvement in the pregnancy process. This course of action requires the total involvement of both heart and mind. To act as an advocate, however, we must be knowledgeable about what we advocate. In other words, we must educate ourselves about pregnancy. Be truthful (with yourself), how many of you have read this book carefully? I know that I knew very little about pregnancy and childbirth before the birth of our first child, despite having attended two home births previously and being married to a midwife. My life was busy; pregnancy was her field. Yet there is no way that I could advocate on behalf of Aviva and our babies if I didn't educate myself about the needs of pregnant women and the prenatal experiences of babies. When your partner puts those books in front of you, don't say "later." Turn off the television, quiet the music, put down your book. With all of the excellent material available today, which our forefathers didn't have access to, we have no excuse. If we remain uninformed, we are choosing to remain ignorant; what we are conveying is nothing less than disinterest.

THE NATURAL PREGNANCY BOOK

As you attune your mind to pregnancy, you can act from the heart with mindfulness. During pregnancy, loving your mate is the best way of loving your baby. In this dance, actions clearly speak louder than words, and it is often the simple, everyday actions that speak the loudest. Support your mate in caring for herself and the baby, for example, by bringing her a glass of fresh juice or water before she asks for it. Keep an eye on the refrigerator and ensure that it is well stocked with a variety of healthful foods. Exercise is something you can do together, whether it's a brisk walk or a session of yoga. Remember that pregnancy requires extra sleep. If your mate is at home full-time, she might need to be reminded that it is okay to let the housework wait—she's not being lazy. Be resourceful: there are countless ways that you can show her that you recognize and appreciate all of her hard work growing your baby.

For those of you who already have children, the challenges can be far greater. I never realized how much easier the first pregnancy was until we experienced subsequent ones. With our first child Aviva could eat and rest when her body signaled; in later pregnancies she had to juggle the competing demands of children and the in utero baby. Fathers often have to be even more energetic in supporting these pregnant moms. There were times when I felt that coming home from work was like going to a second job. Fathers really need to be proactive with later pregnancies. Taking care of the children while your mate rests, preparing evening meals, pitching in with the housework—each of these acts serves not only to give her a break but to remind her that you care.

Be involved with your mate's prenatal care. This means more than just attending the regularly scheduled prenatal visits. Educate yourself about the various complications of pregnancy, and be ready to question a health care provider about any tests that are recommended. Pregnancy can activate many fears for a woman, especially about the well-being of her baby, and a father has a responsibility to deflect unwarranted pressures on his mate to submit to any procedures. The best health care providers welcome questions from fathers who are sincerely trying to become part of the pregnancy.

It is critically important that you continue to nurture your relationship with your mate. While this sounds easy, often you may get so busy with added responsibilities around the house that you forget to connect directly with her. You may even begin to feel imposed upon if, despite your contributions, she still wants to spend more time with you. Intimacy shared during pregnancy creates a reservoir of trust that can be drawn upon when you need it most—for example, during birth or after.

Massage is probably one of the easiest and most effective ways to connect two people, and its value in a healthy pregnancy cannot be overstated. You do not have to be a massage therapist to give a massage. More than anything else, what is required is sensitivity to your partner. Ask her what feels good, work lightly, and let her signal if she wants you to work harder on an area; give her the choice of using a massage oil or not. If you keep the lines of communication open and allow your heart to guide your hands, you will not go wrong. There is nothing that a pregnant mom enjoys more than to feel you loving your baby as you rub her belly. Gently stroke your child, even speak with him or her. What the child feels or hears perinatally is a question of current scientific research. My sense in the matter is clear: with each child I felt a certain familiarity and bonding from the first moments after the birth. If nothing else, rubbing Aviva's belly on a regular basis gave me the confidence that our child felt truly loved and wanted by both of us, and that I knew how to hold and touch him or her in nurturing ways.

By no means is this section exhaustive of the ways fathers can become a part of pregnancy. Needs and life circumstances vary. Through each of our four children I feel that I have grown to be a more supportive and loving partner in pregnancy. But I have made mistakes, stemming primarily from an inability to listen and to yield to Aviva. I share this observation with you both as an encouragement and a reminder. It is possible to grow into the kind of man you envision and value, despite the lack of role models in our culture. In the process you may inspire others and thereby contribute to the evolution of new models of manhood. Just remember that your opportunities to experience pregnancy are limited: most of us have only a handful of chances to be this close to the miracle of life. Cherish the occasion.

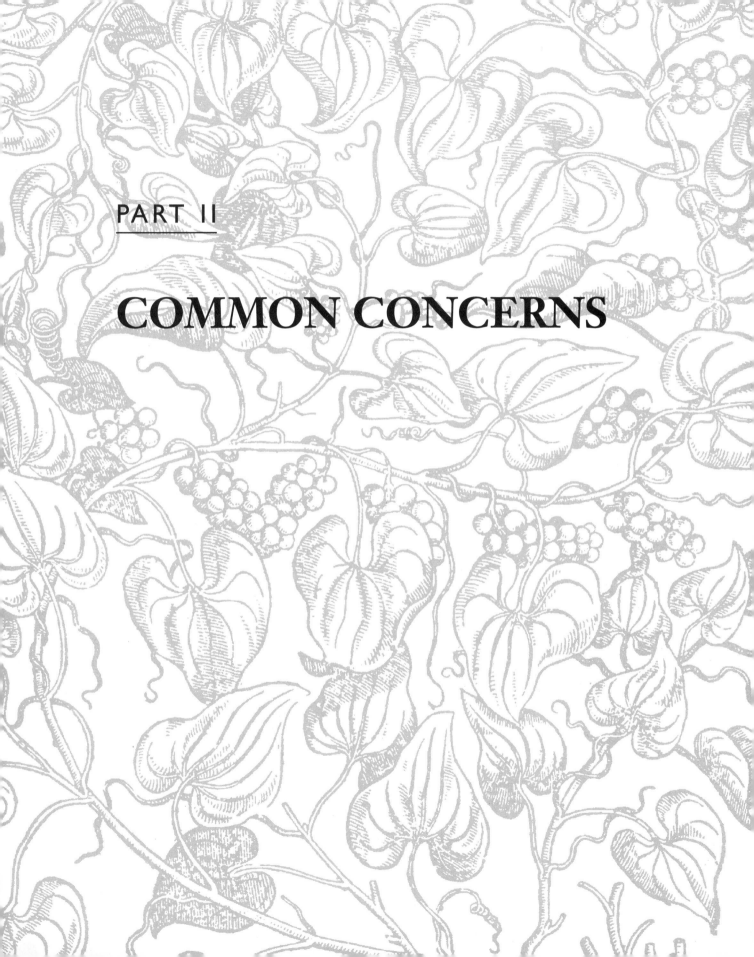

PART II

COMMON CONCERNS

CHAPTER 14

Common Concerns During Pregnancy

Pregnancy is a normal process that our bodies are quite capable of accomplishing. It is also a process that transforms our bodies and our lives, and sometimes these changes can be difficult for a pregnant woman to integrate. For instance, some of the physiological changes of pregnancy can lead to discomfort. Your growing uterus may cause your stomach to be displaced upward. This change, along with decreased gastric motility can lead to heartburn. Or a woman who works on her feet all day may get severe backaches. By means of some suggestions and natural remedies, many such discomforts common to pregnancy can be prevented, alleviated, or at least minimized. It is also true that by paying early attention to some common complaints, such as vomiting or a bladder infection, a woman can prevent these conditions from worsening into more severe problems, such as clinical dehydration or kidney infection.

As a midwife and herbalist, I emphasize natural healing techniques. These are what I have experience using, and I've made every effort to present remedies that have been widely used with efficacy and safety. No deleterious effects are known to occur when the techniques described in this chapter are used as directed. When there may be a risk associated with a health concern, I have noted it and indicated the standard medical protocol currently in use. The descriptions of natural healing techniques in this chapter are also accompanied by any potential side effects. Always remember that any therapy—natural or otherwise—should be used carefully. Of course, every woman is unique, so please always give utmost attention to how you feel when trying anything new, and do consult your health care assistant if you suspect a problem or need help in determining which treatment you should try. Refer to the safety of herbs during pregnancy in Chapter 6 for further information.

May these suggestions assist you in enjoying a healthy and comfortable pregnancy.

ANEMIA

Anemia is a reduction in the number of red blood cells in the bloodstream. Because red blood cells carry oxygen throughout the body, this reduction decreases the efficiency of the body's processes and causes a number of symptoms, including dizziness, shortness of breath, general weakness, paleness (of the skin, fingernail beds, and mucous membranes), loss of appetite, heart palpitations, and gastrointestinal disturbances including constipation and abdominal pain. Frequent colds or infections may also be a sign that you are anemic. Anemia is not a disease; it is a symptom of an insufficient number of red blood cells. The cause of anemia is in most cases a nutritional deficiency. Sometimes anemia is caused by sickle cell disease or a chronic infection. Anemia may also occur as a result of blood loss or hemorrhage, such as with ongoing bleeding gums, which also may be nutritionally related.

Three types of nutritional anemias are most likely to occur during pregnancy: iron-deficiency anemia; folic acid deficiency, known as "megaloblastic anemia"; and pernicious anemia, which is a deficiency of vitamin B12. In most cases, a healthy diet with appropriate supplementation will prevent and rectify nutritional deficiencies. Left untreated, anemia can lead to a variety of discomforts and medical problems for both mother and baby. The childbearing cycle is an excellent time for laying the foundation for a lifespan of nutritional health. Refer to Chapter 5 for further nutritional information. If your condition doesn't respond to dietary improvements, seek medical evaluation.

—Folic Acid Anemia—

Folic acid is one of the B vitamins. It is found primarily in leafy green vegetables as well as in wheat germ, molasses, nutritional yeast, whole grains, root vegetables, beans, milk, and liver. Animal liver contains high concentrations of environmental and systemic toxins, so I do not suggest it for pregnant women. In the case of severe deficiency, I sometimes do suggest it but only if the liver comes from an organically raised animal.

Spirulina, according to midwife and author Anne Frye, is exceptionally high in folic acid as well as other nutrients, including easily assimilable protein.

To obtain the maximum amount of folic acid from vegetables, eat them raw, steamed, or lightly sautéed. When they are boiled, folic acid is leached out in the cooking water and most of it ends up discarded. All pregnant women should be certain to eat at least two large portions of leafy green vegetables daily as well as an ample amount of foods that also contain folic acid.

Symptoms of folic acid deficiency include the mask of pregnancy and other skin pigment changes, appetite loss, vomiting, persistent vaginal infections, and, because other B-complex vitamins may also be deficient, a host of nervous system complaints. Babies are more likely to be born with neural tube defects (such as spina bifida) when mothers are deficient in folic acid.

Herbs that contain folic acid include amaranth, watercress, parsley, chicory, nettle, dandelion leaves, and lamb's quarter greens. Most of these can be eaten as vegetables or steeped to make tea, though parsley should only be used in limited quantities as a vegetable, not as a tea, during pregnancy.

—Vitamin B12 Deficiency—

This deficiency is not common because vitamin B12 is manufactured by bacteria in our intestines. We need only minute amounts daily, and that is usually available in most diets. It is stored in the liver and becomes available as needed by our bodies. Several factors can lead to inadequate intake or absorption of this nutrient:

- A vegetarian diet that contains no dairy products may cause problems. It may take up to five years to use up stores of B12 in the liver, and that long for a deficiency to appear.

- Stored B12 may not cross the placenta (or breast milk) and therefore the baby may be deficient.

- Stomach acids that aid in the breakdown, absorption, and stimulation of B12 production may be insufficient.

- The content of vitamin B12 may be depleted in foods produced by poor agricultural practices and nutrient depletion in soils, particularly of the mineral cobalt, an essential component of vitamin B12. Nutrient loss in soils affects the levels of B12 in both animal and vegetable foods.

Symptoms of vitamin B12 deficiency include weakness and gastrointestinal disturbances such as loss of appetite and diarrhea; a sore tongue; slight yellowing of the skin; nervous system disturbances including soreness, weakness, or coordination problems in the fingers, arms, legs, and feet; diminished reflex response and sensory perception; difficulty in walking and speaking (stammering); and nerve deterioration. If you have these symptoms, you should seek medical diagnosis. Treatment of an existing B12 deficiency includes an injection of vitamin B12 twice in one year. It is considered safe, has no side effects, and is very effective. Left untreated, B12 deficiency can result in permanent mental impairment and paralysis.

You can usually get enough vitamin B12 by eating a wide variety of high-quality foods (particularly organically grown foods where there tends to be attention to soil quality) including ample amounts of whole grains and vegetables, fruits, nuts, seeds, and the regular consumption of some dairy products, preferably yogurt and hard cheeses, on a daily basis. Small amounts of meat on an occasional basis can ensure that you are also getting a concentrated source of the nutrient. Fermented foods such as miso and tempeh may contain small amounts of B12 and may also improve the intestinal production of this vitamin, which grows much like yeast and penicillin. Nutritional yeast can serve as a B12 supplement. Pregnant women need more B12 than nonpregnant women (see Chapter 5). Adequate amounts may serve to prevent infection as well as aid in nervous irritability, memory impairment, depression, and insomnia.

—Iron-Deficiency Anemia—

This deficiency is common in women because we lose blood every month, and also don't always take optimal care of ourselves. Women may begin their pregnancies deficient in iron. Iron is essential during pregnancy for the adequate transport of oxygen through both mother and baby. The baby will store enough iron in its liver during the last couple of months of gestation to last for up to six months after birth. This is nature's way of assuring that the baby has enough iron reserves because breast milk is low in iron. If the mother is anemic, the baby may have insufficient iron stores and may also become anemic. Iron-deficient mothers may also have more difficulty with bleeding during birth than those who are well nourished.

A simple blood test, done by just having your finger pricked by your midwife or

Bonnie had fatigue, skin pallor, and shortness of breath. A blood test confirmed mild anemia. She began to increase her dietary iron, and added herbal iron supplementation to her diet. Within a month her symptoms were relieved and her blood tests normal. Her overall quality of life also improved dramatically as she began to have more energy and feel better.

physician and a quick analysis done, can reveal your hematocrit, telling you whether you are anemic. If you are iron deficient you may experience symptoms including pallor of the skin, fingernail beds, and the lining of the eyelids; weakness; fatigue and irritability; nausea, and appetite loss (particularly when prolonged past the first trimester); constipation; shortness of breath; heart palpitations; pica (cravings for nonfood items such as cornstarch, clay, dirt, and ice); and an uncomfortable, irritable feeling in your legs at night. Hemoglobin is the oxygen carrying portion of the red blood cell. As the amount of blood plasma increases in mid-pregnancy, the concentration of hemoglobin decreases, causing the hemoglobin count to drop slightly, though the actual amount of hemoglobin in the blood has not changed. This is a desirable effect referred to as hemodilution. If the hemoglobin is below 11 in mid-pregnancy, herbal and nutritional approaches can be used to improve the levels. A low hemoglobin count (below 12 mg) in early or late pregnancy is considered indicative of anemia.

During the second trimester, at about twenty weeks, a pregnant woman's blood volume should expand to about 50 percent more than it was before. Most midwives feel that a hemoglobin count of 12 is ideal at the end of pregnancy. In fact, a high hemoglobin (over 13.5 mg) might actually be a sign of a contracted blood volume, in which case you may need to increase your protein, fluid, and salt intake. If this is the case, discuss the situation with your midwife or other care provider, and refer to books by midwife Anne Frye (see "Further Reading") for a complete discussion of this subject.

You don't need to reduce your diet to numbers and milligrams to avoid iron-deficiency anemia. Eating a well-balanced diet based on whole foods provides an excellent nutritional foundation. To ensure that you are obtaining adequate supplies of iron, eat iron-rich foods on a daily basis and choose from the selection of herbs that provide the extra boost you need. You can also use the following suggestions for the prevention and treatment of iron-deficiency anemia prior to conception and throughout pregnancy. You can also use them during the time after birth, especially if you've had any significant bleeding. If you are already anemic, you can expect to see noticeable improvement after two to three weeks of diligent work to build your blood.

DIETARY RECOMMENDATIONS

- Iron supplements are hard for the body to assimilate and should not take the place of nutrient-rich foods. Therefore, it is important to include daily portions of iron-rich foods in your diet. These include dark green leafy vegetables, sunflower and pumpkin seeds, organic unsulphured dried fruits (raisins, prunes, black mission figs, apricots, and cherries), blackstrap molasses, beets, red beans, dark turkey meat, eggs, and organ meats (provided they are from organic sources). Also, many of the plants listed under "Herbal Recommendations" can be used as vegetables.

- Seaweeds, most notably kelp (kombu) and dulse, are very rich sources of iron. They can be eaten as vegetables (refer to macrobiotic cookbooks, available at natural foods stores, for recipes); in powdered or flaked form they can be sprinkled on foods; or, if you can't tolerate the taste, they can be taken in capsules. Take 1 to 2 tablespoons of flakes or powder, or approximately 8 "00" capsules daily.

- Eat foods high in iron with vitamin C (250 to 500 mg of C with each meal but do not exceed 2,000 mg per day).

Vitamin C assists in the absorption of iron. Of course, all nutrients work in concert, so be certain that your overall diet is well balanced.

- Dairy products may inhibit iron absorption, so have iron-rich meals and dairy-rich meals at different times. Don't take your iron supplements with dairy products.

- Caffeine and phosphates in soda interfere with iron absorption (and inhibit appetite, preventing adequate nutritional intake), so decrease your consumption or omit pop from your diet.

- Cooking in cast-iron pots increases the iron content of foods, so use them whenever possible

- Regular exercise increases the body's demand for oxygen. This causes a response in the body that allows iron to be absorbed more easily, as iron occurs in the red blood cells as part of the oxygen carrying capacity.

- If you do choose to take an iron supplement, use a chelated iron. (*Chelated* means that the mineral is chemically bound to another substance that the body can more easily absorb than the mineral itself and thus acts as a vehicle for the absorption of the mineral.) Ferrous gluconate, ferrous fumerate, and ferrous lactate are considered the most easily absorbable forms of iron.

- Iron supplements may be most easily digested when taken with a meal, particularly with dinner if you are prone to nausea earlier in the day.

NOTE: *Commercial and prescription iron supplements may do more harm than good, particularly if they are causing constipation or other digestive upsets. In fact, I have often recommended that pregnant women discontinue iron pills because assimilating them is too taxing on the body. Herbal and dietary approaches to increasing your blood levels of iron are usually more effective.*

HERBAL RECOMMENDATIONS

- An excellent iron tonic for pregnant women is the humble herb, nettle. Not only is this plant rich in iron and other minerals, it also strengthens the blood vessels, the kidneys, and the adrenal glands. You can be take it daily throughout pregnancy to increase your blood count. My own preference is for a very dark green and strong-tasting brew, made by steeping a large handful of the dried herb in 1 quart of boiling water for a couple of hours. If you prefer a milder brew, steep 3 to 4 tablespoons of the herb per quart of boiling water for thirty minutes. Drink between 1 and 4 cups daily depending on your needs.

- Iron Tonic Syrup—This version of yellow dock and dandelion syrup increases iron supplies and encourages iron to be liberated from the liver. It also eases the constipation associated with both anemia and commercial iron supplements. Place 1/2 ounce each of yellow dock and dandelion roots into a quart jar and fill with boiling water. Cover the jar and steep for four to eight hours. Strain the liquid into a small stainless steel or glass pot, and simmer uncovered until the liquid is reduced to 1 cup. Add 1/2 cup of blackstrap molasses (also high in iron), stir well, and turn off the heat. Pour into a jar, cool to room temperature, label the jar, and store it in the refrigerator. It will keep for many months. Dosage is 1 to 2 tablespoons daily. Take each dose with 250 mg of vitamin C for enhanced iron absorption.

- Yellow dock and dandelion root tinctures can be taken twice a day on those occasions when you are unable to carry your syrup with you—for example, if you are traveling. Take 30 drops of each twice daily. However, this is not a long-term substitute for the syrup because the alcohol extract does not contain substantial amounts of iron. The alcohol extract does assist your body in better assimilating the iron that is available and liberates iron stored in your liver, making it more available in your general circulation.

- Liquid chlorophyll, usually derived from alfalfa, is another herbal source of iron. Take 1 tablespoon daily (not more unless so directed on the product label) as a supplement.

- Floradix Iron and Herbs is a supplement made from iron and extracts of dried fruits and herbs. It is delicious, easy to take, and can be purchased at most natural foods stores. Many women have good results when using it along with the dietary recommendations and perhaps another of the herbal recommendations included here.

- Chinese herbal formulas, such as dong quai and peony formula, can be beneficial for women with a history of anemia. Seek the assistance of a person trained in Chinese diagnosis and herbal prescription, and refer to "Resources" for suppliers of Chinese herbal formulas.

ANXIETY

(see Insomnia and Anxiety)

BACKACHES AND SCIATICA

Pregnant women get backaches for many reasons: the weight of the baby and uterine contents placing stress on the lower back muscles, constipation, poor posture, standing for long periods of time, urinary tract infections, and the stress of overwork. Sciatica, a severe back pain that radiates into the legs, can occur from the growing baby and womb placing pressure on the sciatic nerve (located in the space between the hip bone and sacrum). In many cases, backaches and sciatica can be alleviated with the sensible use of exercise, nutrition, and herbs.

Pregnancy adds to the workload of your kidneys, which must filter both your wastes and your baby's wastes and maintain your expanding blood volume. The enlargement of your uterus can add physical pressure on the urinary tract, leading to infection, which in turn can cause backache. If you are experiencing chronic backache, refer to "Urinary Tract Infections."

GENERAL RECOMMENDATIONS

- Good posture can prevent sciatic nerve discomfort and backache. Many pregnant women have a tendency to sway their bellies forward to handle the weight of the baby. This posture, known as "lordosis," allows the lower back to sway forward, straining and eventually weakening the muscles in the lower back, leading to discomfort as well as strain on the abdominal muscles. Likewise, many women will slouch their shoulders forward, which leads to neck, shoulder, and upper-back discomfort.

- To improve your posture, and therefore greatly improve how you feel (your digestion will improve and you will find it easier to breathe and eat), stand up very straight and tall—but not stiffly. Tuck your tailbone under so that your pelvis does not tilt forward and your back doesn't sway. Wear flat, comfortable shoes, and sit up straight in chairs and when you drive. Over time, good posture will become second nature to you because you will have strengthened your muscles. (See Chapter 7: "Exercise and Posture.")

- Take a walk every day and do exercises like leg lifts and lunges. Exercise is a great way to reduce both emotional and muscular tension and can greatly improve back problems. Swimming is a great way to become weightless for a short time and get low-impact exercise. Yoga is useful for many problems. A few excellent yoga and exercise books for pregnant women are *Prenatal Yoga and Natural Birth* by my friend and teacher Jeannine Parvati Baker, *Positive Pregnancy Through Yoga* by Sylvia Klein Olkin, and *Essential Exercises for the Childbearing Year* by Elizabeth Noble.

- Passionate love-making is great for relieving pelvic congestion, and if you rock your hips, you will also reduce lower back discomforts.

- Eliminating constipation is a must, because constipation can lead directly to lower backaches and pelvic discomfort. See "Constipation" in this section.

- Be certain that you are getting enough minerals from your diet. Insufficient calcium and magnesium, for example, can lead to muscle aches and a lowered threshold of discomfort. See Chapter 5 for information on nutrition.

- Elevate your legs periodically, preferably for twenty minutes a day, to improve circulation in your legs. You can put your feet up on a chair or lie down and put them up on two pillows.

DIETARY RECOMMENDATIONS

- If you are experiencing lower backache, try these suggestions. Keep cold foods and raw foods to a minimum in your diet, since they place increased strain on your kidneys. If you've been eating a lot of salads, you might try more steamed greens and other vegetables. Fruits such as grapes, pears, and apples are the least watery of the commonly available fruits and place the least strain on the kidneys. Minimize your use of fruit juices, and eliminate caffeinated items—coffee, chocolate, cocoa, cola—from your diet. While they may give you a burst of energy, they do so in part because the chemicals they contain act

like adrenaline. Overstimulation by adrenaline will aggravate kidney and adrenal problems, and over time cause a weakening of these organs.

HERBAL RECOMMENDATIONS

- Even if you do not have a urinary tract infection, paying extra attention to the health of your kidneys is wise, particularly if you hurt in your lower back or beneath your ribs. If you are tired, overworked, or stressed you could be experiencing adrenal gland weakness. Two excellent herbs for nourishing the kidneys are nettle and dandelion. They are highly nutritive and are safe for pregnant women to drink on a regular basis. Both help regulate blood sugar, and nettle supports the adrenals. Steep 1/2 ounce of the dried herb (1 ounce if fresh) in 1 quart water for up to two hours; strain and drink. To make this tea more pleasant tasting, add 1 teaspoon of fennel or anise seeds and a few pieces of dried orange peel or a tablespoon of spearmint leaves. Drink up to 2 cups daily.

- Many herbs can reduce aches and pains. My two favorite herbs to be taken internally for deep backache and sciatica are skullcap and St. John's wort. Together these herbs form a dynamic duo that can be taken as a tincture, 10 drops of each twice a day over the course of a few weeks, and, if necessary, a similar dose during acute discomfort. These tinctures can be added to a cup of hot chamomile or lemon balm tea for added relaxation and pain reduction qualities.

- Black haw or cramp bark can be taken, 25 drops of either, up to 4 times a day, to relieve backache.

- Apply a combination of arnica and St. John's wort oils externally to relieve tension, promote healing of muscles, and reduce nerve tenderness, preferably having someone massage them into the affected areas. Put a warm water bottle over the treated area, and take time to consciously visualize yourself becoming loose and free of tension. You can do this daily. St. John's wort is said to contain substances that are able to penetrate to the endings of nerve fibers and promote their healing.

• Here are two recipes for external use that you can easily make at home with wonderful results.

Muscle Ache Oil

To 2 cups of olive oil add 1 teaspoon of each of the following: camphor oil, peppermint oil, clove oil, rosemary oil, eucalyptus oil, and lavender oil. Shake vigorously and apply as needed. These oils stimulate circulation in the area to which they are applied, relieving circulatory congestion, promoting warmth, and inducing gentle muscle relaxation.

NOTE: *These herbs burn mucous membranes, so keep them away from sensitive areas such as your eyes. Essential oils are highly toxic if ingested, so store bottles out of the reach of children.*

Flower Oil

This is a fragrant oil that can be used for rubbing your belly as well as other areas where you are experiencing discomfort.

Fill a quart jar with 1/4 ounce each of elder flowers, chamomile flowers, calendula flowers, rose petals, and lavender flowers. Add almond oil to fill the jar. Leave the mixture in the sun for three days; then strain and rebottle the oil. Add 1 tablespoon of vitamin E oil to the jar as a skin nutrient and a preservative.

• Dit Dat Jiao, a liniment used to treat martial arts injuries, is excellent for sciatic nerve discomfort. The recipe for this preparation appears on page 173.

• Take a hot bath to which you have added Epsom salts or any of a number of essential oils or herbal infusions. Some possibilities: wintergreen, lavender, or rosemary oil; chamomile, lavender, or lemon balm; or a combination of these.

BLEEDING AND CRAMPING IN EARLY PREGNANCY

Little is more disheartening than vaginal bleeding. Yet many women experience some bleeding during the first trimester, ranging from mild to heavy spotting, and do not miscarry. Bleeding can occur after sexual activity or merely from a vaginal examination. Other causes include implantation of the fertilized egg in the uterine wall, bleeding caused by fluctuating hormonal levels and occurring when you would normally have your period (some women will experience this for the first month or so of pregnancy and very rarely throughout the entire pregnancy), polyps on the cervix (if necessary, a physician can remove them), polyps, and a condition known as a "friable cervix," in which the tissue of the cervix is easily split (this can usually be improved with a high-quality diet). The amount of bleeding you are experiencing can help you to determine the type of care you should seek. If you are spotting or bleeding mildly, especially if the blood is brown, you can call your health care provider and elicit her opinion. Frequently you will be told to wait and watch for further signs of miscarriage (discussed below).

WARNING: If you are hemorrhaging (bleeding heavily and steadily—for example, soaking a large menstrual pad in a half hour or more), if you have been bleeding for a prolonged period of time, or if the blood is bright red (meaning that it is fresh blood), seek the immediate support of your midwife or physician, or go right to the hospital emergency room.

If you feel your uterus cramping it does not mean you will miscarry. There are other causes of the cramping, including stretching of the round ligaments (supporting the uterus), gas, constipation, and insufficient intake of calcium and magnesium. Cramping occurs in many pregnancies, and even when accompanied by spotting, does not necessarily mean that miscarriage is occurring.

Another lesser-known cause of bleeding and cramping during pregnancy is a urinary tract infection (UTI). I have seen several pregnant women bleed profusely and have regular uterine contractions caused by a UTI. Your lower abdomen or low back may ache, your urine may burn, and you may experience flulike symptoms or malaise (depression and lack of motivation). You can have your midwife or physician check your urine (or check it yourself with urinalysis sticks) for the presence of leukocytes (white blood cells) or nitrites (a byproduct of bacterial breakdown). The appearance of these together is a positive sign for a UTI and is a noninvasive method for testing. See "Urinary Tract Infections," later in this chapter, for treatment suggestions.

Perhaps the most dangerous cause of cramping in early pregnancy, sometimes accompanied by vaginal bleeding, is an ectopic pregnancy, which will be discussed later in this chapter.

GENERAL RECOMMENDATIONS

- Try to calmly assess the situation and seek help if necessary.
- Take a warm bath and relax in bed afterward.

- Contact your health care support person and ask for her recommendations.
- Avoid intercourse and heavy lifting or strenuous activity for several days after bleeding has ceased.
- Light massage may help relieve muscular cramping and spasms.
- If you are troubled by gas and constipation, you should address these complaints.
- If you determine that cramping is due to round ligament pain, gentle stretching can be effective. Touching your toes, lying on your back with your legs pulled up to your chest, or alternating toe touches while sitting with your legs stretched in front of you can all be effective.

DIETARY RECOMMENDATIONS

- Be certain that you are getting enough minerals in your diet, especially calcium and magnesium, which are essential for the healthy functioning of muscular tissue and for preventing spasms. A dietary supplement may be in order if you are experiencing chronic problems, but your first recourse should always be to improve your diet and use beneficial herbs. Helpful foods include green leafy vegetables, almonds, sesame seeds, deep-sea fish (salmon is excellent), sea vegetables (kelp, dulse, hijiki), beans, whole grains, and small amounts of yogurt and hard cheeses. Refer to the section on nutrition for further information.
- Excessive intake of dairy, particularly milk, may actually interfere with optimal calcium absorption and therefore should be avoided. Likewise, chocolate and other caffeinated products (cola, coffee) inhibit absorption of calcium.
- For a cervix that tends to bleed or be lacerated easily or a weakness of the placental bed, add 1,000 mg of vitamin C to your daily diet. Vitamin C plays an integral role in the health and strength of the blood vessels. To improve dietary

Lisa had a history of miscarriages, and very much wanted to have this baby. Nonetheless, she began spotting and contracting 10 weeks into her pregnancy. She began regular consumption of an infusion to prevent miscarriage and by 24 hours later, the symptoms had abated. One week later, she again began to spot and have mild contractions. She resumed the infusion, and confirmed that the baby was still alive by having the baby's heartbeat listened to by a midwife who had a doppler (can detect heartbeat this early in the pregnancy). She continued the infusion for another week, had no further problems, and gave birth to a healthy baby a few days after her due date.

intake of C, eat dark green leafy vegetables, raw cabbage, cantaloupe, strawberries, grapefruits, and oranges. Many of the foods you already enjoy may be rich in vitamin C; refer to the chapter on nutrition earlier in this book for an extensive list.

- Vitamin E (alpha tocopherol) has been said to strengthen the placental attachment to the uterus, reducing spotting. It should be taken in doses of up to 800 IU each day for up to three weeks. Prolonged use may result in the placenta becoming abnormally attached to the uterine wall, a complication in itself. Therefore, do not exceed this dosage, and do not prolong your intake past this time. If you have heart disease, do not exceed 50 IU per day without discussing it with your physician.

- Excessive cramping and bleeding can be caused by overconsumption of foods and beverages that are cold in nature because they cause constriction of blood vessels and poor blood circulation. Examples of cold foods are those coming directly from the refrigerator or freezer as well as those produced in climates that are hotter than the one in which you live. For example, bananas and citrus would be considered extremely cooling for one who lives in New York, even more so in autumn or winter. It is also important to eat foods and drink beverages at room temperature or slightly warmed.

HERBAL RECOMMENDATIONS

- Black haw and cramp bark are excellent antispasmodics that may be used safely during the first trimester. You may make an infusion of either herb, very effective though not pleasant tasting; for taste and convenience take the tincture. To prepare an infusion, simmer 4 tablespoons of the herb in a quart of water for twenty minutes, or steep in a quart of boiling water for one hour (in both

cases, cover the vessel while you prepare the remedy). Sip by the quarter cup as needed, up to every fifteen minutes. Take 10 to 20 drops of either tincture, up to every hour in the lower dosage, every two hours in the higher dosage.

- Chamomile tea makes a wonderful antispasmodic for general cramping, and it is high in minerals. Drink up to a quart a day.

- Red raspberry leaf and nettle are both notably high in calcium and magnesium, making them useful for reducing cramping caused by mineral imbalances, and they also act as mild hemostatics, checking bleeding. Take in infusion, up to 2 quarts a day.

- Carminative herbs may be used to reduce chills as well as gas and bowel problems. Cardamom, cinnamon, anise, and fennel are all examples of carminative herbs. Cinnamon is also used as an antihemorrhagic.

- Other general antispasmodics include lemon balm, passion flower, motherwort (do not use if there is bleeding), and lime blossom. These can be taken alone or added to other teas.

- Here is an example of a formula for cramping that includes many of the herbs just mentioned. You can also use it as a basis to create your own formula of favorite herbs.

Formula for Cramping

1 ounce each of black haw, red raspberry
    leaf, and nettle
1/2 ounce each of chamomile blossoms
    and lemon balm
1/4 ounce each of organic orange peel,
    cardamom pods, and cinnamon
    sticks

Mix all the herbs together; then, using only one handful of this mix, steep in a teapot or jar with 4 to 6 cups of boiling water for

---

twenty minutes (longer than this will yield a bitter tea). Strain, sweeten to taste, and drink up to 4 cups daily.

BLEEDING, LATE-PREGNANCY

With the exception of spotting in early pregnancy and blood-tinged discharge preceding or during labor, **if you begin to bleed, call your midwife or physician immediately. If bleeding is profuse, head to the nearest emergency room!**

Sometimes a woman may see some streaks of blood in her vaginal mucous (on toilet tissue or underwear) after intercourse. This is no cause for alarm. It occurs if the cervix was slightly jarred.

CAUTION: *Heavy or steady bleeding during the first four months of pregnancy usually signals a threatened miscarriage. Call your health care provider. See "Miscarriage."*

Bleeding later in pregnancy may be related to a placental problem, such as a placenta previa, a condition in which the placenta partially or completely covers the cervix, or a placental abruption, in which the placenta separates, to varying degrees, from the uterine wall. These two situations require immediate medical attention. A blood loss that causes you to soak a medium-size sanitary pad within thirty minutes is termed a hemorrhage. All bleeding that occurs during pregnancy should be traced to the cause. Calm your mind, assess the situation, and be certain you and the baby are not endangered.

Always remember that even in an emergency room you can find caring and supportive people and that you can maintain your sense of power and authority over your body. Always bring a support person to act as an advocate for yourself when you seek medical care.

BREASTS, SORE

As early as the first few weeks of pregnancy, you may notice that your breasts are tender, sore, or tingly, and that your nipples are unusually sensitive. This is due to the usual breast enlargement that occurs as a result of hormonal changes accompanying pregnancy. It may remind you of those years in junior high school when your growing breasts were highly tender and sensitive. The hormones of pregnancy also help ready the breasts for breastfeeding. While the acute sensitivity usually subsides after a short time, your breasts, because of their increased size, may feel heavy and tender throughout pregnancy.

GENERAL RECOMMENDATIONS

- When you are reclining, go braless to avoid friction.

- When you are out and about, particularly as you get farther along in your pregnancy, wear a bra that offers you support and helps prevent your breasts from feeling heavy.

- Hot soaks in the tub, with the water at a level over your breasts, can help to relieve discomfort and heaviness.

- See "Preparation for Breastfeeding" in Chapter 11 for more information on breast care during pregnancy.

HERBAL RECOMMENDATIONS

- For tenderness in early pregnancy, massage a soothing oil, such as chamomile, St. John's wort, arnica, or lavender oil, on your breasts.

Visualization is a wonderful tool for gently affecting physical change. Mary had been trying various techniques to change her baby to a head down position, but to no avail. Her baby was consistently in a position where the shoulder was presenting. We decided to try a visualization—beginning with deep muscular relaxation, I then guided her through imagining her baby's head in her pelvis. We also told the baby that this head down position would allow it to be born safely. By the end of the visualization the baby's head had moved downward, and it stayed that way until her baby was born, vaginally at home.

BREECH BIRTHS

Your body knows how to birth, even if the baby is in a bottom-first position. Actually, breech births are not uncommon. Many babies are in breech position until well into the pregnancy, even as late as the eighth month. For example, I recently worked with a woman whose baby didn't turn head down until thirty-eight weeks of pregnancy, just two weeks before birth.

If everything seems normal, but your baby insists on remaining bottom-first, then be as determined as your baby is in your desire for a vaginal birth. Many obstetricians support vaginal births of breech babies, so seek a supportive care provider. Some midwives will assist in breech births at home if the mother has had babies before, if the baby seems healthy and is not too big for the mother's pelvis. Sometimes an ultrasound will be recommended to make sure the umbilical cord is not wrapped around the baby in a way that will interfere with birth. Occasionally a breech is caused by congenital anomalies that prevent the baby from fitting head down in the pelvis or by a deformity or variation of the pelvis or uterus that also prevents a head-down position. A discussion of breech birth is beyond the scope of this book but can be found in other childbirth literature. An excellent video on breech births is available from Ina May Gaskin at The Farm; see the listing for *The Birth Gazette* in "Resources."

Suggestions for — Turning a Breech Baby —

At about thirty-two to thirty-four weeks you can begin taking gentle measures to encourage your baby to turn:

• Spend time each day imagining your baby head down. Put pictures around your home of head-down babies in their mothers' bellies. Tell the baby that it's safe to turn and that it would help you relax if he or she would do so. Look closely at your own fears of birth and motherhood as well as any stresses in your life that might cause tight pelvic or abdominal muscles.

• Pelvic tilts are simple to do and quite an effective method to encourage a baby to turn. Rest a slant board (any sturdy board of sufficient width to support you) at a 45-degree angle, put one end on the floor and the other on the edge of a chair or sofa. Lie on the board with your head near the floor and your feet near the top of the board. Ten minutes in this position twice a day is the recommended length of time. If you practice yoga and can handle them, headstands are also effective. If you are a swimmer, you can do headstands in the water. Of course, you should not attempt headstands unless you are already adept at them.

• Take the homeopathic remedy called Pulsatilla, 30x, purported to encourage babies to turn head down, three times a day for three days. I have no definitive proof that a baby will change position with the use of this remedy, but it is totally harmless and therefore worth a try.

• Moxibustion, a traditional Chinese treatment, is highly regarded for its ability to cause a breech baby to turn. It involves holding a lighted "cigar" made of the herb mugwort above the skin near various points along the energy channels of the body related to the various organ systems. These points are the same as those used in acupuncture and acupressure. The heat stimulates energy in the point which is at the outer end of your little toe on the right or left foot. The Chinese doctor from whom I learned this technique witnessed its effectiveness when his sister's baby was breech. I've since employed it and have found it useful as part of an overall approach but have done no studies on its effectiveness as a solitary treatment. It is simple to do and can be done at home with the following instructions.

You will need to purchase a couple of moxa sticks, available inexpensively from Cascade Health Care Products (see "Resources"). Perform the entire treatment in a well-ventilated room unless you purchase the "little smoke" moxa sticks. Unwrap and remove the outer paper, leaving the inner white paper in place. Next, light the end of the stick with a match or candle and blow on the lit end until it glows like a coal. Hold the lit end about 1/2 to 2 inches away from the outside edge of the little toe, near the toenail. It does not matter whether you begin on the left or right foot. Maintain the heat on the point for twenty minutes; then do the same spot on the other foot. If at any time you feel a burning sensation, simply pull the moxa a bit farther away from the spot. Repeat this procedure twice each day until the baby turns.

- The external turning of the baby to a head-down position is frequently an effective method, but it is not without risks and should therefore only be done by a skilled midwife or physician who can carefully monitor the baby's heartbeat while he or she is being turned. Sometimes an ultrasound will be done before the procedure to be sure the baby will not become tangled in the umbilical cord in the turning process. If he or she is already wrapped in the cord, the procedure will not be attempted to avoid harming the baby.

Remember, if the baby does not turn despite all your efforts, if neither you or the baby seem to have a physical problem causing the breech or inhibiting birth, in all likelihood you will be able to birth your baby vaginally.

COLDS, FLU, AND MILD ILLNESSES

Colds and flu generally pose no threat to the mom or baby as long as the mother remains well nourished with foods and fluids. During a severe illness—for example, with high fever (over 103 degrees Fahrenheit), prolonged fever (longer than two or three days), or symptoms such as frequent and violent vomiting, diarrhea, and persistent coughing—it is wise to consult an experienced midwife or a physician. Herbs that you have used for treating colds when you were not pregnant may not be safe now, so refer to "Herbs to Avoid During Pregnancy" in Chapter 6 before you begin any treatment. Never take any herbs if you are not certain they are safe during pregnancy.

Many women find that they have an increased resistance to illness and infection during pregnancy. Getting adequate rest, eating highly nutritious and natural foods, getting moderate exercise, and maintaining a generally adventuresome, positive outlook on life may go a long way to keep our resistance to illness strong. Yet this may be easier said than done if you are already busy with children, a career, or the many stresses that plague human beings in our fast-paced society. Anxieties about money, relationships, and time constraints can open the door to illness. Treatment of colds and other simple illnesses (such as an intestinal virus, for example) must therefore always include reflection on what is going on in your life that may have left you susceptible and what this illness can show you about your lifestyle that might serve you in the long run. This is not an invitation to blame yourself or anyone else; rather, it is an opportunity to be introspective and aware of your needs. Perhaps you can find practical ways to reduce stress in your life and create the space to care for yourself, your health, and your growing baby.

GENERAL AND DIETARY RECOMMENDATIONS

• As soon as you feel the first signs of illness—fatigue, chills, loose bowels, or constipation—try to excuse yourself from your daily responsibilities and *get some rest*. This is the perfect time to turn off your telephone, ask for help with your kids, take a sick day (what I refer to as a "health day"—a day off to prevent yourself from getting really sick), and nurture yourself. Do what is comforting: take a warm bath with a few drops of relaxing oils such as lavender or rose and a few drops of antiseptic oils such as rosemary, thyme, or eucalyptus. The latter help clear respiratory congestion. Then put yourself to bed with a cup of hot herbal tea (see page 145) and perhaps a book you've been wanting to read (if it is relaxing), soothing music, or just a soft pillow and a cozy blanket and let yourself sleep. Fatigue is a prime reason for illness to occur, so let yourself rest as long as you feel you need to without feeling guilty.

• Often when we are ill we lose our appetite. Indeed, this is the body's way of resting the digestive system and sending healing energy to other areas in your body. However, you still need to grow your baby. So if you don't feel much like eating, try broths, soups, and simple buttered toast. A well-made vegetable soup, miso soup, or chicken soup can be as medicinal as any herbal remedy and is worth preparing. Add some rice or pasta and you will have a nourishing, yet light food to sustain you until your appetite returns in a day or so.

• You must drink fluids, even if you must force yourself to do so. Your baby needs amniotic fluid, and your kidneys will be taxed if you don't drink adequately. In fact, you can even begin to have contractions if you get dehydrated. A full glass of clear fluid, broth, or tea every two hours if you are not feverish, and more if

you are, is adequate. Keeping yourself well hydrated is essential when you are pregnant and is moreover an important component of healing from illness.

• Be certain to dress appropriately for the weather. If you are chilled, dress warmly, but don't become overheated. Wear breathable cotton clothing and cover yourself with natural-fiber blankets if at all possible. If your fever breaks in a heavy sweat and your clothes are wet and clammy, change them swiftly so you don't get chilled.

• Take about 250 mg of vitamin C every two hours, but don't exceed 2,000 mg daily during the first trimester; after that, don't exceed 4,000 mg daily. And discontinue either dosage of vitamin C after five days.

HERBAL RECOMMENDATIONS

• Echinacea root tincture is a gentle but effective remedy for either a viral or bacterial infection. Combined with vitamin C, it is probably one of the best cold and flu preventions and treatments. It encourages the body's immune system to resist illness. Begin taking it at the earliest sign of sickness. Dosage is 1 drop of tincture for every 4 pounds of body weight (that is, if you weigh 120 pounds you would take about 30 drops of tincture) every four hours for general prevention and mild colds. For more acute symptoms, you can either take the tincture every two hours or you can increase the dosage to 1 drop per 2 pounds of body weight. As you recover, slowly reduce the amount and frequency of the dosage.

• Garlic lemonade is one of my family's favorite cold and flu remedies. An excellent general bactericide, garlic is effective in treating all manner of general illnesses including colds, intestinal and stomach viruses, and strep throat. It can be taken in conjunction with echinacea and vitamin C.

Garlic Lemonade

Steep 4 to 6 cloves of chopped raw garlic in 1 quart boiling water (cover the jar while you steep) for thirty minutes. Then add the juice of 1 or 2 lemons and honey or maple syrup to taste. Drink warm, up to 1 cup every two hours. If you don't find this tea palatable, try steeping the garlic as above, but add a couple of bouillon cubes or 1 tablespoon of miso to the tea instead of lemon and honey. This is a warming tea if you have chills but can be used at any time of the year.

• Ginger tea is also an excellent cold remedy that produces a warm feeling, preventing your temperature from getting too high and reducing tension. It has properties similar to that of garlic. When made into a mild tea sweetened with honey, it has a very pleasant taste.

Ginger Tea

Steep 1 teaspoon of freshly grated raw ginger in 1 cup boiling water for fifteen minutes. Steep covered to retain the volatile oils, which are antiseptic. Sweeten and add lemon if desired. You can take a hot cup of this tea every two hours. It is also soothing for a sore throat and eases respiratory congestion.

CAUTION: *Ginger can induce miscarriage in susceptible women; therefore, do not prepare it any stronger than directed and avoid during the first trimester if you have a history of miscarriage.*

• Kudzu, an intruder into the southeastern landscape particularly here in Georgia where I live, yields a root high in starch, similar to arrowroot but more nutritious. This starch, available in small chunks and powder, makes an excellent tea that reduces fever, relaxes the muscles, eases stomach discomfort, and soothes inflamed mucous membranes in the throat and bronchial passages. Because of its high starch content, it is also nutritive. You can prepare kudzu root as a tea in a number of ways. I'll give you a couple of ideas, and you can choose what sounds appealing, even creating your own recipes as you go along.

Garlic-Onion-Ginger-Kudzu

This is really more of a soup, taught to me by an acupuncturist friend, and is one of my personal favorites when I feel a cold coming on or if I feel chilled. Sauté half an onion, 2 cloves of fresh chopped garlic, and 1/2 inch of fresh chopped ginger root in 1 tablespoon of olive or sesame oil for two to three minutes. Add 3 cups of water, cover, bring to a boil, and simmer for about twenty minutes. Then add 1 tablespoon of miso paste and stir. In a small cup, dilute 2 teaspoons of kudzu starch in 1/4 cup cold water (if you try to do this in hot water, it will form gelatinous clumps that will not dissolve). Add the starch to the broth, stirring constantly for two minutes. Turn off the heat and drink when it is warm but not hot. Use this freely throughout the day, preparing more as needed.

Kudzu Apple Juice

Bring a cup of apple juice to a boil; then add 1 teaspoon of kudzu starch diluted in 2 tablespoons of cold water. Stir constantly for two minutes; then drink. Pear juice may be substituted; a pinch of cinnamon improves digestion and warms you if you are chilled.

Molly began working with a midwife 30 weeks into her pregnancy. At the time of her first midwife visit, her skin had a yellowish-green hue, her blood pressure was 120/90, she was nauseous, had severe and incapacitating headaches, and hadn't had a bowel movement in 2 weeks. She agreed to quit her iron supplement and began to use gentler, more assimilable forms of supplementation, such as chlorophyll, spirulina, and Floradix each day, in addition to dietary improvements and prunes (for iron and as a laxative) with bran as a drink in the mornings. She added fresh fruits and vegetables to her diet, as well as fresh fish and more water. Within three weeks she was having daily bowel movements, and all of her other symptoms completely resolved. Her blood pressure stabilized at 118/70.

- Other teas that can be used effectively for reducing fever, aches, digestive discomfort, restlessness, or irritability during colds include teas made with lemon balm, catnip, chamomile, or lime (linden) blossom. You can drink these herbal teas either in a single infusion or with the herbs in combination. Sip them freely as needed.

- If you have an illness accompanied by diarrhea, you must be certain to drink enough fluid. Rehydration Drink (see page 211) is good for this. In addition to remedies already mentioned, you can drink a strong infusion of raspberry leaf tea made with 1 ounce of the dried leaves to 1 quart of water (steep for twenty minutes), taking 1/2 cup every thirty minutes to one hour depending on the severity of the diarrhea. Raspberry leaves are notably astringent, tonifying the intestinal lining and reducing bowel discharge. For extreme diarrhea or dysentery symptoms you can take 2 "00" capsules of goldenseal powder every four hours until the symptoms abate, but don't take these for more than twenty-four hours.

CAUTION: *Goldenseal, a uterine stimulant, can stimulate contractions. If you notice any contractions, discontinue goldenseal immediately. Don't use at all if you have a history of miscarriage.*

CONSTIPATION

This is a very common problem for pregnant women because (1) it is widespread in our society; (2) pregnancy hormones cause decreased bowel activity and tone; (3) the growing baby and womb place pressure on the intestines and rectum, sometimes making bowel movements more difficult; (4) iron deficiency, common during pregnancy, leads to constipation; and (5) commercial iron supplements can cause constipation because they are so hard to assimilate.

Constipation is at the root of many other pregnancy complaints, including indigestion, nausea, headaches, skin problems, and poor mineral absorption. It can be a contributing factor in toxemia and even in a difficult birthing, since an impacted rectum takes up the very room that the baby needs for descent and birth. Constipation is avoidable and, with direct attention, easily remedied.

GENERAL RECOMMENDATIONS

- Get more exercise. A brisk walk each day, especially at the same time, can be a great boost to your digestion and promote regular evacuation. Many yoga exercises are also beneficial. See "Further Reading" for recommended yoga books.

- Give yourself time each day to sit on the toilet. Relax and wait patiently, breathing deeply and possibly tightening and relaxing your anal muscle a few times to stimulate a bowel movement. The body has regular intervals for elimination, and if you don't go when you get the urge, the urge will pass and the stool will be retained. The longer it sits in there, the harder it will be to eliminate later on. Avoid straining as it will lead to hemorrhoids.

- Squatting is the physiologically natural position for bowel movements; therefore, getting up and squatting on the seat (no kidding!) can facilitate the process. If you can't handle this idea, at least put your feet up on a low stool or on the side of the bathtub while you try to go.

- Recline on your bed or, if possible, in a warm bath. Massage your abdomen deeply in a clockwise direction, starting at the "six o'clock" point and circling back around to it. Do this for ten or fifteen minutes before you return to the toilet.

- Eat an abundance of fresh vegetables, particularly the various lettuces, kale, and collard greens. Eat raw vegetables with meals and snacks. You should have at least two large portions of raw vegetables each day.

- Eat fresh fruit regularly, at least one to two pieces a day.

- Choose breads, crackers, and pasta made from whole grains. They have a higher fiber content and aid elimination.

- Cut back on cheese, meat, and highly fatty foods.

- Drink a lot of water, about a half gallon daily (herbal teas are also fine). Warm liquids at room temperature improve elimination; cold liquids hinder bowel movements.

- While caffeinated beverages seem to be the most common American drink, they are not healthy for pregnant women or babies; avoid them completely during pregnancy.

- Eating bran for a long time can *decrease* bowel tone and irritate the intestinal lining. However, bran is an excellent remedy for a bout of constipation. Soaked or stewed prunes are also useful and they can be used on a regular, long-term basis.

Constipation Remedy

A delicious way to make use of these two remedies is to soak four prunes and 1 tablespoon of bran in 1 cup of warm apple juice for thirty minutes. Eat and drink all of the juice, bran, and prunes. This can be done either once or twice daily, preferably in the morning and evening. You can substitute black mission figs, also rich in iron and excellent for promoting evacuation.

- Bran muffins are another nutritious and delicious way to use bran. You can eat them as part of a meal or as a snack.

Here is a basic recipe:

Bran Muffins

2 cups whole-wheat flour

1 1/2 cups bran

1 teaspoon baking powder (non-aluminum)

1 teaspoon baking soda

1/4 teaspoon salt

1/4 cup oil (sunflower, walnut, safflower, or canola)

1/4 cup honey

1/4 cup molasses

1 tablespoon tahini or peanut butter, or 1 egg

1 cup raisins

1/2 cup chopped walnuts

1 cup yogurt

1 cup water

Mix all ingredients very well and pour into an oiled muffin tin. Bake at 375° F for twenty minutes or until golden brown and firm.

- Oatmeal, especially when cooked with some raisins, is an excellent laxative and is also highly nutritious. Starting your day with a bowl of warm oatmeal is likely to encourage healthy bowel movements.

- Yogurt (live culture) with fruit as a snack or light meal can also help eliminate constipation and populate the intestines with flora necessary for healthy bowel functioning.

- The most effective and safest remedy for use by pregnant women is a syrup of dandelion and yellow dock roots in a base of blackstrap molasses. Ironically, this same preparation is used for treating iron-deficiency anemia. Unlike typical iron supplements, which are constipating, the natural remedy is iron-rich and also treats constipation—itself a sign of anemia. These herbs help move the energy of the bowels gently downward without stimulating the uterus.

Iron Tonic Syrup

To prepare Iron Tonic Syrup, steep 1/2 ounce each of yellow dock and dandelion roots in 1 pint boiling water for eight hours. Strain into a saucepan and simmer until the liquid is reduced to 1/2 cup. Add 1/4 cup blackstrap molasses, stirring well. Pour the mixture into a glass bottle, cool to room temperature, and store in the refrigerator. It will keep for many months. The dosage is 2 tablespoons along with 1/2 to 1 cup of warm water in the morning or early evening.

CAUTION: *Herbal laxatives like senna, buckthorn, aloes, and castor oil, etc. can cause labor to begin as they stimulate the bowels. Some may also be harmful to the baby's development, affecting the central nervous system. Therefore, avoid the use of all purgatives during pregnancy.*

CRAMPING

(see Bleeding and Cramping in Early Pregnancy)

ECTOPIC PREGNANCY

Ectopic pregnancy means a pregnancy where the baby does not lie within the uterine cavity. Most commonly it occurs in a fallopian tube but also may occur elsewhere, including in the abdomen or ovary. Ectopic pregnancies are extremely dangerous, because when they rupture they can lead to sudden, life-threatening hemorrhage and shock. Part of what makes them so dangerous is that the symptoms may be subtle until rupture occurs, and then the situation becomes an emergency. Before this, a woman may not even realize that she is pregnant, let alone that the pregnancy is ectopic.

Certain factors may increase the likelihood that an ectopic pregnancy will occur, including pelvic infections (especially PID, pelvic inflammatory disease), abortions, endometriosis, prior pelvic surgery, use of an IUD (intrauterine device), previous ectopic pregnancies, or any condition that may have caused scarring or adhesions in the pelvic organs.

Possible symptoms alerting you to an ectopic pregnancy include an unusually early, late, missed, or spotty period; abdominal pain that can be dull or intensely sharp; and irregular vaginal bleeding. When there is a rupture the pain usually becomes severe, gets progressively worse, and most often is located on only one side of the lower abdomen. Other signs may include pain on only one side that may radiate into the arm, shoulder, chest, or upper back; scanty brownish bleeding that is intermittent; and eventually signs of shock, which include dizziness, anxiety, shortness of breath, clamminess of the skin, fainting, and pallor.

WARNING: *Ectopic pregnancy is a life-threatening emergency requiring immediate medical care.*

Usually surgery will be required, and ideally it can be done before the rupture occurs. Most physicians make every effort to repair the tube or ovary, but it may need to be removed; ask whether surgery is the only option.

It is important for you to explore and allow whatever feelings arise because this a frightening medical emergency and it may mean the loss of your baby. Two helpful books that address pregnancy loss are *When Pregnancy Fails: Families Coping with Miscarriage, Ectopic Pregnancy, Stillbirth, and Infant Death*, by Susan Borg and Judith Lasker, and *Empty Arms: Coping with Miscarriage, Stillbirth, and Infant Death* by Sherokee Ilse.

EMOTIONAL SWINGS

Pregnancy is certainly a time of great change for women, both in its physical challenges and the new responsibilities it brings. It is a time when our bodies are circulating high levels of hormones and when our bodies demand a very good diet. Combine all of these factors and it is not surprising that pregnant women find themselves experiencing highs and lows with great rapidity, even in the course of minutes. Add fatigue, the possibility of an unwanted pregnancy, anxieties about the baby's health, the prospect of motherhood, worries about how to maintain a job and care for a baby, an increasing body weight and a changing body shape in a culture that values thinness, not to mention the general discomforts of pregnancy, and it is even less surprising that pregnant women feel bouts of depression and insecurity. I'm always amazed at how easily I cry over sappy sentimental songs when I'm pregnant, and at

how joyful I feel when I see buds opening in the spring and other simple miracles of life.

Pregnancy seems to be a key that unlocks doors to old experiences and feelings, particularly those regarding relationships that have had great impact on us, most notably our relationships with our mothers. For some women the availability of their mothers as a source of support and information is comforting and valuable, but for others proximity to our mothers can be a source of pain and conflict. For all women, pregnancy causes us to reflect on how we were raised and how we may want to raise our children similarly or differently. Reflecting on childhood can be confusing or painful, but it also offers new opportunities for personal growth. Finding ways to heal painful feelings can be productive, enabling us to move into motherhood with a fresh perspective. Moreover, such reflection may allow you to enjoy extended family support. I highly recommend *The Dance of Anger* by psychologist Harriet Godhor Lerner for women locked in conflict with their moms or other family members.

How your partner reacts and responds to your pregnancy can influence how you feel about yourself, particularly if you are dependent on your mate for financial (or other) support. Even if you are not financially dependent, if your partner finds your changing body unattractive, for example, you are likely to feel very hurt. If your partner seems disinterested in feeling the baby move, or if he refuses to share in your joy, you may experience rejection, sadness, or a sense of being "in it" alone.

Pregnant women are culturally expected to, and thus "allowed to," have periodic emotional outbursts, be subject to strange whims and cravings, and to be somewhat irrational, but we are also expected to be in

Audrey's baby was still breech just a week and a half before it was due. This was her third baby, but a breech birth was not ideal—she had anxieties about it. During this time she was also experiencing a lot of personal stress—her husband's business wasn't going well, she was over- whelmed by her two children, both under four years old, and had recently been told some birth horror stories by a neighbor. At a prenatal visit she opened up and shared all of these worries, and had a healthy cry. Within a day her baby changed to a head down position, and was born after a labor of a few hours. Perhaps this was coincidental—or perhaps letting go of her tensions, which were affecting her pelvic and uterine muscles, provided more room for her baby to change position.

a state of joyful anticipation about the coming baby—to have a certain pregnancy "glow." Our culture also characterizes feelings of sadness, depression, anger, and anxiety as negative and even as symptoms of emotional problems. As a result, a pregnant woman may feel obligated to keep these feelings to herself or dismiss them as "normal emotional outbursts." The problem is that we may be disregarding issues that need some attention. We should tell our mates that we feel rejected when they are disinterested in the baby, or when they do not find our growing bodies attractive. While we may still feel these heightened emotions after such a discussion, we probably will be better able to cope. In addition, when we assume that extreme emotional sensitivity is normal in pregnancy, we may overlook nutritional or other physical factors that can contribute to the unpleasantness of being on an emotional roller coaster.

GENERAL RECOMMENDATIONS

- I cannot overstate the importance of excellent nutrition from both food and herbal sources, as well as adequate rest and exercise. Read Chapters 5 through 8 thoroughly for a full discussion of these topics.

- Accepting, not dismissing your feelings is important. This means that you recognize and acknowledge what is bothering you. If you feel worried about birth, you don't have to dwell on gruesome details of rare complications or imagine yourself in some horrible scene from a television emergency room. You can say to yourself, "Okay, I am afraid about birth." Try to find a source for your fear, ask yourself where this anxiety arises from. Perhaps as a young child you knew someone who had problems or you've heard frightening birth stories. By recognizing the source of your fear,

you can separate it from your own personal experience.

- If you are afraid of a particular complication, you can ask your midwife or physician how she deals with it. Becoming more educated often will decrease your anxiety. If your issues relate to other matters, such as relationship problems with your mate, body-image anxieties, or financial worries, try to find constructive ways to address and resolve them. Midwives often help women work through a wide variety of issues, so speaking with your midwife, if you have one, can be helpful and comforting. A close friend or a counselor can also be a good listener and help you get to the bottom of your fears.

- Be true to yourself and deal with your problems to the best of your ability. If you find yourself in a situation that makes you feel bad, it is fair either to change the situation or extricate yourself from it. For example, if other women start to tell you awful stories about birth, it is perfectly reasonable to excuse yourself from the discussion or make it clear that the discussion disturbs you and you don't wish it to continue. You can't always wait for people to read your mind—sometimes you must make your needs known and stand up for yourself.

- Keeping a journal is an excellent way to give voice to your emotions. It can also provide a time of quiet reflection on a regular basis. You can create a nice ritual for yourself: drink a cup of relaxing herbal tea in your favorite cup, listen to soothing music, and write your thoughts, feelings, and impressions. This can be a welcome release from which you emerge refreshed. The act of writing can help you work out and resolve concerns. There are several books available on journal writing, some written specifically for women; inquire at your local bookstore for titles.

- Allow yourself to be human, accepting all the ups and downs we must go through. Don't give yourself the double whammy by feeling bad about feeling bad. Guilt doesn't get you anywhere in this situation. Feel what you feel, and move on—you don't have to psychoanalyze yourself or have to explain or justify your feelings. How you feel is simply how you feel.

- Try to appreciate your heightened sensitivity. Being attuned to subtle emotional nuances in your interactions with others and to your own emotions can give rise to a deep empathy that will help you understand the subtle messages and feelings that your baby will need you to interpret after birth. When babies' subtle cues are heeded, they frequently have less need to resort to crying to get their message across. Many times crying is a strong way of expressing something that wasn't picked up through more subtle communications. Daily time for reflection and journal writing enhance your consciousness.

- Creative forms of expression can provide a welcome outlet for your emotions. Painting, drawing, sculpting, dancing, or singing can transform inner tensions.

DIETARY RECOMMENDATIONS

- Depression and other difficult emotional states can result from nutritional deficiency as well as lack of exercise. Low blood sugar can cause extreme irritability, sadness, anxiety, or depression. Read the chapter on nutrition earlier in this book and be sure you are meeting all of your nutritional requirements.

- Depression can also result from dehydration. Drink plenty of fluids, herbal teas, and *fresh* fruit and vegetable juices. Insufficient fluid intake can contribute to lower blood volume and indeed a state of depression. Pay attention to your thirst, and try to drink about 6 to 8 glasses of fluid a day.

HERBAL RECOMMENDATIONS

While herbs cannot remove emotional or other problems, they may reduce stress so that you can relax and develop strategies. In addition, herbs can directly help your hormones, act as nerve tonics, and support the functioning of your organs, especially the heart and liver. Herbs will help you so that you don't become bogged down by the increased volume of blood and hormones that you must circulate each day. The following suggestions, in addition to the recommendations discussed above, may help improve your emotional outlook during pregnancy.

- To calm your nerves as well as benefit digestion, prepare the following tea:

Calming Tea

1 teaspoon chamomile flowers, 1 teaspoon lemon balm, 1/2 teaspoon lavender flowers, and 1/2 teaspoon fennel seeds steeped in 1 cup boiling water (covered) for ten to fifteen minutes. Strain and drink warm, with milk and honey if you prefer, as often as you wish throughout pregnancy for stress, indigestion, sleeplessness, and anxiety. You also can take this tea during labor to help you ease discomfort from contractions. A worthwhile additive to your medicine pantry, it is simple to prepare and delicious.

- Oatstraw is another herb that nourishes the nervous system, particularly when taken over an extended time. Add 1 teaspoon of oatstraw to the above tea or make an infusion of it alone or with other herbs of your choice.

- Motherwort can be used in small doses up to 20 drops occasionally, not to exceed a few doses a week unless directed by a midwife or herbalist during pregnancy. It is a wonderful bitter tonic for the heart, and as its name implies, is a healing herb for mothers. Its Latin name, *Leonorus cardiaca*, means "lion-hearted," implying the herb imparts strength and courage. It is particularly useful when you feel irritable, bothered, or overwhelmed. Take a tincture of this herb (it's too bitter for tea) in doses of 10 to 15 drops up to three times a day for a few days only. Also, do not exceed three doses daily.

NOTE: *Because motherwort is an emmenagogue, avoid it in early pregnancy if you have a history of miscarriage or have had any bleeding.*

- Skullcap nourishes the nerves and brings about gentle relaxation when you feel irritated or restless. It is not indicated for depression or weepiness; it is, however, an excellent nerve tonic. Dosage is 1 to 2 cups of tea daily, or 10 to 20 drops of tincture two to four times a day. The herb or the tincture can be added to other teas.

- Valerian has marked benefits for pregnant women with extreme mood swings. It is known to reduce anxiety, curb aggressiveness, and diminish irritability with no known side effects. Take it as a tea, up to 2 cups daily made by steeping 1 teaspoon of the dried root in a cup of boiling water for fifteen minutes, or use a tincture, 10 to 20 drops up to three times daily.

- Bach Rescue Remedy, now also known as Bach Calming Essence, has brought many people relief from stress and feelings of being overwhelmed. Available at local natural foods stores and herb shops, it contains Star of Bethlehem, Rock Rose, Impatiens, Cherry Plum, and Clematis. Take 4 drops of the essence, repeating every fifteen minutes for up to one hour, and repeat later on if necessary. It is good for acute stress.

- Dandelion root is an herb that I find effective for moderating mood swings. It promotes improved liver functioning, regulating hormones, and thus helps reduce intense emotional swings. When it is taken over time, its nutritive blood-building qualities, along with its slightly cooling nature, may combine to reduce irritability. In addition, dandelion root helps regulate blood sugar, preventing drastic dips that can cause mild to severe mood swings. It can be taken as a syrup, 1 to 2 tablespoons daily, in a nutritive base of blackstrap molasses; as an infusion, up to 2 cups daily; or as a tincture, 20 drops up to four times a day.

- The general comfort of a warm bath enhanced with a few drops of essential oil of rose or lavender, or a massage with diluted oils of rose, lavender, St. John's wort, and chamomile are very helpful. To promote a more restful sleep and to reduce irritability when you wake, try sleeping on an herbal pillow stuffed with chamomile or lavender blossoms, or sprinkle a few drops of these oils on your pillow or put them in a diffuser next to your bed.

EDEMA

(see Swelling)

FATIGUE

It is completely normal to need more sleep during pregnancy. Your body is working overtime. As my close friend, also a midwife, says, "It's a time of heavy construction." By the end of your first trimester you have helped your baby develop all of his or her body parts, and that is an incredible accomplishment! In addition to all this building work, your own body and psyche are undergoing great changes and adjustments.

GENERAL RECOMMENDATIONS

• Getting more sleep now that you are pregnant is important. Your emotions will be steadier, your digestion easier, and you will be less susceptible to infections, constipation, headaches, and morning sickness. Lack of sleep can lead to depression, irritability, and weepiness.

You may, in fact, find yourself taking naps or dozing off in a chair at eight o'clock in the evening. Learn to listen to your body and your need to rest. Try not to worry about all that you are "not getting done."

• Stress, a job outside of the home, or older children to look after can further increase your fatigue. Women who have had children close together and are still nursing a toddler or keeping up with the needs of a family are particularly prone to exhaustion. This fatigue sometimes will ebb and flow. To minimize this permit yourself to rest when you can, and prioritize your activities. For example, if housekeeping can wait, rest when you might otherwise be cleaning.

• Exercise, especially in the fresh air, is an excellent way to increase your oxygen intake, improve your circulation, appetite, and bowel function. Your depression will lift, insomnia and restless sleep will lessen. Even a brisk walk at least three times a week can make a tremendous difference in your well-being. A gentle toning exercise such as yoga can help wash away fatigue. Getting a massage can be relaxing and invigorating. If you can't afford a professional massage, have your mate or close friend give you one (or ask your midwife to massage you at prenatal sessions).

• When you need help be sure to ask for it.

DIETARY RECOMMENDATIONS

• If you find yourself persistently irritable and exhausted, this may be a symptom of a nutritional problem. Frequently this type of deep exhaustion is accompanied by some of the following symptoms: general weakness, pallor, shortness of breath, nausea ranging from mild to severe, dizziness, heart palpitations, lack of appetite. See "Anemia" for natural therapies that can help you obtain enough iron in your daily diet. When there is insufficient iron in your diet, your body is not getting enough oxygen.

• Be certain that you are eating regularly and getting enough protein and complex carbohydrates, nutrients that provide your body with a steady source of energy. Excessive reliance on sweet foods (including fresh fruit) without adequate intake of these other nutrients will lead to feelings of fatigue.

HERBAL RECOMMENDATIONS

• Herbs can help you improve your energy by improving your nutrition. However, stimulants—even herbal ones—should not be used during pregnancy. They can give a false sense of energy when what you really need is rest or nourishment. "Super foods," concentrated food supplements like spirulina (a blue-green algae) and kelp (a dried sea vegetable), can boost your nutrient levels, and thus your energy. Unlike stimulants, you can take these daily.

• Take spirulina in pill form, according to the recommended dosage, or up to a tablespoon of the powder daily. It can be taken in smoothies, in juice, or in capsules.

• Sprinkle kelp powder onto food; take it in capsules, up to 10 daily, steep the whole vegetable in water and drink it as a tea. Cook a 6-inch piece with beans or squash or in soup. Macrobiotic cookbooks are an excellent source of seaweed recipes.

• Refresh yourself with teas of peppermint, chamomile, nettle, oatstraw, and ginger or tinctures of yellow dock and dandelion roots (15 to 30 drops of each, or either, three to four times daily).

- Herbal baths can be invigorating, refreshing the mind and spirit and reducing fatigue and depression. Add 3 to 5 drops of an essential oil to your bath. Good choices are peppermint, eucalyptus, lemon, sandalwood, and rosemary. Splash mildly cool water on your body after the bath and settle in for a peaceful rest.

CAUTION: *Never use essential oil internally.*

FIBROIDS, UTERINE

Uterine fibroids are benign—that is, non-cancerous—growths that may occur on the uterus (subserous myomas) or in it (intra-mural or submucous myomas). Because a fibroid is an outgrowth of the myometrial, or muscular layer, of the uterus, they are actually encapsulations of your own tissue. They are known to increase in size in the presence of high levels of estrogen, as occurs during pregnancy, or when women are on birth control pills, or in women with high levels of body fat and fat intake. The fact that they are noncancerous and not dangerous is often confusing because they are frequently referred to as "fibroid tumors," and of course the word *tumor* (which simply refers to a growth) conjures up fearful images.

Fibroids occur in up to 30 percent of all females, in nearly half of all women of menopausal age, and very common in younger women, especially those who have not borne children. Small fibroids are almost always completely painless and asymptomatic; however, fibroids can grow to become quite large, as big as a grapefruit or more! A fibroid is generally described in relation to the size of a pregnant uterus (even in nonpregnant women)—for example, a woman may be said to have a fibroid the size of an eight-week pregnancy.

Large fibroids may cause bleeding, irregular menstruation, and pain; they may prevent conception or cause miscarriage; and they may cause other symptoms such as urinary frequency if the uterus becomes quite enlarged and puts pressure on the bladder. A hysterectomy is commonly recommended for women with large fibroids, but this is a very serious surgery with long-term consequences, and one of the most frequently unnecessary surgical procedures performed in the United States. It is also an option most pregnant women would not want to consider. Given the low risk of fibroids and the efficacy of dietary and herbal therapies for addressing the problem, and the tendency of fibroids to shrink as estrogen levels go down at menopause, any woman considering a hysterectomy should research the problem, seek second—if not third—opinions, try natural approaches, and determine if the problem is worse than the solution, or vice versa.

Small fibroids generally cause absolutely no difficulty during pregnancy and birth; large fibroids on rare occasion may obstruct the baby's passage out of the uterus, make it difficult to control bleeding immediately after the birth, and sometimes can interfere with the baby's nourishment, as was the case with one pregnant mother I worked with who had a fibroid rapidly growing under her placenta. I note that she successfully curtailed its growth with the following series of recommendations despite her obstetrician's belief that it would become dangerously large.

The following suggestions may be used by any woman with fibroids: all the herbs may be safely used during pregnancy.

Because fibroids grow in the presence of estrogen, the high estrogen levels of pregnancy may precipitate their growth. Therefore, in order to prevent them from growing and interfering with your pregnancy or birth, it is sensible to follow some or all of these recommendations. Give yourself at least two months before you will notice obvious changes. As estrogen levels decrease after pregnancy, the fibroids will likely decrease in size as well.

GENERAL AND DIETARY RECOMMENDATIONS

- Milk, eggs, cheese, and butter may contain significant levels of estrogen from the hormones fed to chickens and cows to increase their production of eggs and milk. This exogenous estrogen increases our own levels of estrogen that will stimulate the growth of fibroids. Therefore, try to obtain these foods from organic sources only. Reducing your use of eggs and dairy products, whether or not they are organically produced, is optimal, however, because they tend to lead to mucous congestion and excess fat in the body, both of which can cause fibroid growth.

- Eat a diet rich in whole grains, vegetables, fresh local fruits in season, and high-quality vegetable protein in the form of nuts, seeds, beans, and tofu. Eat animal products occasionally but not as staple parts of the diet. If you are regularly a heavy meat eater, gradually reduce the amount. Drastic changes are not advisable during pregnancy.

- Add sea vegetables to your diet, particularly kelp. Seaweeds are highly regarded for their ability to soften and reduce tumors and growths. In traditional Chinese medicine, foods and herbs of a mildly salty nature are said to do just this. Kelp is also an excellent nutritional supplement. Use kelp on foods or as tea or add it to soups or beans. Or steep

a 4-inch long strip of kelp in 1 cup of water for about thirty minutes, and then drink the liquid; or take 2 "00" capsules of kelp powder four times a day.

- A juice made from a combination of freshly juiced apples, carrots, and beets makes an excellent lymphatic cleanser and mineral supplement, nourishes the immune system, and reduces tumors. It has a sweet taste and a lovely pink color. I use predominantly apples and carrots, adding about half a beet to an 8-ounce glass of juice. You can adjust the proportions to your taste. Make it fresh each day, and take one 8-ounce glass daily at least five days a week.

- Activities that promote pelvic circulation are beneficial in reducing blockages and congestion in the pelvis, both physically and psychologically. Yoga, brisk walks, belly dancing, making love—whatever rocks your boat, so to speak—do it at least three times a week for optimal pelvic health. Once or twice a week you can take a cool (not cold) hip bath to increase pelvic circulation.

- Visualization, the art of deliberately imagining your desired outcome as something actually happening, can be a useful tool for letting your body know what you want to do. You can imagine your womb filled with warm light, imagine the fibroids actually shrinking, or imagine the wall of your womb as healthy and vibrant. See Chapter 8 for more suggestions on creative visualization.

HERBAL RECOMMENDATIONS

- The best way to reduce fibroids is to use a combination of strategies. Basically, you want to strengthen the functioning of your liver so your hormones are effectively moving through your body in appropriate amounts and being transformed and eliminated. In addition, consider using herbs that help promote healthy blood and facilitate bowel elimination. The following formula, taken on a regular basis, is very effective for helping your body perform all of these tasks.

Liver Strengthening Tea

Mix equal parts of burdock root, dandelion root, yellow dock root, red clover blossoms, cleavers, and nettle. Steep 1 ounce of this mixture in 1 quart of boiling water for two hours. Strain and discard the herbs. Drink 2 cups of this brew daily.

- In addition to the tea, take 20 drops of chasteberry tincture two to three times a day. The tincture can be added to the tea. Chasteberry is indicated in the case of uterine fibroids and other gynecological problems.

- Avoid licorice, as it increases estrogen levels.

FLU

(See Colds, Flu, and Mild Illnesses)

HEADACHES

Headaches can stem from a number of causes, most commonly stress, tension, low blood sugar, constipation, dehydration, inadequate protein intake, or dietary insufficiency of other minerals, particularly calcium and iron. Women prone to headaches before pregnancy may continue to have headaches during pregnancy, and women who are unable to nurture themselves adequately may develop headaches.

Severe headaches beginning suddenly after the sixth month of pregnancy can signal toxemia, so check with your midwife or physician and care for yourself accordingly (see "Toxemia" later in this chapter). Untreated, toxemia can become a life-threatening condition. Severe headaches that increase in frequency and pain or occur in women who are not prone to them can be a sign of a serious problem requiring medical assistance. The following discussion does not address headaches of pathological origin.

GENERAL RECOMMENDATIONS

- Stress causes you to contract your muscles, reducing blood flow, and causing your body to function less effectively. Sometimes fatigue can cause tension headaches, so be sure that you are sleeping enough, and whenever possible, take a nap.

- Creative visualization will be useful. Begin by choosing a comfortable spot in which you can sit or stretch out for as long as you are able, or a minimum of ten minutes. Get comfortable. Close your eyes and allow the tension to melt away, beginning at your feet and slowly working up your body until you reach your head. The different parts of your body should become progressively looser, as if you are floating on water. You can imagine hands massaging you deeply, lightly, however you prefer. Imagine yourself basking in this relaxed state. Allow your mind to travel then to an environment that comforts, relaxes, and nourishes you. Choose a favorite image—walking on the beach, floating in a luxurious bath, or sinking deeply into a featherbed. When you feel calm and relaxed, open your eyes and slowly come back.

- As you relax, specifically focus on any images that may tell you the cause of the headache or possible remedies. When we enter deep states of relaxation, we are often able to access information that is not immediately available to us in our waking consciousness. You may see images of tension or experience fears about pregnancy or birth. By becoming aware of tension and its source, we can take steps to resolve it. If you want to address pregnancy and birth fears and anxieties, refer to *Pregnant Feelings* by Baldwin and Palmarini, *Silent Knife* by Nancy Wainer Cohen, and all of the books by Gayle Peterson and Lewis Mehl listed in "Further Reading." Relaxation tapes for pregnant women are available, or make your own using the visualization suggestions in Chapter 8.

- Constipation is a common cause of headaches. Substances that your body needs to eliminate are reabsorbed. At least one bowel movement daily can relieve headaches as well as prevent other health problems. See "Constipation" later in this chapter for more information.

DIETARY RECOMMENDATIONS

- Poor nutrition with resulting hypoglycemia can cause headaches. High-protein, high-carbohydrate snacks can help.

- Dehydration can also cause headaches, so drink enough fluids throughout the day, at least a tall glass of water or a nutritious beverage every few hours. You may feel parched, depressed, or hot if you aren't drinking enough. You may notice that you have some contractions, known to occur when pregnant women become dehydrated. You can reverse all these symptoms by eating and drinking adequately throughout the day.

- Caffeinated beverages, such as coffee and cola, and chocolate can cause headaches. Try to avoid them.

- Iron deficiency may lead you to have headaches, as will protein deficiency.

- You may need to add more calcium and magnesium to your diet. Refer to Chapter 5 for dietary recommendations and consider adding a supplement containing 600 to 800 mg of calcium and 300 to 400 mg of magnesium.

HERBAL RECOMMENDATIONS

- Many nervine herbs are effective for soothing tension headaches. You will notice that some of these herbs recommended elsewhere in this book have a high calcium content. Calcium is necessary for healthy nerve functioning and promotes relaxation.

- Herbs that can be used as teas include chamomile, lemon balm, catnip, oatstraw, meadowsweet, lavender, rosemary, passion flower, and skullcap. You can take these herbs singly or in a combination of two or three. For more severe headaches, you can use herbal tinctures, 20 to 30 drops added to an herbal tea or 1/4 cup of warm water.

Relaxation Tea

A formula that I enjoy for relaxation during pregnancy contains 1 teaspoon cham-omile flowers, 1 teaspoon lemon balm, 1/2 teaspoon lavender flowers, and 1/2 teaspoon fennel seeds. Steep this mixture in 1 cup of boiling water for ten minutes (covered) and drink hot. You can add milk and honey for flavor. To add calcium, add milk or take 2 calcium lactate capsules with the tea.

- Herbs that can supplement your nutrient intake include oatstraw, nettle, red raspberry leaves, alfalfa, dandelion leaves, and slippery elm bark. Kelp can be taken in capsules as a supplement, up to two "00"-size capsules four times daily.

- The best herbs for nourishing the liver include dandelion root and leaves, yellow dock root, wild yam, chasteberry, false unicorn, and burdock root. For convenience, you can take any of these as tinctures, up to 30 drops (individually or combined) three to four times daily.

HEARTBURN

(see Indigestion and Heartburn)

HEMORRHOIDS

(see Varicose Veins and Hemorrhoids)

HERPES

This section discusses Type II, genital herpes, though the recommendations are also applicable to Type I, oral herpes.

Herpes is a viral infection that once contracted stays dormant in the nerves located at the base of the spine. This infection will flare up when triggered by stress, fatigue, and dietary deficiencies. A woman who becomes infected with herpes for the first time during pregnancy, and particularly when she is close to the time of birth, may miscarry, or the baby may develop congenital anomalies, or become very sick. It is therefore essential that you know whether your sexual partner has ever been exposed to or had herpes. People think that only promiscuous people, poor people with poor hygienic habits, or drug addicts have sexual diseases. I have met many wealthy, educated people who have had herpes, gonorrhea, crabs, and other sexually transmitted conditions. Most people are embarrassed to admit that they have herpes, but it is very common. A cesarean section is a standard procedure for women in the United States with active herpes at the end of pregnancy.

Women who had herpes before becoming pregnant are at minimal risk for passing the infection on to the baby prenatally because they have developed antibodies to the virus that protect the baby. In fact, it is becoming more common for women to give birth vaginally even with mild herpes as long as it isn't a primary infection. This is a matter of debate among obstetricians: European physicians claim that herpes is a fairly low risk for the baby compared to the higher risk of a cesarean section. But most American doctors are not yet convinced of the safety of vaginal birth with active herpes lesions. See Anne Frye's *Understanding Lab Work in the Childbearing Year* and Nancy Wainer Cohen's *Open Season* for a discussion of this issue. Obviously, this will be a decision that requires a good deal of thought and the support of your birth attendant. Because of the potential risks, you should investigate the risks and benefits of both vaginal birth and cesarean for you and your baby.

The symptoms of a herpes outbreak usually begin three to five days before the sores appear: flulike feelings, aching in the genital area, tingling or itching where the sores will erupt, emotional irritability, and sometimes painful urination or swollen lymph nodes. The lesions begin as small blisters that turn into small sores that then crust over and heal. There can be one lesion or many, and they can appear either on the external or internal parts of the genitals, including the cervix. The infection is contagious during the entire range of symptoms, so sexual activity should be discontinued at the earliest sign of any symptom until the sores are completely healed and are no longer visible. This can take up to a couple of weeks.

Herpes is quite common. I've worked with a number of women with a history of herpes, including one woman who had two previous cesareans. She went on to have her third baby at home with no lesions present. Most people have a "body barometer," a physical symptom or syndrome that pops up at times of stress. It could be an old injury site that begins to ache, a headache that develops when you have a deadline, or herpes that flares up. These are messages that you are dealing with too much internal pressure. By learning to recognize the early signs of stress we can learn to slow down. If you anticipate a stressful time coming, you can take measures that prevent an outbreak; and if you do notice prodromal (pre-herpes) symptoms, you can begin to use herbs, address the stress, and improve your diet. You can get to the point where you rarely, if ever, have another herpes outbreak.

If you are troubled by regular herpes outbreaks, it is very important to take an honest look at your beliefs about your body and your sexuality. For example, are your outbreaks an excuse (conscious or otherwise—look deeply) to avoid sexual intimacy with your mate? Are you feeling unclean, unworthy of being loved, of experiencing sexual pleasure? Learning to feel comfortable about yourself sexually can heal herpes.

GENERAL AND DIETARY RECOMMENDATIONS

Sexual partners with herpes can also follow the recommendations here.

- Stress reduction will help prevent herpes outbreaks. Make sure you are resting enough, and address any sexual issues that may be causing you anxiety. Refer to the sections on relaxation and creative visualization in Chapter 8, and incorporate some of these practices into your life on a regular basis, especially during stressful times. Take up an activity such as yoga or Tai Chi.

- Learning which foods to emphasize and which to avoid can be a step toward a life without outbreaks.

Identify the processed foods in your diet and replace them with healthful foods. Eat plenty of fresh fruits and vegetables. Refer to "Further Reading" for natural foods cookbooks.

Nadine had 2 prior cesareans for active herpes lesions at the time of birth. With this pregnancy she chose to eat well, avoiding foods that aggravate herpes and increasing those that prevent it. She chose to follow an herbal program, drinking echinacea and burdock root infusion daily for her third trimester, and she planned for a home-birth. She had no outbreaks and gave birth, at home, vaginally of course!

HIGH-ARGININE FOODS	HIGH-LYSINE FOODS
Reduce these in your diet:	Emphasize these in your diet:
nuts	*fresh fish*
seeds	*chicken*
wheat	*beef*
brown rice	*milk*
oats	*cheese, milk, and yogurt*
raisins	*beans*
chocolate, coffee, and caffeinated teas	*eggs*
coconut	*sprouts*
carob	*nutritional yeast*
eggplants	*fresh vegetables*
green peppers	
tomatoes	
mushrooms	
garbanzo beans (chickpeas)	
sugar	

Arginine and lysine are two of the many essential amino acids our bodies require as part of our overall protein intake. However, arginine is known to contribute to herpes outbreaks whereas lysine helps to prevent them. Therefore a diet higher in lysine and lower in arginine is part of a herpes prevention diet.

This list does not imply that you should completely avoid all high-arginine foods, but common sense dictates that those foods not essential for health be avoided, such as chocolate and coffee. Whole grains, for example, should be eaten in moderation with a dietary emphasis on high-lysine foods.

- Some people find that a lysine supplement of 500 mg daily prevents outbreaks. According to Anne Frye, as much as 5,000 mg of lysine during prodromal symptoms may be necessary. If you are close to your due time and sense an outbreak, this higher dosage may be a good idea.

- 1,000 mg of vitamin C daily for prevention of an outbreak, and 2,000 mg daily during an outbreak, can enhance your immunity. Vitamin C is a reputable antiviral remedy.

HERBAL RECOMMENDATIONS

For the prevention and treatment of herpes, you can take herbs that nourish, tonify, and calm the nerves (remember, this is where the virus actually resides in the body); herbs that have antiviral capacity internally and topically, that strengthen immunity, reduce moist heat in the body, and "purify the blood," as old-time herbalists would say.

- To reduce stress and tonify the nervous system, include 1 to 2 cups daily of any of these herbal teas alone or in a combination (1 to 2 tablespoons of the herb to a cup of boiling water), or use tinctures of these herbs: chamomile, lemon balm, lavender, lime (linden) blossom, oat-

straw, valerian, passion flower, skull-cap, lady's slipper, wood betony, catnip. Take tinctures in warm water, directly under the tongue, or add to one of the teas just mentioned. Average dosage is 10 to 15 drops of any of these (or that amount of a combination), two to three times a day.

- The following remedy has proven consistently effective in my practice for preventing herpes outbreaks during pregnancy. It has immune-enhancing properties as well as antiviral potential and it reduces dampness and heat in the pelvis. Place 1/2 ounce each of *Echinacea angustifolia* root and burdock root in a quart jar; fill the jar with boiling water, cap tightly, and let steep for eight hours. Strain and drink, storing the next day's portion in the refrigerator. You can carry this brew with you in a jar or insulated container. Dosage is 2 cups daily, preferably 1/2 cup four times a day. You should take this remedy throughout pregnancy if you have regular outbreaks; otherwise, begin taking it if you notice prodromal symptoms and continue until all symptoms are gone. It will reduce the frequency and duration of outbreaks. For every week you take these herbs, take a three-day break (for example, seven days on, three days off) to avoid sensitization to the herbs, and therefore decreased effectiveness. To prevent outbreaks toward the time of birth, take regularly throughout the third trimester (with the recommended breaks).

Echinacea and burdock can also be taken in tincture form: 30 drops of each taken four times daily in place of the infusion, following the same recommended course as above.

- Other herbs can be *added* to this infusion (do not substitute any herb for echinacea or burdock) or taken as tinctures, including cleavers, a well-known blood cleanser; chickweed, an anti-inflammatory herb; yellow dock root;

dandelion root; and spearmint leaves. Add 1 to 2 tablespoons of the dried herbs to the echinacea-burdock brew at the beginning of steeping.

- Astragalus tincture, 20 to 30 drops three times a day, is a specific immune-system enhancer and can also be added to your daily brew.

- You can heal herpes blisters in a number of ways: a paste of myrrh powder, made by mixing a teaspoon of myrrh with enough water to make a sticky paste and applying it to the affected areas; a tincture of calendula or calendula oil dabbed onto the affected areas with a cotton ball or swab; St. John's wort (hypericum) oil dabbed on the affected area during the prodromal phase; or a paste of green clay applied to dry up the sores.

- Take sitz baths made with a strong infusion (steep 2 ounces of dried herbs per quart of water, for four hours) of equal parts of burdock root, echinacea, calendula, comfrey root, and myrrh.

- Significant improvement of symptoms and accelerated scabbing of sores in herpes patients has been shown with the topical application of an extract of *Melissa officinalis*, lemon balm. Though the preparation was highly concentrated, you may find it beneficial to add this herb to sitz baths and to dab extracts of lemon balm onto the affected area. As it is both relaxing and potentially antiviral, you may want to add a few tablespoons of the dried herb or a handful of the fresh leaves to your burdock and echinacea infusion. To be effective, the study concluded, the treatment must be begun during the early stages of infection.

These recommendations are also applicable for oral (Type I) herpes (cold sores). Herpes is spread through skin contact; careful hygiene is essential if you have either type and are caring for a newborn. Up to six months of age babies are highly susceptible to the herpes virus, with up to a 50 percent fatality rate.

CAUTION: *If a baby shows any signs of illness when there is a family member with either a history of herpes or active herpes, seek immediate medical care for the baby.*

HIGH BLOOD PRESSURE

There are two kinds of blood pressure: essential hypertension, high blood pressure that pre-exists pregnancy, and pregnancy-induced hypertension (PIH), which usually shows up after twenty weeks' gestation. The general criteria for the diagnosis of any hypertension is a blood pressure of 140/90 or above, or any rise in systolic pressure (the top number) of 30 points or more and/or a rise in diastolic pressure (the bottom number) of 15 points or more. The rise must be seen in two readings at least six hours apart to be considered conclusive because blood pressure is variable throughout the day and can change according to your mood, environment, and interactions. Therefore, any singular incidents of high blood pressure can be disregarded if you generally have a blood pressure within a normal range.

What I look for in pregnant women is a steadily rising blood pressure over the course of two or more prenatal visits to indicate that the woman is developing what may be problematic hypertension. Of course, physicians, hospitals, and midwives may see women whose health history they do not know and must determine whether those women are at risk for problems associated with high blood pressure. For example, a woman who shows up at the hospital in labor, or a woman who chooses a midwife very late in pregnancy, can have a blood pressure of 130/80. This can be considered within the normal 140/90 range, but if her blood pressure is normally 100/60, it may be hypertension. The optimal situation, if you

Beth began experiencing elevated blood pressure—from an initial reading of 106/60 to a steady 128/74. She began a program of motherwort and hawthorn extract, as well as reducing her work load and increasing her fluid intake. Her blood pressure did not continue to rise and stabilized at an average of 124/68.

are planning to use a care provider for your pregnancy and birth, is that you do so early in the pregnancy to establish your "baseline" vital signs. Only in seeing the whole picture can deviations from your normal pattern become apparent.

Many health care providers fear high blood pressure in pregnant women because it is one symptom of pre-eclampsia (toxemia), which has other symptoms: not feeling well; slow growth of the baby; swelling of the ankles, face, and hands; visual disturbance; upper abdominal pain; headaches; kidney, heart, or thyroid problems; and the presence of protein in the urine. While pre-eclampsia is very serious and needs both thoughtful prevention and careful treatment, not all high blood pressure results in complications. Treatments such as the use of aspirin, diuretics, medications, salt restriction, along with a lack of attention to lifestyle and diet, leave any true imbalances unresolved and predispose pregnant women to other problems such as hemorrhage and kidney problems. This does not mean that medical treatments should be avoided—it does mean that you should fully explore other approaches beforehand, or that you should use them only in emergencies. Hypertension can be a symptom of kidney infection, kidney disease, and rarely, tumors, vascular disturbances, nervous-system disorders, hydatidiform moles, and liver disease, all requiring medical diagnosis and treatment (with the exception of a urinary tract infection, which can usually be treated quite successfully with natural therapies). If you are attempting to treat hypertension naturally, it is important to rule out more serious causes which require medical attention. Consult with a midwife or physician to help you determine whether it is safe for you to try a natural approach.

The greatest contributors to high blood pressure are stress, poor nutrition, and lack of exercise. Improvement in these areas will almost always reduce blood pressure if it is high. If the mother has elevated blood pressure but seems otherwise in excellent health, I simply keep tabs on her blood pressure for a few weeks or more (depending upon how far along she is in her pregnancy), and I provide clear instructions on eating well, getting more exercise, and reducing stress. I might suggest herbs that can assist in the reduction of blood pressure. I don't make a big fuss about high blood pressure unless it becomes consistently elevated and doesn't respond to any of my suggestions. In this case a home birth becomes contraindicated. I've not had this happen, perhaps by luck, or perhaps because of the body's wonderful ability to heal itself when it is given support. Of course, if the mother were to develop symptoms of toxemia or any other complications, a medical evaluation is essential.

The general risks of hypertension in pregnancy are lack of adequate oxygen flow to the baby, the potential for low birth weight and possible stillbirth, and, because of the force of the blood behind the placenta, the risk of a placental abruption, a situation in which the placenta prematurely separates from the uterine wall, a potentially dangerous situation for mother and baby. It is up to you, along with the educated assistance of your care provider, to determine when high blood pressure seems to be problematic, and to decide whether to try to reduce elevation by attempting to normalize circulation, or to use medication to control it. The following suggestions may assist you in preventing high blood pressure if you are prone to it, and for lowering blood pressure should it become elevated.

GENERAL AND DIETARY RECOMMENDATIONS

- If you are pregnant and have hypertension, you need to evaluate your diet. Keeping a diet diary is the best way to do this (see Chapter 5). After completing it, you can ask your midwife to review it for the content, quality, and quantity of the foods you are eating. If you are working with a physician or other practitioner who is not well versed in the nutritional needs of pregnant women from the standpoint of dietary intake, be sure to read the nutritional information in this book or books in "Further Reading." Highly processed, refined foods with their plethora of chemical additives tax the liver, kidneys, and bowels, placing unnecessary burdens on the whole circulatory system, possibly contributing to hypertension. Preparing homemade foods and salting them to taste and inviting more natural foods into your diet, especially whole grains, high-quality protein from beans, moderate consumption of hard cheeses and yogurt, nuts, seeds, and fish, can help prevent and reduce hypertension.

- High salt intake has long been associated with the development of high blood pressure in both pregnant women and the general population. In addition, pregnant women have long been told to reduce their salt intake to prevent water retention. However, a great deal of contemporary research has shown that inadequate salt intake during pregnancy can be dangerous, contributing to the development of both high blood pressure and edema. This is because salt helps keep blood volume adequately expanded, which is essential during pregnancy. Lack of salt causes the blood volume to contract, the heart must work harder to circulate less blood volume, and the blood vessels also constrict, leading to higher blood pressure. You do need adequate

amounts of salt during pregnancy. The key is what type of salt you are getting. Regular table salt, which is used in most prepackaged foods, fast foods, and as table salt, is high in chlorine as well as stabilizers, sometimes even sugar, and can contribute to high blood pressure.

The key is to lightly salt your foods using sea salt, tamari (natural soy sauce), or earth salt, available at health-food stores and in many supermarkets. Cut down on oversalted packaged goods and fast foods, and eat freshly prepared vegetables. In the summertime you may need to replace extra salt lost through perspiration by salting your food to taste and perhaps even drinking an electrolyte replacement such as Recharge or Third Wind if you've been sweating a great deal.

A tasty and nutritious salty condiment that my family has used for years is called "gomasio," a mixture of sesame seeds and salt (*goma* means "sesame"; *sio*, "salt"). It is said that the combination makes salt more usable by the body's cells. To prepare it, simply roast about a cup of raw, unhulled sesame seeds in a skillet on low heat until they begin to "pop" and turn light brown. Stir continuously to avoid burning the seeds. Just before they are done, add 1 tablespoon of sea salt and stir for a minute more. When slightly cool, grind in the blender or in a traditional Japanese mortar and pestle called a "suribachi" (available at many Asian grocery stores) until the mix is mostly ground but not powdered. Gomasio can be sprinkled liberally on grains, beans, cooked vegetables, and salads. It can be kept unrefrigerated for up to two weeks but is best used within a week.

- Be sure you drink enough water throughout the day to help you maintain an expanded blood volume, important for preventing high blood pressure. Frequently women do not drink enough fluids or drink sodas or coffee, which, even though they contain water, do more harm than good. Caffeinated and sugared fruit beverages do not belong in a healthy pregnancy diet. The way I remember to drink enough of the right kind of fluids throughout the day is to place a full half-gallon jug of water on my table each morning, and drink as close to all of it as I can by that evening. You can use the water to make tea as well, and you can include in that half gallon other fluids such as broths and freshly made fruit or vegetable juices.

• Here are some foods that may reduce blood pressure by improving general circulation and kidney function, and by supporting the circulatory system.

Foods for Blood Pressure Reduction

Watermelon and cucumbers (two slices of watermelon or one whole cucumber, preferably slightly overripe) and parsley (a few sprigs with a meal, once daily)

Buckwheat, the grain, can be eaten for its high rutin content, and vitamin C with bioflavonoids, up to 2,000 mg daily can be taken during pregnancy.

Raw onions and garlic eaten in large amounts each day. Chop the onions into salads, in pasta dishes, or on sandwiches. To use raw garlic, mince one clove, put it on a teaspoon with honey, and swallow without chewing by chasing it with water. This technique reduces virtually all side effects associated with eating raw garlic such as nausea, headache, and garlic breath. You can also use garlic "perles" (encapsulated garlic extracts) available at natural foods stores.

• Insufficient intake of essential fatty acids (EFAs) in the diet is also associated with hypertension. It may be improved by using walnut oil and safflower oil added to raw salads and other dishes in place of oils high in saturated fats. EFAs help enlarge blood vessels, thereby reducing high blood pressure. Fatty, deep-water fish such as salmon and tuna are high in EFAs. You can supplement your diet with 1 tablespoon of raw flaxseed oil added to a daily salad (do not cook the oil as heat destroys the EFAs). Or take two 500 milligram capsules of evening primrose or black currant seed oil daily.

• Raw olive oil is associated with low levels of heart disease in Italian women who use it on a daily basis. In Germany, an extract made from the leaves of the olive tree is used to treat essential hypertension. Although the leaves are not indicated during pregnancy, the addition of raw olive oil to the diet on a daily basis may be beneficial for women with high blood pressure (and may work as a preventative). Rather than sautéed vegetables or fried rice, you may want to prepare simple steamed veggies dressed with olive oil and other seasonings, or a rice or pasta salad. One of my favorite meals is a big raw salad with a half cup of garbanzo beans on top, sprinkled with a dash of tamari soy sauce, some olive oil, and Parmesan cheese. You could even add some chopped raw onion or minced raw garlic.

A practical way to use raw garlic is to keep on hand a batch of garlic oil for seasoning your foods. Simply peel and mince a whole bulb and place it in a jar with 1 cup of olive oil. Let stand on your counter or in the refrigerator for a couple of days before beginning to use it once a day, garlic and all, on top of salad, beans, pasta, or whole wheat bread. A delicious traditional accompaniment to Italian meals is bread spread with olive oil and garlic.

- Daily exercise helps to improve circulatory functioning and therefore is an essential part of any program to reduce high blood pressure. A brisk walk for twenty minutes, working out on a stationary bicycle, swimming, or any exercise that you like that stimulates your circulation is excellent.

- As important as exercise is the time set aside each day for relaxation, stress reduction, meditation, whatever you call it. This is what I alternately call my sacred time, my sanctuary time, my retreat time, or simply taking space. It is a time devoted to unwinding, letting go of worries and worldly concerns, finding a peaceful place within yourself, feeling centered, breathing deeply, and letting go of physical tension. Occasionally, if you are able, include a full body massage from a professional massage therapist, your mate, or a close friend. This deep relaxation experience is particularly effective if it directly follows your exercise time or a yoga session. Your body's restlessness is reduced from the activity you've just done, and your blood circulation and oxygenation are at a peak, which actually promotes deep rest. (Can you remember how well you slept when you played outside all day?) Refer to Chapter 8 for further suggestions on relaxation, creative visualization, and exercise.

- Taking twenty minutes or so to rest on your left side can help reduce blood pressure because it eases the effort on your heart and circulatory system. This is an excellent position during labor if you already have elevated blood pressure.

- Be honest with yourself, your midwife, or other care provider about your anxieties. This is very important, simply because the effort of damping down your anxieties can contribute to high blood pressure. For example, I once worked with a couple who intellectually seemed to want to have a home birth, but who, on a lot of levels, seemed very afraid of birth. Despite my efforts to help them address their anxieties, they insisted that they were comfortable with birth and wanted to have the baby at home. When the woman finally went into labor, a couple of weeks past due, her blood pressure rose dramatically. We chose to go to the hospital for the birth, where her blood pressure normalized upon arrival. When I mentioned this phenomenon to the attending nurse-midwife, the head of a large midwifery teaching program at a well-known university, she confirmed it, remarking that women can and do psychologically create symptoms that land them in the hospital if that is where they truly feel safer. In our culture, where a technologically advanced birth is considered to be the safest, we cannot dismiss high blood pressure as merely a "psychological factor." For similar reasons, blood pressure should be checked at a prenatal visit only after you have had a chance to take your coat off and relax rather than when you first come in. Incidentally, make sure your blood pressure is checked with the appropriate size cuff, as a cuff that is too tight will cause your blood pressure to appear high.

- Funny movies are great for stress reduction. Whoopie Goldberg always gets me laughing and feeling more relaxed! Internal emotional pressure is reflected in high blood pressure, so do things that you enjoy and find ways to let off steam.

HERBAL RECOMMENDATIONS

- When a rise in blood pressure is related to stress and anxiety, herbs may help. These include teas of lemon balm, chamomile, lavender, hops, oatstraw, lime blossom, skullcap, valerian, passion flower, lady's slipper, and wood betony. Drink a tea of any of these herbs alone or in combination twice a day to prevent high blood pressure, or sip up to a quart throughout the day to reduce elevated blood pressure. Many of these herbs can also be used as tinctures (although lemon balm and chamomile are best as teas) at a general dosage of 10 to 15 drops taken two to four times a day. Use hops only during the last trimester of pregnancy. The unusual smell and taste of valerian makes it best suited for use as a tincture.

- This is an excellent herbal combination for the reduction of tension and hypertension: cramp bark, hawthorn (berries, leaves, and flowers), and motherwort. Cramp bark eases physical stress by reducing muscular and nervous tension; hawthorn is a cardiotonic that dilates peripheral blood vessels and improves cardiac output and reduces strain on the heart, thereby reducing blood pressure; motherwort, a gentle antispasmodic and nervine, reduces muscular tension and emotional stress, contains bitter glycosides that have hypotensive properties—they help reduce blood pressure. This combination can be taken as a tincture beginning after the first trimester.

CAUTION: *Motherwort has the potential of acting as a uterine tonic and can therefore stimulate contractions. This doesn't usually occur, but it is advisable to wait until after the first trimester to use this herb. Of course, discontinue it if you notice increased contractions before you are due.*

If you are showing slightly elevated blood pressure which continues to rise, try 15 drops of cramp bark and 10 drops each of motherwort and hawthorn twice daily. If you are late in pregnancy (after thirty-five weeks) you can increase the dosage to four times daily and, if necessary, to 20 drops of cramp bark and 15 to 20 drops of each of the others. You may also take this tincture combination during labor if you have hypertension.

- Another herb with a reputation as a hypotensive is black cohosh, which relaxes the nerves and the muscles and dilates the peripheral blood vessels. It should be taken only during the last four to six weeks of pregnancy. It is best taken as a tincture because its properties are best extracted in alcohol. The dose is small, 5 to 10 drops twice a day. You can add it to the above tincture combination.

- I've never tried this. I came across the mention of kelp in reducing high blood pressure in Daniel Mowrey's book *The Scientific Validation of Herbal Medicine.* In repeated studies, he reports, drinking it (presumably in the form of tea) caused "a significant improvement in blood pressure readings, subjective well-being, and cardiac efficiency without any side effects." It is quite safe for use during pregnancy. Chinese medicine recommends it to resolve obstructions to the flow of energy. Therefore, it seems reasonable to drink a cup or two daily if you have high blood pressure or need to prevent it if you've had pregnancy-induced hypertension in the past.

To prepare the tea, place a 4-inch piece of kelp in a mug, and cover with 1 cup boiling water. Let it steep for one hour; then drink the water and eat the leaf as well. Alternately, boil a piece of kelp in 1 1/2 cups of water for 30 minutes; then drink the water and eat the leaf. Kelp is available in capsules, but Mowrey does not indicate whether the capsules are as effective. If you are unable to find kelp, order it from The Maine Seaweed Company, listed in the "Resources." The owner, Larch Hanson, harvests the most delicious, highest-quality kelp I've ever tried.

INDIGESTION AND HEARTBURN

Indigestion and heartburn (burping, gas, occasional stomach upset) are common in pregnancy for a couple of reasons. The increased level of progesterone that softens smooth muscles also slows digestion and sometimes causes incomplete closure of the valve in the upper portion of the stomach, making stomach acid reflux more likely. The baby's growing size puts great upward pressure on the stomach. This is more common in women who are already prone to digestive complaints. Sensible eating habits and gently soothing herbs usually reduce these problems, as will foods and herbs that help stimulate digestion. Do not use over-the-counter antacids or baking soda: these are generally contraindicated during pregnancy.

GENERAL RECOMMENDATIONS

- Because the dietary recommendations (given below) are the most important part of this approach, follow all those that are relevant to you.
- If lying down causes heartburn, sleep with extra pillows under your head.
- Deep relaxation exercises (see Chapter 8) before bed may also allay nighttime heartburn.
- Physical symptoms are sometimes a manifestation of psychic and emotional imbalance. You might take a look at what's "burning you up" or what you just can't digest in your daily life. Do you feel overwhelmed or angry? This is a good time to deal with any issues that are blocking the free flow of your energy. Writing out issues that are weighing on you is a good way to take stock. You may come up with ways to lighten your burdens.

DIETARY RECOMMENDATIONS

- Oily, heavy, rich, and spicy foods that are hard to digest are major heartburn culprits. Avoid foods that aggravate you, especially at your evening meal.

- Eat small, frequent snacks rather than large meals. A large amount of food consumed at one time can sit in your stomach and disagree with you.
- Have supper at least two hours before you go to bed, and eat a light snack if you are hungry late in the evening. Yogurt is a traditional heartburn remedy.
- To improve digestive activity, try to eat slowly, taking time to enjoy your food thoroughly.
- Some women find that drinking liquids with their meals aggravates them; for others, a glass of water during the meal or a cup of grapefruit juice just before the meal aids digestion. Try it both ways to see what works for you.
- A substance in raw almonds (cyanogenic glycoside) increases the activity of the parasympathetic nervous system, which in turn increases vagal tone (a response of one of your nerves, known as the vagus nerve), slows the heart rate, and improves digestion. A small handful as a snack or after a meal will do the trick. Chew them slowly. Raw cashews may have a similar action.
- Baked potato is sometimes helpful. With a pat of butter or a small amount of cheese and a bit of salt it makes an excellent snack or small meal.

HERBAL RECOMMENDATIONS

- According to Ayurvedic medicine, an ancient Indian system of medicine, there are three "humours," elemental influences in the body: *kapha*, the fluid substance; *pitta*, fire; and *vata*, wind. It is said that too much vata in the intestines causes nervous difficulties. Interestingly, herbs that can be used to reduce "wind" in Ayurvedic terms can also reduce general digestive complaints. Prepare and drink the following tea after a meal, or take it before bedtime to ease your digestion:

Digestion Tea

In a teapot place 1 teaspoon each of catnip or lemon balm, meadowsweet, chamomile, spearmint, fennel or anise seeds, and organic orange or tangerine peel. Pour 2 cups of boiling water over the herbs, cover the pot, and let it steep for fifteen minutes. Strain, sweeten with 1 teaspoon of honey, and drink warm.

- Dandelion is an excellent bitter tonic that pregnant women can use for indigestion. Take 20 drops of tincture four times a day or when you are having a spell of heartburn.
- Slippery elm bark is wonderful for relieving heartburn. It is best taken on a regular basis or during a bout of heartburn. It can be taken a few different ways, depending upon your preference:

Slippery Elm Bark for Heartburn

1. Stir 1 level teaspoon of the herb into a cup of boiling water or warm milk; add a teaspoon of honey and a pinch of cinnamon.

2. Boil 1 tablespoon of slippery elm bark pieces and 1 cinnamon stick in 1 1/2 cups of water (covered) for twenty minutes. Strain, sweeten, and drink.

3. Mix 1/4 ounce of slippery elm bark powder, 1 heaping tablespoon of licorice root powder, and 1 heaping teaspoon of ginger root powder. Place into capsules and take 2 capsules as needed, up to 8 a day. These three herbs reduce acidity and inflammation from indigestion.

4. Suck on slippery elm lozenges, a sore-throat remedy available at natural foods stores.

CAUTION: *Avoid any lozenges that contain coltsfoot or comfrey root while you are pregnant.*

You can also make your own lozenges:

Slippery Elm Lozenges

Take 1/4 cup of slippery elm powder and mix with enough honey to make a dough that is neither dry nor sticky. For additional flavor, add 2 to 5 drops of peppermint oil, lemon oil, or vanilla flavoring. Dust a small cutting board with some extra powder. Now roll your dough in this powder to form a long, thin roll (like a snake made out of modeling clay). Next, cut the roll into small pieces the size of a pea or slightly larger. Roll these into little balls and place on a cookie sheet and bake at 250° F for about an hour. When done these are great to suck on for indigestion (and sore throats).

- Kudzu root tea seems to reduce stomach acidity.

Kudzu Root Tea

To prepare, bring 1 cup of water to a boil in a small saucepan and then reduce heat. Meanwhile, dissolve 2 teaspoons of kudzu starch in 2 tablespoons of cold water. Add the starch to the simmering water and stir continuously for two minutes. Kudzu has a completely bland taste, so you may wish to add 2 teaspoons of soy sauce, a bouillon cube, or honey to taste. Drink while still warm.

- Activated charcoal is a great emergency remedy for severe heartburn. It absorbs and eliminates poisons and is effective in relieving stomach acidity. Take two activated charcoal tablets if you have a bad case of heartburn. Repeat only on occasion, when absolutely necessary.

INSOMNIA AND ANXIETY

Insomnia is a common problem during pregnancy. It can be difficult to go to sleep, and if we have to get up to urinate or if the baby's movements wake us up, we may find it hard to go back to sleep. This section will provide you with suggestions for treating insomnia as well as techniques you can use to relieve your anxieties.

GENERAL RECOMMENDATIONS

- Try to give yourself a wind-down time in the evenings before you go to bed. If you are pushing yourself all day, your body cannot be expected to suddenly switch gears. Instead, induce your body and mind into a quieter state by slowing down your activity level in the evening, reducing stimulating influences (television, phone calls, the newspaper). Read a pleasant book, take a bath or a walk, read poetry or a story to your children. By slowing down, you will be closer to the relaxed state needed for sleep.

- Regular exercise increases the body's calcium utilization. You will greatly increase your ability to sleep if you practice mild aerobic exercise at least three times per week, for twenty minutes each time.

DIETARY RECOMMENDATIONS

- One of the most common reasons for insomnia is *hunger*. You may feel restless, hypersensitive to touch, and slightly nauseous. Perhaps you may even have a vague sense of hunger but are too tired to fix a snack. If this is the case, your problem may be simple to resolve: eat a high-protein snack before bed, especially one that is also calcium rich. For some women (myself included) you may occasionally need to eat again when you wake in the middle of the night. You can ask your mate to get up and get a snack for you. Or you can anticipate hunger and keep a snack beside your bed. A cup of yogurt, a banana, a handful of almonds, melted cheese on toast, or a cup of soup—really anything that strikes your fancy is fine. One late evening during my fourth pregnancy I couldn't come up with an appetizing snack, so I called a friend for an idea. She came up with a super snack (it probably sounds like a gastronomic disaster to anyone who isn't pregnant) from *Moosewood Cookbook*: slice up an apple and some walnuts, grab a few raisins, and put them all on a piece of whole-wheat bread; then put cheddar cheese on top of the whole deal and melt it under the broiler. Believe it or not, it really hit the spot. *If it's nutritious* and it strikes your fancy, go ahead. Just avoid foods that give you indigestion. See *What to Eat When You're Expecting*, listed in "Further Reading."

- Calcium helps insomnia and also gets the muscles to relax. A deficit of calcium can induce anxiety and tension. Adding high-calcium foods to your diet, such as almonds, dark greens, broccoli, hard cheese, yogurt, kelp, beans, carrot juice, oats, beets, fish, and blackstrap molasses, can help. High-calcium herbs can also help. The latter include nettle, oatstraw, red raspberry leaves, chamomile, and dandelion greens prepared as infusions. Drinking cow's milk is not an optimal way to obtain calcium because it is high in fat and is hard to digest but a cup of warm milk before

Stacy was having insomnia, nightmares, occasional heart palpitations, and feelings of being overheated. She began taking tinctures of motherwort and skullcap in lemon balm tea, several times each day. Within a week her nightmares and palpitations had ceased, and her feelings of being overheated subsided. She was no longer experiencing insomnia.

bed with a pinch of cinnamon added is very relaxing. A calcium lactate supplement (preferably a calcium-magnesium blend to maintain the proper 2:1 ratio of these minerals in your body) is best taken before bed as calcium is most readily absorbed by the body while you sleep. You can take approximately 600 to 800 mg of calcium and 300 to 400 mg of magnesium a day.

- Caffeinated foods, coffee, chocolate, and cola can interfere with calcium absorption because they bind to calcium receptor sites in the body. Plants that are high in oxalic acid, beets, and spinach should be eaten in moderation.

HERBAL RECOMMENDATIONS

- Herbal nervines are relaxing to the nervous system and mildly sedating; some are calcium rich. They can be used to help you sleep. Chronic insomnia may indicate underlying worries and nutritional deficiencies, so you should address these possibilities by improving your diet and exploring your concerns even while using nervines.

- Chamomile is a prime example of a nervine that is calcium rich and aids digestion. You can take it regularly to bring about a peaceful feeling.

Chamomile Tea

To prepare, steep 1 tablespoon of chamomile blossoms in 1 cup boiling water for ten to fifteen minutes; cover the cup while steeping to preserve the volatile oils.

- Oatstraw is another nutrient-rich herb that you can use on a regular basis. Used over time it will help reduce nervous tension. It is best prepared as an infusion rather than as a tea.

- Skullcap, a gentle nerve tonic, promotes restfulness, stress reduction, and sleep. I prefer to use it in tincture form, about 15 drops at a time, but it can be prepared as a tea or in infusions. You can take it up to four times a day during periods of acute stress or twice before bedtime with a fifteen-minute interval. Skullcap tincture can be added to chamomile tea.

- Lavender blossoms promote a sense of calm. They make a mildly bitter tea that is best steeped for a short time and then sweetened with 1 teaspoon of honey. Use 2 teaspoons of the herb to 1 cup boiling water and steep with a cover on the cup for ten minutes. My own favorite is to use equal parts of lavender and chamomile blossoms to make a tea, add 10 drops of skullcap tincture, and drink hot.

- You can drink a tea of hops to induce sleep, or, if you wish, add 1 teaspoon of hops to chamomile or lavender tea. Hops tincture can be used, 15 drops in warm water or tea.

CAUTION: *Because of its estrogenic effects, avoid hops during the entire first trimester of pregnancy.*

- Other relaxing herbs include lime (linden) blossom, passion flower, lemon balm, catnip, motherwort, St. John's wort, and valerian.

- Herbal baths help you sleep. Create a nightly bedtime ritual: a cup of your favorite relaxing tea to drink, quiet music, perhaps a candle, and a warm bath. To the bath add 1 quart of lavender or chamomile infusion or 5 to 10 drops of lavender essential oil. Soak for a while, feeling the baby's movements in your womb, and consciously relaxing your muscles. Let the water ease your tension away. (Take care not to fall asleep in the bath, and take fire safety precautions if you use a candle.)

- For more relaxation techniques to reduce anxiety, refer to Chapter 8.

ITCHINESS AND SKIN TROUBLES

Many women notice that their skin improves during pregnancy. However, you may notice some itchiness. The skin stretches over the belly, breasts, and thighs; extra sweating and decreased bowel functioning causes the skin to work harder in eliminating toxins. The liver, which must now process an increased hormonal load, may be overworked and cause the skin to itch. With a natural diet and herbs, you can prevent as well as reduce skin discomfort during pregnancy. Itching can also be related to stress. Itching can be a signal that something is "getting under your skin." Take a look at whether you are manifesting stress as a skin problem.

WARNING: *If itching is persistent or progressively worsening, seek medical evaluation. Rarely, that is a sign of liver disorders specific to pregnancy.*

GENERAL RECOMMENDATIONS

- Clean your skin with a mild natural soap or just a warm cloth with no soap. Be certain that the soap you use has no additives and no strong perfume. A loofah sponge or a soft body brush can stimulate circulation and clean away dead cells, leaving your skin cleaner and softer.

- Daily exercise gets your circulation moving, bringing a healthy glow to your skin. As your circulation improves, so will your bowel functioning, reducing the burden of elimination on your skin, and the resulting itching.

DIETARY RECOMMENDATIONS

- Eat plenty of fresh fruit and vegetables daily, as well as whole grains, nuts, seeds, and beans. Eliminate processed foods and reduce your intake of saturated fats, butter, and fried foods.

- Drink a lot of water. About a half gallon a day is ideal for most pregnant women.

- You will have to work on promoting healthy bowel functioning as part of clearing up skin complaints. See "Constipation," earlier in this section.

HERBAL RECOMMENDATIONS

- My favorite herbs for healing skin complaints are dandelion root, burdock root, and chickweed. These herbs reduce heat in the body. Dandelion root is a mild bitter digestive tonic that promotes bowel health, and burdock provides moisture to the body and blood, reducing dryness as well as heat and irritation. You can eat burdock root sautéed with onions and carrots; you can eat dandelion greens sautéed with lemon, butter, garlic, and tamari soy sauce; and you can use all three herbs alone or, preferably, combined in infusions—steeping about 1 ounce total of dried herbs or 2 ounces total of fresh herbs in 1 quart of boiling water for two hours. Strain and drink up to 2 cups daily for a week at a time.

- Nettle infusion used regularly will tone the whole system, contributing to healthy skin. Cleavers can also be used safely.

- Rub cocoa butter on your body each day to reduce itching. Cocoa butter is also purported to prevent stretch marks, though to some degree these do seem either hereditary (women of Italian descent in my practice seem to have the fewest) or related to the length of the torso (women with longer torsos seem to develop fewer). You can also use coconut oil, or the following blend that one of my clients came up with: to a base of almond oil add a few drops each of essential oils of lavender, rose, and tangerine, and rub on your belly each day.

- Calendula oil can be used to reduce itching and irritation.

Neesa was having severe leg cramps during the night. She began taking a calcium and magnesium supplement and within a few days the cramps ceased. She continued the supplement throughout her pregnancy and had no further problems with cramps.

- Slippery elm bark powder or marshmallow root powder can be sprinkled in the creases, such as on the "ledge" between your breasts and belly, to reduce chafing or rashes from heat and increased sweating.

- You can reduce stress-related itching with the use of nervine herbs as discussed under the topics "Fatigue," "Emotional Swings," "Insomnia and Anxiety," and "High Blood Pressure."

KETONES IN URINE

(see Urine Testing for Protein, Sugar, or Ketones)

LATE-PREGNANCY BLEEDING

(see Bleeding, Late-Pregnancy)

LEG CRAMPS

Leg cramps usually indicate that you need more minerals than you are getting: the muscles spasm because of inadequate calcium or magnesium or from inadequate oxygenation caused by lack of iron. In addition, lack of exercise not only contributes to leg cramps, but also decreases your body's mineral absorption. Overly vigorous exercise during pregnancy can also cause cramping. Leg cramps tend to be most annoying at night. Improve your mineral intake, get appropriate amounts of exercise, and learn to release tension in your muscles consciously. Not all women will experience obvious cramps but instead may have a vague, uncomfortable, restless, fidgety, pulling, or aching feeling in their legs. These are all symptoms of the same condition.

- When you get a leg cramp, stand up and place your feet flat and firmly against the floor, as if you are pushing your heels into the ground; then massage the cramped area vigorously and firmly. Another method is to flex your foot gently by holding onto it, curling your toes up toward your knee, and massaging your calf. This can be done either while standing or lying down. If you have varicose veins in that area, don't massage it.

- Avoid pointing your toes during pregnancy—it can start a cramp.

- Exercise daily by walking and doing leg exercises such as leg lifts and lunges. If at all possible, swim or exercise your legs in a pool of water.

- Elevate your legs periodically, preferably for twenty minutes a day, to improve circulation. You can put your feet up on a chair or lie down and put them up on two pillows.

- Be sure you are getting enough calcium and magnesium in your diet (see Chapter 5). There are herbs that can increase dietary calcium intake: nettle, dandelion leaf, oatstraw, chamomile, and all seaweeds, but especially kelp and hijiki. If your cramping is severe, add a calcium magnesium supplement to your diet in a 2:1 ratio, that is, about 600–800 mg calcium to 300–400 mg magnesium.

- Lack of salt can cause muscle cramps, so salt your food to taste with sea salt, and replenish salt lost through perspiration in hot weather or after exercise. Also take care to drink enough fluids.

- Vitamin E is also said to reduce cramping. Take 200 IU daily unless you have a heart condition or high blood pressure, in which case you should begin with 50 IU daily and gradually, over the course of a couple of months, work your way up to 200 IU daily. Foods high in vitamin E include whole grains, sunflower seeds, cold-pressed oils, eggs, molasses, wheat germ, and organ meats (obtained from organic sources only). Cooking destroys the vitamin E in foods, and eating cooked foods increases your body's need for vitamin E, so try to eat some foods daily that are rich in vitamin E and uncooked—for example, sunflower seeds and olive oil in a raw salad.

- Vitamin C deficiency may also be associated with leg cramps. You can take up to 2,000 mg in a supplement in addition to your food sources of this nutrient.

HERBAL RECOMMENDATIONS

- Include calcium-rich herbs as mentioned above as part of your daily diet. Here is a recipe for a high-calcium brew:

High-Calcium Tea

Mix 1 ounce each of nettle and oatstraw with 1/2 ounce of alfalfa and 1/4 ounce of slippery elm. Prepare an infusion, adding 1/4 ounce of the mix to 1 pint of boiling water, and steep for thirty minutes to one hour. To assist in assimilation of calcium, add 1 tablespoon of apple cider vinegar and sweeten to taste.

- Herbal foot baths can relieve muscular tension. Soak your feet (and calves, if possible) in a very warm bath to which you add 5 drops of wintergreen oil, 2 drops of camphor oil, and 2 tablespoons of ginger juice (grate about a 2-inch section of fresh ginger root and squeeze until the juice comes from it).
- Foot and leg massage promotes muscular relaxation, improved circulation, and the release of nutrients stored in the muscles, all of which make it useful as prevention and first aid for leg cramps.

The optimal time for a deep foot and leg massage is at bedtime, but it can be given anytime. Use massage oil that contains arnica, St. John's wort, and chamomile, or use a Chinese herbal liniment such as Dit Dat Jiao, an old remedy used for martial arts injuries and prepared as follows (credit for this recipe goes to Michael and Lesley Tierra):

Dit Dat Jiao

6 parts angelica root
6 parts comfrey root
4 parts cinnamon bark
4 parts valerian root
3 parts hyssop
3 parts safflower petals
3 parts calendula blossoms

Place the herbs in a wide-mouth jar and cover with 80–100 proof liquor (I use vodka) until the liquid rises two inches over the herbs. Cover the jar, store in a warm, dark place, and shake the jar daily for two weeks. Strain and bottle for use. This liniment is absolutely for external use only and should be labeled clearly. It warms the skin, dissolves clots and congestion, stimulates circulation, soothes, and heals. Be aware that it may stain fabrics.

- Black haw or cramp bark tincture can be taken to reduce leg spasms. Take 15 drops of either as needed, or up to three times a day. In addition, drink teas made from any of these herbs: chamomile, lemon balm, catnip, lavender, and skullcap.

NOTE: *Persistent leg pain, especially when accompanied by local heat or varicosities (swelling) can be due to phlebitis and merits the attention of an experienced health practitioner. If you suspect this problem, do not massage the area.*

MINOR ILLNESSES

(see Colds, Flu, and Minor Illnesses)

MISCARRIAGE

Miscarriages, pregnancies that end spontaneously usually before twenty-eight weeks' gestation, occur in about 20 percent of all pregnancies in the United States. As cited in *The Encyclopedia of Childbearing* (Rothman, 1993), each year in the United States between 600,000 and 800,000 women miscarry. Many women miscarry very early in pregnancy, without ever realizing they were pregnant, having what appears to be a heavy period. Miscarriage rates are highest for young teenagers and middle-aged women (especially when pregnancy has been accomplished with the use of reproductive technologies), and they are more common in early pregnancy than after the first trimester. For women who want to be pregnant, particularly those with a history of repeated miscarriage, losing the pregnancy and the baby is a devastating experience. Many women fear that something is wrong with them as women or that they did something to harm the baby. Because of our culture's refusal to talk about miscarriage, few women know what to do or what to expect when it happens.

If you are experiencing cramping and/or bleeding because of a threatened miscarriage, you can do a number of things to prevent the miscarriage from becoming inevitable *if the baby is healthy*. The recommendations that follow are in no way harmful to the baby if the baby is otherwise healthy. As blunt as this may sound, miscarriage is nature's way of preventing unhealthy babies from being carried full term. This is painful for the woman to accept, but it may spare the baby a life full of adversity. Our bodies have a wisdom of their own. It is important to realize that attempts to prevent miscarriage will not be effective if the baby is not healthy.

Other causes of miscarriage include hormonal imbalances, cervical looseness (called an "incompetent cervix" in the medical world, I detest this term), infections, and nutritional deficiencies. Many of these conditions can be improved naturally.

Preventing a —Threatened Miscarriage—

A miscarriage is threatened when you experience spotting, bleeding, or cramping, often with a low backache. These symptoms may begin abruptly or slowly and will usually persist for hours or even days. You may experience some spotting or bleeding and that is the end of the whole episode, or the symptoms may be so severe you will fear you are going to lose the baby. At this time the cervix will be closed, but an internal exam is best avoided, as it is unnecessarily intrusive and may stimulate the uterus further. Chances are you will still feel pregnant, with continuing breast tenderness and nausea, but you may feel anxious and question whether you are really feeling these signs or you just want to feel them. Most often, if you still feel pregnant, then you are. While I am opposed to the routine use of the doppler (an electronic device used to hear the fetal heartbeat), in this situation it can be very reassuring. Usually at about ten to twelve weeks the baby's heartbeat can be heard with the doppler. A midwife can do this test at home. Of course, if the doppler is tried earlier, the heartbeat may not yet be audible and could unnecessarily discourage the mother. An ultrasound can also confirm the baby's wellness or indicate otherwise.

GENERAL RECOMMENDATIONS

- You may have to come to terms with whether in your heart of hearts you really want to be pregnant or whether you or your partner have fears, anxieties, or ambivalence about having a baby. We can influence our receptivity to a baby in our wombs. In no way does this mean that all miscarriages are a result of ambivalence, because the baby's health certainly influences its ability to maintain life. But your desire to continue the pregnancy will support your efforts.

- On a spiritual level you can communicate your desire to have the baby, also giving the baby permission to go if he or she needs to. Both partners can place their hands on the mother's belly, directly over the womb, and speak to the baby, either aloud or silently. Let your hearts flow with your feelings of love for the baby and for each other, particularly if there is strain between you. Your bond as a couple can strengthen the bond between you and the baby and can aid your efforts to arrest a miscarriage. This can be a strong time of healing.

- As part of making clear your intention for the baby to stay, you can set up a small pregnancy altar in your home on the top of a dresser or bed table or even on a sunny windowsill. You can go to this special place to send loving thoughts to your baby and visualize your womb surrounded with protection. On this altar place objects that remind you of healthy babies, healthy pregnant mothers, and families: pictures, small statues or figurines, a healthy plant, a stone egg, candles, or anything else that arises from your imagination.

- Treat yourself with the utmost love and care. This is a trying experience that may also challenge your faith in your body. Try to love your body and don't blame yourself for miscarrying.

- If you are having contractions or bleeding or spotting, get off your feet and rest. Try to get up only if you need to use the bathroom. Take time to visualize the baby as healthy, your placenta as strongly connected to your uterus, and your body providing love and nourishment to the baby. Avoid lifting heavy objects and abstain from sexual activity until all signs of miscarriage have been gone for a week. Think positively and use relaxation techniques to help you rest and to reduce anxiety-ridden thoughts.

- Warm baths (not hot) can reduce uterine irritability and bring some relief to low backache. A warm bath is also a great place for relaxing and having a good cry to release pent-up feelings.

DIETARY RECOMMENDATIONS

- For the prevention of miscarriage it is very important that you avoid all cold-natured and cold-temperature foods, including foods that have just come out of the refrigerator, cold or iced beverages, fruit and vegetable juices, all tropical fruits, including citrus (unless you live in an environment where they are grown locally), and all foods out of season, including fresh salads when locally grown produce is not available. I've seen a consistent connection between the intake of "cold" foods and the onset of threatened miscarriage. In traditional Chinese medicine there is a notion of cold as a downward moving, heavy force, so perhaps it is not unreasonable to think that such substances could cause an excess of downward flow in the pelvic region. As a practical matter, it takes a certain degree of warmth in the womb, not unlike incubating eggs until they hatch, to create the conditions necessary for the optimal health of a baby. Cold-natured substances may cause warmth needed in the womb to fluctuate, destabilizing the environment.

Marley had been having aching in her bones all night, had dark puffy circles under her eyes, and vomited in the morning. She had no appetite, severe leg cramps, pelvic pressure, aching in her lower back beneath her ribs, and a temperature (oral) of 99.2° F. She is 30 weeks pregnant (third baby) and was having mild, irregular contractions. She began taking echinacea at a high dose, along with an infusion of uva-ursi, increased fluids, vitmain C, and cranberry juice. Within 24 hours all symptoms subsided, and there was no recurrence. Marley gave birth at home at 40 weeks, gestation.

- It follows that it is preferable to eat foods of a warmer and nourishing nature, such as soups. Miso soup, prepared from a protein-rich paste of aged soybeans, is excellent, as are chicken soup and bean soups. Also, emphasize whole-grain stews and hot cereals, root vegetables, and dark greens until your symptoms have been gone for at least a week. Warm tea or water at room temperature can be taken as a beverage.

- Vitamin E (alpha tocopherol) has been said to strengthen the placental attachment to the uterus, thereby reducing spotting and the likelihood of miscarriage. It should be taken in doses of up to 800 IU each day for up to three weeks. However, prolonged use may result in the placenta becoming abnormally attached to the uterine wall, a complication in itself. Therefore, do not exceed this dosage, and do not take vitamin E for longer than three weeks. If you have heart disease, do not exceed 50 IU per day without discussing it with your physician.

- Vitamin C plus a bioflavonoid complex—that is, along with the whole group of vitamins that naturally occur with vitamin C in foods—is reputed to strengthen the capillaries, reducing the likelihood of miscarriage. You can take up to 1,000 mg daily, including the amount that is in your prenatal multiple vitamin. High doses of vitamin C—in excess of 2,000 mg—can cause a miscarriage, so do not exceed the recommended amount.

- Be certain that you are getting adequate protein, carbohydrates, vitamins, minerals, and fluids. Thoroughly read the section on nutrition in Chapter 5.

HERBAL RECOMMENDATIONS

- The following remedy seems to be so effective in preventing miscarriage that midwives across the nation recommend it in one formulation or another. Following is a miscarriage brew par excellence. Variations on the theme follow the basic recipe.

Miscarriage Prevention Tea

Mix 1 ounce each of *Mitchella repens* (partridge berry), cramp bark or black haw, false unicorn root, and wild yam, as well as 1/4 ounce of lobelia and 1/8 ounce of dried ginger root (you may have to break the root into small pieces so it mixes evenly throughout the blend).

Take a total of 1 ounce of the mixture and place it into a quart-size jar. Next, completely fill the jar with boiling water, cover the jar, and let the tea steep for four hours. (If you need it quickly, you can begin to drink it after two hours.) After steeping, strain the liquid and drink between 1/4 and 1/2 cup every two hours. If you are cramping a lot, you can drink this brew by taking a mouthful every fifteen minutes.

Partridge berry tones the uterus while also causing uterine relaxation, reducing cramps and contractions. It also supports the nervous system, perhaps helping to reduce the anxiety and apprehension associated with a threatened miscarriage.

Cramp bark and black haw have very similar actions on the uterine muscles, relaxing them and reducing the severity of contractions. They also have some relaxing effects upon the nervous system, making them appropriate choices in a formula for preventing miscarriage. One herb may be substituted for the other or the two may be used together.

False unicorn root contains steroidal saponins, precursors or building blocks of our sex hormones. For this reason it is an excellent hormonal balancer as well as a specific uterine tonic, making it applicable for threatened miscarriages. It may be particularly helpful to women whose progesterone levels are low, but it can be taken by anyone who is bleeding and cramping in the first trimester.

Chasteberry (vitex) helps to regulate reproductive hormones so that the pregnancy can be sustained, most probably by causing the pituitary gland to increase the progesterone levels so necessary for the maintenance of pregnancy.

Lobelia, a strong, sedating herb, is used in this formula specifically for reducing uterine contractions, and also for calming the nerves. In high doses, however, it is potentially toxic. It is important to avoid exposing the developing baby to excessive doses of this herb. In the amount in this formula you are unlikely to experience side effects. If you do notice nausea, strange feelings, scratchy throat, or low blood pressure, immediately reduce the amount of lobelia in your formula by half or omit it completely.

Ginger root is added for its mildly stimulating and warming properties, and also for the taste it imparts to the infusion, which is not particularly delicious.

You can if you wish take some or all of these herbs in tincture form. This may be necessary if you are also suffering from nausea or vomiting. Take 10 to 15 drops of each of the first four herbs plus 5 drops of the lobelia in a quarter cup of warm water every fifteen to thirty minutes. Omit the ginger root. If symptoms are very acute continue the dosage, but only if there are no signs of hemorrhage. For less intense symptoms, take this same dosage every one to two hours, tapering off to every four hours, then every eight hours, over the course of a few days as symptoms subside.

Another variation is to add the tinctures to a cup of red raspberry leaf tea, a uterine tonic and an astringent (astringents help to control bleeding).

—*When Miscarriage Continues*—

Not every miscarriage can be stopped. My heart goes out to those of you whose baby is unable to stay with you right now. It is my hope that you will find peace and inner strength in this experience and not blame yourself.

When a miscarriage is inevitable, the bleeding and cramping will not stop until all the products of conception (the tissue that was the developing fetus, the placenta, and the uterine lining that is shed) pass from your body. If the pregnancy ends in the first couple of weeks, it will seem like a normal to heavy period. The further advanced the pregnancy, the more noticeable will be the signs of miscarriage and the more effort you will need to make to clear everything out. Inevitable miscarriage can be suspected when cramping becomes more intense and inconsistent, and the bleeding becomes heavier, to the point of soaking through your clothing or pads. At this time the cervix will usually be dilating, will be shorter than usual, or will be slightly bulging. It is not necessary for you to check your cervix—I offer this information to those who are familiar with how their cervix feels.

How you choose to handle a miscarriage is a very personal decision. Most women who allow nature to take its course and who receive support through the process will miscarry with no complications. However, miscarriage should not be taken lightly, carrying as it does risks of hemorrhage and infection. The follow-up procedure at the hospital is generally a dilation and curettage, which carries the risk of damaging the womb, or a vacuum suction. Any time you enter the hospital, you are exposed to a host of pathogenic germs unlikely to be encountered in most homes. Also, certain exams and interventions are routine in hospitals. Each woman and each situation must be evaluated on an individual basis and with an open mind, common sense, and a healthy dose of caution.

Your vitality and coherence as well as how long and how much you've been bleeding are good indications of how you are doing. If you feel very weak, strange, or spaced out, or have been cramping heavily (experiencing strong pain, much more than a normal period) and bleeding steadily for more than two hours without emptying the contents of your womb, then going to the hospital is probably warranted. If you are having a lot of cramping but are *not* bleeding heavily, you can probably continue to take a wait-and-see attitude until you complete the miscarriage or unless bleeding becomes heavy.

WARNING: *If at anytime you become spaced out, fuzzy, incoherent, unusually anxious, sleepy, clammy, or begin to look pale, you need to get to the hospital immediately. These can be signs of shock, which is life threatening.*

If everything seems normal and you choose to stay at home, or if you are unable to reach medical services, the following information will often help to complete a miscarriage at home. Again, if at any time you notice the above signs, seek emergency medical care.

A miscarriage is similar to any birth in that the uterus, in the effort to empty its contents, goes through contractions that build in intensity until it completes the process. However, a normal miscarriage tends to have more continuous bleeding than a normal birth. Women who are miscarrying have not yet experienced the blood volume expansion that usually occurs at about twenty weeks, and therefore are not protected against blood loss. The amount of bleeding in a miscarriage can vary from mild to severe, and depending upon a woman's health reserves, she can become very weak from blood loss.

Therefore, **if you are miscarrying, you should not remain alone**. Always have with you someone who can get you to the hospital—and stay in close contact with someone who is knowledgeable about the process, such as a midwife or nurse practitioner.

At some point during the process you will pass the tissue that was the fetus as well as the placenta and the sac of membranes that surrounded the fetus. Since you will also be passing clots, you will want to save any such matter for a closer look, in order to determine if you have in fact emptied your womb. A womb not fully cleared out predisposes you to continued bleeding, cramps, and the risk of serious infection. You can look at the tissue yourself (it can be fished out of the toilet if necessary) and try to determine if you see any tissue that looks like a small sac (ranging from about the size of the bowl of a teaspoon to the bowl of a tablespoon, depending upon how early in the first trimester you are). It will be milky white or clear, with some light pink tinges. Clots are more like gelled masses of blood, with some stringiness from the clotting factors that cause the blood to bind. You may find other matter as well, such as small vesicles that look like grapes—a sign that a baby never developed after conception. (This requires medical attention.) Saving any material that you pass for analysis by your midwife or physician can help you and them determine whether the miscarriage was complete.

A miscarriage may build up for several days or even weeks before it actually is complete, with cramping and spotting building in intensity. The actual miscarriage, with regular cramping and heavier bleeding, usually takes place within a couple of hours. After the tissue has been passed, cramping and bleeding will subside, though you may have some more contracting and will definitely bleed some afterward. This will be about the length of time of a regular period, about five days. Heavy bleeding at any time (soaking a pad within thirty minutes is very heavy bleeding) or bleeding persisting for more than five days may mean that pieces of tissue are retained in the uterus. Until the womb is emptied, it cannot completely clamp down, hence the continued cramping is an effort to do so, and the bleeding is a sign that something is preventing this from happening.

WARNING: *Retained tissue can cause serious, life-threatening infection. If natural treatment recommendations (below) for completing a miscarriage are not effective in the first days after the miscarriage, or if at any time your temperature becomes elevated or you notice a foul-smelling vaginal discharge, you should seek immediate medical help.*

In some cases a D & C (dilation and curettage) is the best recourse. Sometimes a physician can simply prescribe Methergine (an ergot-rye fungus derivative) used historically by midwives but now available only by prescription. An antibiotic may be warranted if infection is present.

GENERAL RECOMMENDATIONS

- Have an experienced or a very responsible person with you at all times until your miscarriage is definitely completed. A miscarriage is completed when bleeding and cramping stop and the uterus has passed the products of conception.
- Take it very easy throughout the miscarriage, but do not go to sleep if you are bleeding—drowsiness can be a signal of shock.
- Drink fluids regularly, a cup of liquid every one to two hours, to keep your blood volume expanded. Rehydration Drink (see page 211) can keep your electrolytes and minerals in balance, as well as such drinks as Recharge, Third Wind, and Gatorade. Remember to urinate regularly; a full bladder can aggravate cramping and prevent effective emptying of the uterus.
- Keep yourself warm and comfortable.
- Visualize your cramps effectively emptying your womb. Surround your uterus with light, and imagine the placental tissue releasing from your uterine wall and from your body.
- Have somebody massage your feet or your lower back, especially applying firm pressure to the area over your sacrum. A hot-water bottle applied to this area can also be comforting.
- As painful as this is for you emotionally and physically, try to remember that your body knows how to do this job. Listen to what your body is telling you.

HERBAL RECOMMENDATIONS

Often midwives, to facilitate miscarriage, encourage complete emptying of the uterus, to prevent hemorrhage and infection. Herbs can be used to help reduce anxiety during the process and promote healing afterward.

- Perhaps the most widely recommended herbs for facilitating a miscarriage are blue and black cohosh. These herbs help regulate uterine contractions, reducing spastic muscle contraction and promoting an effective labor. Black cohosh is also an effective nervine, reducing anxiety as well as physical tension. During a miscarriage, tinctures are probably the most effective and convenient form for taking these herbs. Dosage ranges from 10 to 15 drops of each tincture every one hour to every four hours, depending upon the severity of the symptoms. Discontinue after the acute phase of the miscarriage is complete, and do not exceed five doses.

- A combination of bayberry bark, shepherd's purse, and witch hazel in the form of tinctures or infusion can be taken to prevent or offset heavy bleeding during a miscarriage. Take 20 drops of bayberry and 5 to 10 drops of each of the others every thirty minutes to one hour, or 2 to 4 tablespoons of the infusion with similar frequency.

NOTE: *Herbal remedies may help prevent excessive bleeding but are not a substitute for medical care during hemorrhage.*

- Bethroot is another excellent herb for promoting uterine contractions while preventing hemorrhage. Take 10 to 15 drops of tincture as often as every fifteen minutes during the acute stage of the miscarriage, less frequently if things already seem to be happening on their own.
- You can sip a tea of basil or of cinnamon throughout the miscarriage to promote contractions and prevent excessive bleeding. Steep 1 teaspoon of either herb in 1 cup of boiling water (cover while steeping) for ten minutes.
- If the miscarriage is proceeding efficiently and the main problem seems to be anxiety, sip a tea of chamomile or lavender blossoms (1 teaspoon of herb to 1 cup boiling water, steeped covered for ten minutes).

—After a Miscarriage—

When the miscarriage is complete your immediate concerns are infection and bleeding. Much healing needs to occur in the first weeks, then a longer-term physical healing over the following months, and, for some women, an emotional healing that can take years. When you miscarry, your body must make a hormonal adjustment from a pregnant to a nonpregnant state, and you must make an adjustment in your view of yourself. It is important that you give yourself the time to treat yourself gently during the transition. Essentially, you have gone through a birth without getting a baby.

During the first few days after your miscarriage you can expect to bleed as if you have your period, and you may pass some small clots.

WARNING: *If after four or five days you are still bleeding, or if at any time you are soaking a medium-size sanitary pad in thirty minutes, you must seek immediate medical attention. Also, if you are passing large clots, having a lot of cramping, or notice any foul-smelling discharge, you probably have retained tissue and possibly have an infection, and need prompt medical attention.*

After a miscarriage it is advisable to use herbs that work to prevent infection, facilitate the discharge of retained tissue, and promote the healing of your uterus. A general program for the first three days after miscarriage is as follows:

- Check your temperature three to four times each day. It should be normal, which for most of us is 98.6 degrees Fahrenheit.
- Get plenty of rest, eat nourishing foods such as hearty soups and stews, and drink plenty of fluids. If you have lost a considerable amount of blood, refer to "Anemia."
- Take 2,000 mg of vitamin C over the course of each day as a preventative measure against infection.
- Take 25 to 50 drops of echinacea tincture (depending on your body weight—heavier women should take a higher dose than lighter women) four times daily to stimulate your immune response and as a preventative against infection. Other herbs

that can be used in conjunction with echinacea to prevent infection include calendula tincture (10 drops with each dose of echinacea) or infusion, thyme tea, fresh garlic (garlic perles can also be taken), or goldenseal tincture (10 drops with each dose of echinacea) or capsules (two "00"-size capsules four times daily). Both calendula and goldenseal also promote uterine contractions and act as astringents to prevent hemorrhage.

- Angelica has a reputation for helping to clear the uterus of any retained fragments and is also a warming uterine tonic. Take 10 to 15 drops three times daily to ensure complete uterine emptying, and increase that dosage to as frequently as every two hours if you are having cramps and are passing clots. Ground ivy is another tincture with this reputation, and though I've not used it for these purposes, herbalist Susun Weed recommends it highly for retained placenta after birth. Do not use it to prevent miscarriage, but if you are still cramping and passing clots, take 20 to 30 drops of fresh ground ivy tincture every two to three hours.

- Change your menstrual pad every couple of hours to avoid infection from bacteria in the pad. Be sure to wipe from front to back after you have a bowel movement to prevent rectal bacteria from entering the vulva and causing infection.

- Refrain from all sexual activity until the bleeding has completely stopped. If anyone needs to examine you (your midwife or doctor) make sure that he or she does so with sterile hands. Do not bathe (you can shower) for the first few days.

- It is essential that you seek a trusted person to help you work out your grief, disappointment, and guilt.

- While you cannot use any substances, including herbs, to heal your grief, a few herbs can help you steady your emotions. If you are unable to rest, you can drink warm teas of chamomile and lavender combined, adding, if you wish, up to 20 drops of

motherwort, hops, or skullcap tincture (or a combination of these to equal 20 drops total). You can also take these as tinctures, up to three times a day. Other herbs that support the nerves and promote gentle relaxation include oatstraw, rosemary, lemon balm, catnip, and valerian.

After the first week you will probably begin to feel more like your pre-pregnant self, with all signs of pregnancy gone, particularly if the miscarriage was early. Herbs that nourish the female reproductive system, including those that help to regulate the hormones and the menstrual cycle, can be used to assist you in this transition: red clover leaves and blossoms, red raspberry leaves, chasteberry, false unicorn root, wild yam, calendula, dong quai, ginseng, and licorice. A small amount of ginger root or cinnamon bark can be added to infusions to facilitate the actions of the herbs, while warming your pelvic region and promoting healthy circulation.

You may want to try this mix:

Feminine Nourishment Tea

1/2 ounce each of false unicorn root, chasteberry, and wild yam with 1/8 ounce of ginger root. Store this dry mixture in an airtight jar or plastic bag.

To prepare the tea, place 1/2 ounce of the mixture in a jar, add 2 cups boiling water, and let it steep for two hours. Strain and drink 1/4 to 1/2 cup of this brew three to four times a day for six weeks after the miscarriage.

You may also drink teas or infusions of red raspberry and red clover. If the infusions are difficult to prepare or seem like a job each day, you can take tinctures of these herbs instead. Prepare a mixture of equal parts of false unicorn root, chasteberry, wild yam, and dong quai, and take 15 to 25 drops four times daily in warm water.

This is naturally a painful time for many women. People who are unaware that you miscarried may ask how the pregnancy is going. You will have to adjust your view of the future, which recently included the expectation of a baby. This can be an especially difficult time if this was your first pregnancy, or if you have had a history of miscarriage. Miscarriage can also add stress to your relationship with your mate. At the time most women miscarry, the pregnancy may not have felt "real" to the father. He may not take your emotional response to the miscarriage seriously, saying that you can simply try again. For many women, these responses are, in the least, insensitive. The idea of trying again and possibly experiencing such disappointment again is unbearable. For the sake of the relationship, the dad needs to be deeply sensitive to and supportive of his partner. He must listen to you and offer love without dismissing your pain. If you are both deeply grieved and disappointed, this can be a time of holding each other closely and reaffirming your commitment to being a family. If this miscarriage makes the relationship more difficult, intensifies, or makes more apparent the stresses you were already having, you may want to consult a professional to help both of you work through the crisis together.

—*Preventing Future Miscarriages*—

After having miscarried once, many women are eager to conceive, yet fearful of miscarrying again. In the vast majority of cases, repeated miscarriage is not likely, but it is best to wait until you've had *at least* three

regular periods in a row before you conceive again. By doing so, you allow your uterus to regenerate fully at the implantation site and replenish your blood supply if you bled a lot during the miscarriage. The delay will allow you to experience your next pregnancy as a fresh experience. It really is better not to try to fill the void of your lost pregnancy with another one, but to heal your loss and then embrace your new experience. Some excellent books and resource groups (see "Further Reading" and "Resources" at the end of this book) can assist you in integrating your miscarriage into the experience of your life.

Whether or not you went into your previous pregnancy well prepared, now is a time for getting yourself into excellent health. Creating a pregnancy altar, for example, can give you a place to affirm your desire to have a healthy pregnancy and a healthy baby. The work of creating a gift for your baby, such as a quilt, can give you a concrete way to manifest your intention.

If you don't have children, this is a time to be completely honest about whether you want to become a mother right now. If you already have children, be honest about whether you want another child. Discussing these issues openly with your partner can clear the air and help you make the decision.

If you decide that you do want to become pregnant again, you can use herbs to support the pregnancy and prevent miscarriage. These are basically the same herbs used to prevent a threatened miscarriage and may be taken both before you conceive (begin taking them up to a month before you try) and then into your first trimester, preferably until two or three weeks after the time of your last miscarriage or throughout the whole first trimester. This is the basic formula: 1 ounce each of wild yam, partridge berry, and false unicorn root; 1/2 ounce of cramp bark or black haw; 1/4 ounce of red raspberry leaf. Combine all of these herbs and store in an airtight jar or plastic bag. Place 4 to 6 tablespoons of the mixture in a quart jar, fill with boiling water, and steep until the tea is cool enough to drink. Strain out the herbs and drink 1/4 cup four times daily. (If you begin to miscarry, refer to "Preventing a Threatened Miscarriage," earlier in this section.) If you find it difficult to prepare or carry these herbs with you each day, use tinctures. Mix together (in a small bottle with a dropper) equal parts of wild yam, partridge berry, false unicorn, and cramp bark, and take 20 drops two to four times daily, the frequency depending upon your miscarriage history. If you've had more than one miscarriage, take the herbs four times daily. Also, if you have such a history, begin taking these herbs for up to two months prior to conception, and consider seeking an experienced doctor of traditional Chinese herbal medicine and acupuncture. The combination of both approaches can be very effective for preventing miscarriage and strengthening you for a healthy pregnancy.

MORNING SICKNESS

Women experience different degrees of morning sickness ranging from no problem at all to very mild discomfort, to nearly constant nausea and vomiting during the first trimester or longer. I once heard it said that the reason it is called "morning sickness" is because it starts in the morning and lasts all day. Actually, morning sickness can occur at any time of the day or night. Generally, this nausea begins around six weeks into pregnancy and persists until the fourteenth week. It is triggered by different factors:

- Empty stomach, hunger, low blood sugar (hypoglycemia)

- Strong smells (fumes, food cooking)
- Hormonal surges and imbalances
- Normal pregnancy-related changes in the digestive system
- Oily foods
- Very sweet, sugary foods (which for some women may include fruits)
- Vitamin or mineral deficiencies
- Lack of exercise
- Fatigue
- Stress
- Constipation
- Ambivalence or anxiety about pregnancy

Nausea that persists much longer than the fourteenth week is usually related to insufficient nutritional intake, unresolved emotional issues, or rarely, a health problem. If you are experiencing persistent nausea past your first trimester, please seek the help of an experienced health care practitioner who is knowledgeable about the nutritional needs of pregnant women.

There is much speculation as to what actually causes morning sickness and why some women experience it while others don't. Theories include hormonal fluctuations, emotional reactions to pregnancy, nutritional factors, and biological mechanisms that cause women to reject substances that may cause the babies harm. It has been suggested that women who do experience morning sickness have a greater likelihood of a healthy pregnancy and a healthy baby and a decreased incidence of miscarriage. But as yet no one has come to a definitive conclusion. Medical attempts to reduce morning sickness through medication have not proven safe for the fetus. The only advice I can give is to avoid eating stuff that prompts nausea, and at the same time improve your eating habits.

Pregnancy-related nausea is not dangerous, but if you are vomiting excessively, you

Nancy was very nauseous all of the time and was unable to find appetizing, easy to digest foods that satisfied her hunger. She'd been a vegetarian for many years, but I had a strong feeling that chicken might settle her stomach and satisfy her. I asked her if she'd consider eating chicken soup, and at this point she was ready to do just about anything. Her husband prepared her a pot of chicken vegetable soup. The chicken broth was immensely satisfying, she ate the meat and vegetables, and began to feel much better. Occasionally, such flexibility can make a tremendous difference in morning sickness.

(and the baby) run the risk of dehydration and severe malnutrition. The condition occasionally requires hospitalization and rehydration with intravenous fluids (see the next section for a specific discussion of hyperemesis).

- Normal physiological changes of early pregnancy, such as increased levels of estrogen and progesterone, hormones that maintain pregnancy, cause body tissue to become soft and more engorged, and promote such changes as breast enlargement and milk production, and also cause the entire digestive system to slow down and become "softer." The processing of these hormones (equivalent to one hundred birth control pills a day) in addition to these changes can lead to nausea. Moreover, the softening and slowing down of the digestive tract increases the likelihood of constipation, which aggravates nausea; and the incredible amount of work being done by the body causes first-trimester fatigue, which can reduce the likelihood of your eating well, also instigating nausea. By staying well rested, eating well, and taking other precautions to prevent constipation, you can minimize nausea.

- Avoid smells that nauseate you. Don't walk near busy roads if exhaust nauseates you; ask someone to fill your gas tank; let your husband, friends, or relatives help you in the kitchen; and don't prepare those foods that are distasteful to you (by smell, sight, or taste). Often just the smell of a particular food (or a few foods) will completely turn the stomach of a pregnant woman.

- Lack of cardiovascular stimulation—exercise—can contribute to nausea because greater levels of acids and carbon dioxide will build up in the blood. A brisk walk in fresh air or with some form of exercise daily can reduce the severity of nausea. Regular exercise also reduces fatigue and prevents constipation. Eating a snack about a half hour before you plan to be active will help prevent nausea or low blood sugar. It is also essential that you eat well after exercising to replenish lost calories, particularly if the exercise is strenuous. If exercising triggers nausea, try regular massage, a form of passive exercise.

- You can reduce nausea by getting plenty of rest, using relaxing herbs, and asking for help with your responsibilities if you are fatigued. Perhaps you can think of at least one or two people who will watch your older kids or help with household chores.

- Ambivalence about the pregnancy can cause internal tension that may exacerbate feelings of nausea, and vice versa. Even women who are completely thrilled to be pregnant may have misgivings. It is important to acknowledge and accept your feelings rather than feel guilt for these emotions. Worrying that you are harming your baby with your negative thoughts only adds to your tension. Talk to friends, other pregnant women, or a midwife or counselor; use a journal as an outlet for your concerns. It is perfectly normal to go through a time of uncertainty—children are a great responsibility. Perhaps there are steps you can take to enjoy your pregnancy. If your ambivalence is triggered by the nausea, know that this too shall pass and you will soon begin to enjoy your pregnant body much more.

- Eat small, frequent snacks that contain complex carbohydrates and protein. A simple snack of a cheese sandwich on whole-wheat toast will quell hunger, prevent blood sugar from dropping with ensuing nausea, and is quick and easy to prepare. Other suggestions: tofu sandwiches, bean or chicken noodle soup, pasta dishes, yogurt with granola, peanut butter on toast with a topping you enjoy, hummus on toast, chips, crackers, or vegetable sticks. Eating snacks about every two hours is less likely to trigger nausea and vomiting than a few large meals a day; in doing so you will prevent your stomach from becoming empty. Eating a snack such as crackers or toast when you first wake in the morning can reduce the nausea caused by stomach acids in an empty stomach. Some women find that a grapefruit or a small cup of fruit juice just before a meal gets the digestive juices going just enough to help food go down. Breakfast, or its lack, can set the tone for your entire day, so be sure not to skimp on it.

- Many women wake in the night and find themselves unable to return to sleep. This is frequently due to unrecognized hunger; the baby takes nourishment from you even while you sleep, causing you to become hungry at odd hours. Try eating a snack before bed and, if necessary, in the middle of the night. This may seem odd, but you'll find yourself sleeping more restfully. Yogurt makes an excellent before-bed or middle-of-the-night snack, as does toast, a banana, a handful of almonds, any food that you enjoy and that digests easily.

- Always carry nutritious food with you whenever you go out. Skipping food for as little as two hours during early pregnancy can cause you to feel extremely nauseated and depleted. Hypoglycemia—low blood sugar—can trigger not only nausea but also dizziness, headaches, hot flashes followed by cold sweats, anxiety, and fainting. A mix of nuts and seeds, a container of yogurt, or even small containers of food can keep you feeling well. Don't tide yourself over with caffeinated beverages or candy bars—you won't be providing yourself or your baby with any nutrients, and you'll still end up feeling nauseous in the long run. There is no need to feel embarrassed about eating in public

wherever you are, even if no one else is eating.

- Many pregnant women find that drinking fluids aggravates nausea, but actually dehydration causes worse problems. You need to drink plenty of liquids throughout the day. If you are vomiting you are losing fluids, so you must replenish them. Water with a squeeze of lemon, natural grape juice, grapefruit, or orange juice, or carbonated water with a squeeze of lemon are all choices that may be palatable and settle your stomach. Avoid coffee, soda, and other caffeinated or sugar-laden drinks. Taking sips of liquids throughout the day may be easier than drinking glassfuls at a time.

- Oily foods are hard to digest. Sweet foods may lead to a quick blood sugar drop after their initial energy boost, leaving you feeling nauseous and drained. Choose foods that are prepared by steaming, water-sautéing, or baking; choose foods that contain complex carbohydrates. These will sustain your energy level in a more balanced way and are also easier to digest, helping you avoid nausea. See Chapter 5 for a discussion on nutrition.

- Nutritional deficiencies—too little iron, vitamin B-complex, magnesium, or calcium—as well as too little protein or complex carbohydrates can cause morning sickness. Perhaps you didn't really notice these deficiencies until your body had the increased nutritional demands of pregnancy. Consider taking a vitamin and mineral supplement designed for pregnant and lactating women. See Chapter 5 for more information.

Unfortunately, supplements may aggravate nausea in the first trimester. If this is the case, avoid taking supplements on an empty stomach; instead, try taking them while eating. Some women have found that taking between 50 and 200 mg of vitamin B6 daily can alleviate nausea because it helps regulate blood sugar levels. This is safe. Once you have gotten past the nausea stage, you should take vitamin B-complex, not just B6 by itself. Another remedy is to take 50 mg of vitamin K once daily, and 250 mg of vitamin C twice daily.

HERBAL RECOMMENDATIONS

During my pregnancies I would try something for nausea and that would work for a few days. But I would quickly become tired of a certain herb and keep changing. Play around with different approaches to see what works for you.

- Dandelion root is one of my favorite herbs. It seems to sweeten the sour feeling, calms and strengthens the stomach, improves the appetite, and supports the liver, which must work overtime during pregnancy to process the increased quantity of hormones surging through you. Dandelion root is also highly nutritive. All of these functions of dandelion root plus its safety during pregnancy make it an excellent choice for morning sickness. To prepare an infusion, use 4 to 6 tablespoons of the dried roots or twice that amount of the fresh roots in 1 quart of boiling water, and steep for four hours. Strain and take mouthfuls at a time, up to 2 cups daily. Or take 30 drops of tincture three or four times a day. You can also use dandelion leaves in infusion or tincture, or preferably, as a vegetable.

- Ginger tea can quell nausea by improving sluggish digestion and gently warming the digestive tract. It is pleasant tasting when sweetened lightly with honey. Steep 1 teaspoon of freshly grated ginger root in 1 cup of boiling water for ten minutes and sip throughout the day. Or take powdered ginger in capsules, up to 2 every few hours, but do not exceed 10 capsules per day. Sucking ginger-flavored hard candies can also be helpful. Look for these in a health food store that carries macrobiotic products.

CAUTION: *Ginger is an emmenagogue, that is, it induces or hastens menstrual flow, and excessive use in early pregnancy may cause miscarriage. Do not use if you have a history of miscarriage, and do not exceed the dosages mentioned above.*

- Chamomile tea is another of my personal favorites. It relaxes the stomach, reduces acidic feelings, supports the liver, stimulates the gallbladder, and improves appetite. It also reduces anxiety and tension. Prepare by steeping 1 tablespoon of the herb in 1 cup of boiling water for ten to fifteen minutes. Cover while steeping to retain the volatile oils in the blossoms. You can sip it throughout the day or drink up to 2 cups daily.

- Many herbs in the mint family, including peppermint, spearmint, catnip, and lemon balm, will reduce digestive upsets. To prepare any of these teas, steep a heaping teaspoon of the dried leaves or 2 teaspoons of fresh leaves in 1 cup of boiling water (steep with the cover on to retain volatile oils) for fifteen minutes. Occasionally women find that strong mint teas actually aggravate nausea. This is probably due to the nature of the plant, which causes a strong rising up of the body's energy. Most women find the scent of peppermint beneficial, however. You can place 1 or 2 drops of peppermint oil on a small piece of cloth and smell it periodically, or if you have access to the fresh plant, crush a few leaves between your fingers and smell it as needed. I always found this to be helpful on long car rides, which terribly aggravated my nausea during pregnancy.

CAUTION: *Pennyroyal, also a member of the mint family, causes miscarriages and is dangerous to use during pregnancy.*

- Wild yam is an herb that balances the hormonal system and reduces irritation and irritability. It is an excellent herb for reducing nausea and relieving vomiting. The dosage is up to 30 drops, four to six times daily. You can also use false unicorn root and chasteberry; a combination tincture combining equal parts of these three herbs may be taken at the same dosage.

Other remedies that can be useful for morning sickness include

- Miso broth
- Chicken soup
- Peach leaf infusion, sipped as needed
- Umeboshi (sour plum) candies, available at natural foods stores (the sweet-and-sour taste of umeboshi can allay nausea)
- Activated charcoal, 2 capsules when you feel queasy, up to twice a day
- Homeopathic sepia, nux vomica, or ipecac (all 30x)
- A warm bath to which you add essential oils such as lavender and rose or a few drops of sandalwood

In addition, some women gain relief from Chinese herbs and acupuncture or acupressure treatment. For information on Chinese therapeutics for pregnancy, you may wish to consult *The Path of Pregnancy* by Bob Flaws, listed in "Further Reading."

PROTEIN IN URINE

(see Urine Testing for Protein, Sugar, or Ketones)

SCIATICA

(see Backaches and Sciatica)

SKIN TROUBLES

(see Itchiness and Skin Troubles)

STRETCH MARKS

Silvery jewelry draped on the belly of Woman, adorning her and reflecting her ability to grow and change—this is how I view stretch marks. Some women develop stretch marks; others don't. Various factors may be involved: heredity, nutrition, tissue strength, the elasticity of your skin. There are no definitive answers.

Most women do not want stretch marks any more than they want sagging breasts. Our society tells us that flat bellies, perky breasts, and tight flesh are sexy and beautiful. Unfortunately, these characteristics are present in young women who have not borne children. They are associated with a sexual ideal that few women actually approach even before childbearing. The body after childbearing is typically not considered beautiful in our culture, although in others, for example the Mbuti pygmies of Africa, pendulous breasts are respected because they reflect the fact that a woman has nourished her community through her very flesh. In fact, the more a woman's breasts sag, the greater her status in the community. It is time that we, as active participants in our culture, take pride in our individual form, shape, and markings, and help change society with our values.

Women are often advised to massage their bellies with cocoa butter or other oils to prevent stretch marks. This is all well and good. It may be effective, but it is not loving yourself to rub your belly with the intention of preventing stretch marks. To love yourself, rub your belly and breasts with awe at the amazing accommodation your body is giving to your growing baby. Babies can feel this attention and they love it! Praise and admire yourself, and you will be rewarded with self-respect, whether or not you develop stretch marks.

Lydia was having mild swelling in her right hand and right foot, as well as heart palpitations. She had no history of heart disease, and the swelling seemed to be associated with sleeping on her right side. She began to sleep on her left side and take a combination of Motherwort and Hawthorn extracts. Within three weeks the swelling ceased to occur, and the heart palpitations also stopped.

Oils and herbs that are nourishing for the skin include cocoa butter, pure almond oil or wheat germ oil, and herbal oils made with chamomile, lavender, calendula, rose petals, and comfrey. You can make a wonderful belly and breast massage oil for your breasts and belly by mixing a few handfuls of any of these herbs in a pint jar with 2 cups of an oil of your choice. If you wish to use cocoa butter, use half oil and half cocoa butter, and carefully cook the mixture over a double boiler for twenty to thirty minutes because cocoa butter is hard at room temperature. Cover the jar tightly and let sit on a sunny windowsill for one week. Strain the oil into another jar, and it is ready for use. You can add a few drops of an essential oil for fragrance, if you wish, and 400 IU of vitamin E as a preservative and skin nutrient. See Appendix I, "Herbal Preparations," for further instructions on making herbal oils.

SUGAR IN URINE

(see Urine Testing for Protein, Sugar, or Ketones)

SWELLING

Mild swelling of the feet and ankles is considered normal as pregnancy advances and may actually signal that blood volume has expanded enough to meet the needs of the pregnancy. Some women do not swell at all, and as long as they've gained weight adequately, have plenty of amniotic fluid, and anemia is not a problem, that is also fine.

I pay attention to the severity and constancy of the swelling. "Healthy" swelling is usually mild, occurs mainly in the feet and ankles, and tends to come and go—appearing more after you've been on your feet a lot

or at the end of the day, and going down a good deal after you rest and in the morning when you've just awakened. Swelling that is present all the time, swelling that leaves an impression on your leg a few seconds after you press on it, or swelling that particularly occurs in your face and hands that is visible the first thing in the morning, may be signs of toxemia. This section addresses only normal physiological swelling, but you can use these suggestions in conjunction with other therapies for more specific conditions.

GENERAL RECOMMENDATIONS

- Elevate your feet for twenty minutes, three to four times each day. Put them on pillows to get them above the level of your heart to improve circulation. The weight of your uterus on your blood vessels impedes venous return, causing blood and fluid to collect in your lower body. Allowing this circulation to freely return to your heart not only reduces swelling but also can be invigorating and lift depression.

- Lying on your left side while you sleep or rest can also improve circulatory function, thereby lessening swelling.

- Exercise for thirty minutes a day. Pelvic rocks, leg lifts, and gentle yoga can enhance circulation and reduce swelling. See "Further Reading" for books on yoga and exercise during pregnancy.

DIETARY RECOMMENDATIONS

- Be certain that your diet contains plentiful amounts of high-quality protein and adequate salt plus all the other nutrients you need. Inadequate intake of protein and salt is linked to toxemia. Without this adequate intake, your cells cannot retain fluid, and you will have swelling from the seepage of fluid into the interstitial spaces (the spaces between the cells). Pregnancy is a time to eat foods salted to taste. Be certain to compensate for salt lost in perspiration either in hot weather or after exercise, and use only sea salt available at natural foods stores.

HERBAL RECOMMENDATIONS

- Soak your feet in a warm bath, using 1/2 cup of Epsom salts in a basin, or 1 cup in the bathtub, high enough to cover your feet. To the Epsom salted water, you can add lavender flowers, rose petals, sprigs of rosemary, or drops of wintergreen oil.

- Get a regular foot massage. Arnica oil rubbed into swollen areas reduces soreness and aching in muscles and joints. Your mate or friend can easily give you a foot massage as you sit together. Perhaps have your partner rub your feet before you go to sleep at night (lie on your left side to enhance effectiveness).

- Drink a nettle and dandelion infusion (1 to 2 cups) daily, or take 15 to 20 drops of each of these tinctures twice a day to improve general circulation, help the kidneys remove and retain the appropriate amounts of fluids for your body, and improve your overall nutritional status.

If you have persistent swelling, speak with your care provider for further suggestions. Do not accept diuretics and salt restricted diets as your solution as they are almost always inappropriate for pregnant women. See books by Anne Frye and Gail and Tom Brewer (see "Further Reading") for further discussion of the problems associated with these treatments.

TOXEMIA

I would like to thank midwife and author Anne Frye for her remarkable work to educate and enlighten midwives and other related health professionals on the key issues underlying toxemia and on the very real ways we may address and prevent this serious health problem with excellent prenatal care. I am also indebted to her commitment to restore healing and empowerment to all women whether pregnant or in their work as midwives, and her gracious permission to incorporate her research into this section.

Toxemia, formally called "metabolic toxemia of pregnancy," or "pre-eclampsia," is a serious condition, the consequences of which include placental insufficiency (insufficient nutrients get to the baby, resulting in undernourishment and low birth weight), placental abruption (the placenta separates prematurely, which predisposes the mother to hemorrhage and is often fatal for the baby), premature birth, complicated births, and, if untreated, eclampsia, a complicated stage of the disease that can lead to seizures and liver damage for the mother, even her death. In short, it is not a condition to be ignored or taken lightly.

The causes of toxemia have been related to a few factors, including heredity and faulty implantation of the placenta, but the most probable factor is poor nutrition.

Toxemia is usually diagnosed when three main symptoms—high blood pressure, swelling, and protein in the mother's urine—occur together. Women can have one or two of these signs and may or may not be at risk. In fact, women who exhibit only one of two of the symptoms may be at risk for toxemia but it may be overlooked as a possibility, in part because toxemia symptoms often do not become apparent until the third trimester. Other symptoms may indicate toxemia: severe and persistent nausea past the first trimester, poor appetite, headaches, poor weight gain, upper abdominal pain, blurry vision or seeing flashing lights before your eyes, feeling "lousy," and persistent hypoglycemia.

If your baby seems small for its gestational age and you have symptoms of toxemia, you certainly should consult your health care provider. It is always wise to determine the origins of your symptoms. If you are eating an excellent diet and feel otherwise healthy and vibrant, and the baby is growing steadily, you are unlikely to have or develop toxemia.

Any woman who is having trouble obtaining high-quality nutrients (meaning adequate protein, carbohydrates, vitamins, minerals, fluids, and salt) is at risk for toxemia. Pregnant teenagers, poor women, underweight women, and exercise-conscious women are at higher risk. If you fit into any of these categories, you should eat well and you ought to discuss any eating problems with your midwife or obstetrician.

While all of this may seem rather grim, the good news is that toxemia appears to be preventable if you get excellent prenatal care, both the care you give to yourself and the care you receive from others.

The guidelines in this section are for the prevention of pre-eclampsia, and therefore you would be wise to read them carefully *before* you exhibit symptoms.

WARNING: *Should toxemia develop, begin following these suggestions immediately, and get medical help.*

Remember that even the public health department provides prenatal screening. For more information about toxemia, consult the books by Gail and Tom Brewer and Anne Frye listed in "Further Reading."

DIETARY RECOMMENDATIONS

- Inadequate nutrition is the common denominator in toxemia. Read the information on nutrition in Chapter 5, and follow the suggestions for creating an ideal diet diary.

- Make sure you get between 60 and 100 grams of protein per day. (See Chapter 5 for a full discussion of protein and nutritional sources.) Protein is essential for healthy cell functioning and proper kidney functioning. It is also essential to help the body maintain fluid in the cells. Women who get enough protein rarely develop toxemia.

- Complex carbohydrates are essential for energy, blood sugar stability, and healthy weight gain. Eat whole-grain foods at all meals and as part of snacks during pregnancy.

- You must obtain enough salt to maintain the blood volume you and your baby need. Salt-restricted diets can actually lead to toxemia. You need extra salt as well as extra protein and carbohydrates if you exercise regularly.

- Vitamins and minerals are also essential. You should get them from organic foods and herbs, and take nutritional supplements when necessary.

- Junk foods are an express ticket to poor health. They keep you from eating nutritious foods because their high sugar or fat content causes you to feel full. Teach yourself about healthy eating. Your health and your baby's health depend upon it!

- Healthy absorption of nutrients is as important as healthy eating. Regular constipation or frequent diarrhea is a sign that your intestinal health needs direct attention. For constipation, refer to that topic on page 146. For diarrhea, mix equal parts of slippery elm bark powder, marshmallow root powder, licorice root powder, and cinnamon powder. Place in "00" capsules and take 2 three times a day, preferably just before meals. Try this for one week and discontinue when your bowels are no longer loose.

- An excellent nutritional supplement for pregnant women is spirulina. This super-food is a blue-green alga with high protein, vitamin, and mineral content. It is harvested from lakes where it occurs naturally. The dosage is 2 tablespoons of powder or 15 to 30 tablets (depending on the particular brand you choose) daily. Powdered spirulina can be added to smoothies to disguise the taste (it will turn your smoothie an interesting shade of green!). Here is a nutritious smoothie recipe even kids will drink:

Spirulina Smoothie

In a blender place 1 cup of naturally sweetened vanilla yogurt; 1 tablespoon of spirulina; one or two bananas; 1 tablespoon of peanut, almond, or sesame butter; and if in season, a handful of blueberries or a few strawberries. Optionally, you can add 1 tablespoon of brewer's yeast or 1 teaspoon of bee pollen as well as 1 teaspoon of honey if needed for taste. Blend well at a high speed and enjoy.

HERBAL RECOMMENDATIONS

- The liver and kidneys are the two organ systems most likely to need support for preventing toxemia. Weakness of these organs seems to play a role in the development of toxemia, and these organs are likely to be further damaged if it arises. The following formula can be taken daily for toxemia prevention and for liver and kidney wellness (take 1 cup daily) or for restoring health if you seem at risk for this condition (take 2 cups daily).

Liver and Kidney Wellness Formula

Mix together 1 ounce each of nettle and oatstraw; 1/2 ounce each of dandelion root, yellow dock root, burdock root, false unicorn root, and wild yam; 1/4 ounce each of passion flower and skullcap; and 1/8 ounce of chopped ginger root (dried). Steep 4 to 6 tablespoons of this mix in a covered vessel with 1 quart of boiling water for one to two hours. Strain and drink a quarter cup at a time throughout the day. This formula strengthens the liver and kidneys, provides minerals, supports relaxation, and assists in stabilization of both blood sugar and blood pressure.

- Nettle infusion can be taken as well. Drink 2 cups as a beverage in addition to the above formula. Dandelion greens can be added to the diet as a lively tasting green, steamed or used in salads, that is highly nutritious and beneficial to health.
- Kelp powder is a mineral supplement that can be taken daily throughout pregnancy for optimal wellness. Take 2 "00" capsules twice a day, or eat as a vegetable (in dried or fresh form it is known as "kombu").

URINE TESTING FOR PROTEIN, SUGAR, OR KETONES

These are not complaints specific to pregnancy, but this section is included here because urine tests for these substances are an almost-universal routine part of the prenatal exam and every woman should know what they reveal.

In urinalysis, chemically coated test strips are dipped in a sample of urine (that's why a midwife or a nurse in a physician's office will ask you to urinate in a cup). After about thirty to sixty seconds the colors on the strip will change according to the reaction of each chemical with substances in your urine. Most commonly looked for are protein, sugar, and ketones, as well as a few other substances such as leukocytes and nitrites, both of which can indicate a urinary tract infection. In my practice I usually have mothers check their own urine at their prenatal visits rather than handing it over to a technician. I want to give the women a better opportunity to understand the results. This section explains the significance of the three main substances I have mentioned and provides recommendations should you come up with "positive" test results.

Urinalysis is a simple, noninvasive method for evaluating kidney functioning as well as dietary intake of carbohydrates and proteins. It can be an excellent tool for detecting an imbalance before a disorder arises. At this point, an emphasis on excellent nutrition and natural therapies can strengthen the mother, thereby averting a later health problem. Nevertheless, these tests are no substitute for the common sense and intuitive awareness you should bring to your observation of your health. This advice should hold for your health care practitioner, too. If an imbalance shows up it should lead to further investigation and to a decision as to what care would be beneficial.

During pregnancy our bodies are working much harder—we are literally eating and eliminating for two. This places an increased load on the kidneys, which control blood volume and remove wastes from the blood. According to the philosophy of traditional Chinese medicine, the kidneys play an important role in fertility, conception, pregnancy, and longevity; therefore, the child's healthy development, as well as the mother's continued wellness, will be influenced by the healthy functioning of the kidneys. This is one of the primary areas revealed when protein or sugar is identified in the urine.

—Protein in the Urine—

Usually the urine of a healthy pregnant woman will not contain protein. A trace of protein from vaginal discharge may have gotten into the urine. This is not uncommon. Protein occurring in conjunction with dark, concentrated urine indicates that the mother is not drinking enough fluids. Pregnant women need to drink close to 2 quarts of fluid a day to keep their blood volume expanded, their kidneys from becoming taxed, their bowels from becoming constipated, and, of course, the baby adequately surrounded by amniotic fluid. Adequate fluid intake even helps prevent depression.

A urinary tract infection may also cause the presence of protein in urine. Usually there will be nitrites (a byproduct of the breakdown of bacteria in the urinary tract) and leukocytes (white blood cells) as well. Often the mother will have symptoms such as lower back or lower abdominal pain, contractions, flulike feelings (chills, achiness, mild depression, or fatigue), soreness beneath the back ribs, frequent and possibly burning urination, and occasionally even vaginal bleeding. A urinary tract infection is usually highly responsive to natural remedies (see page 197), but kidney infections often require medical attention.

Other possible contributions to the presence of protein in urine are heavy physical activity, long periods of standing up, carrying twins, severe high blood pressure, and toxemia. If you must do heavy physical labor during pregnancy, it is very important to wear some form of abdominal support and to be certain you are eating enough. If at all possible, you should cut back on heavy work. If you are carrying more than one baby, you must also be certain to eat adequate amounts of protein and carbohydrates, and you may also want to wear a body support designed for pregnant women (see "Resources"). The symptoms of toxemia are high blood pressure, swelling, and protein in the urine (usually an amount of "plus 2"), but these signs in themselves do not necessarily indicate pre-eclampsia or toxemia. However, one can have toxemia without classic signs. Where toxemia is not the problem, herbal remedies may improve kidney functioning and reduce excessive swelling and the amount of protein in your urine.

—Sugar in the Urine—

The greatest medical concern regarding the presence of sugar (glucosuria) in the urine of a pregnant woman is its indicator of diabetes. There is an enormous amount of debate in the medical and midwifery communities over this condition, which is linked with high levels of blood sugar, very large babies and the attendant risks of birthing larger babies, and "unexplained" fetal deaths. Nevertheless, it is perfectly normal for pregnant women to have a lower kidney threshold that allows more sugar to be spilled in the urine. Sugar in the urine leads many health care practitioners to insist upon testing blood glucose levels. But this test does not necessarily mean that a woman is diabetic. In fact, even a slightly high result from a blood sugar test (glucose tolerance tests or one-, two-, or three-hour postprandial or after-meal testing) does not always imply diabetes. A common cause of glucosuria (sugar in the urine) is the recent consumption of foods with a high sugar content, even those containing natural sugars like fruits and juices, and even sweet, high-carbohydrate items like granola or pancakes with syrup. Consequently, a practitioner is left with the question of how to interpret the sugar in the urine, and what

to do about it if it is consistently present, especially if it is high.

In my own clinical experience I have seen mothers who have had consistently high levels of glucose in their urine (up to "plus 4" at three successive prenatal visits) but who reduced their levels of urinary glucose to zero simply by making dietary changes. All these women, when tested in a medical setting for blood glucose levels, had normal levels according to a one- or two-hour postprandial (after eating a high sugar meal, their blood levels were tested after either one or two hours) test and had normal pregnancies and babies with no unusual difficulties at the birth. This is not to say that health care practitioners should ignore the possibility of diabetes. It does indicate that there may be factors that influence its development, and therefore factors that can prevent it. Of course, if you find that you consistently see high glucose levels despite preventative measures, and the baby seems exceptionally large, you may choose to investigate further with a *nonfasting* blood glucose test, particularly if you have evidence of regular yeast or urinary tract infections that are also unresponsive to treatment or reoccur despite dietary and other measures. Other common symptoms of diabetes include frequent thirst and lack of weight gain or actual weight loss in spite of a voracious appetite.

There is overwhelming evidence that the use of routine glucose testing for pregnant women is an unnecessarily invasive procedure that is best reserved for situations in which the need for the test is clearly indicated. Fasting or loading up on concentrated amounts of sugar, as in a glucose tolerance test, is not good for a pregnant woman. Speak with your midwife or physician about alternatives if a blood test seems

Ruby was having high levels of glucose appearing in her urine test (+3 sugar) at several consecutive prenatals. Prior to her fourth visit she agreed to eliminate most sugars from her diet, including fruit and natural sweeteners, and she daily took a strong infusion of nettles. Within one week her urinary sugar levels were completely normal, with not even a trace of sugar present.

necessary to rule out gestational diabetes. Request that a first morning blood sugar be drawn or a one-hour postprandial done early in the morning after you consume a high-carbohydrate meal (like a large amount of pancakes with maple syrup for breakfast). These methods put the least nutritional stress on both you and the baby. I encourage you to read the sections on gestational diabetes in Anne Frye's books *Understanding Lab Work in the Childbearing Year* and *Holistic Midwifery* and bring the well-researched, thoroughly documented information in her books to the attention of your care provider. In addition, you may want to try the nutritional and herbal suggestions later in this section, which can be effective in preventing gestational diabetes and will strengthen your kidneys and improve your general wellness.

—*Ketones in the Urine*—

The body of a well-nourished pregnant woman is supplied with energy by the regular intake of a high-carbohydrate and protein-rich diet. When the intake of food becomes inadequate, the body must burn fat to supply energy until food sources again become available. Ketones are a product of the metabolism of fat and occur when the body suffers nutritional deprivation, such as from fasting or inadequate nutritional intake, or when a great deal of physical energy is being expended and not replenished, such as during vigorous exercise and labor. If you have ketones in your urine (ketonuria), you are not eating enough or you are not eating frequently enough. This condition is often signaled by symptoms of hypoglycemia (low blood sugar): extreme and sudden hunger accompanied by shakiness, nausea, cold sweat, feelings of faintness, slurred speech, a vague sense of dread, and

extreme exhaustion. After you eat you may feel the need to rest or even sleep. If these symptoms continue, serious health problems can emerge for both you and the baby.

The treatment, quite logically, is to *eat more high-quality foods, eat more often, and drink plenty of fluids!* The exception is when ketones and glucose are occurring together, which is an indication of diabetes. Although this condition may also be nutritionally related, it does require further consideration and testing. In either case, it is essential that you focus on learning more about your nutritional needs during pregnancy and take steps to improve your diet—not just what you eat but how much and how often. In addition to the suggestions given below, see Chapter 5 and refer to "Further Reading" for books on prenatal nutrition.

GENERAL, DIETARY, AND HERBAL RECOMMENDATIONS

- If you have only a trace of any of the above substances on just one test, then really nothing needs to be done other than to consider the possible causes. For example, if you have a lot of vaginal discharge, you may have a trace of protein show on the "pee stick" (as they are fondly called). If you ate a sweet breakfast or a large cup of juice before an early-morning visit, that could easily account for sugar in your urine. Similarly, if you worked out or skipped a meal before your urine-check, that is the likely explanation for ketones. In this case, you need to eat extra food before and after your workout to compensate for the extra burning of calories so you don't develop ketonuria.

- A trace of protein occurring on a regular basis could be due to an abundance of vaginal discharge, a urinary or vaginal infection (see appropriate sections in this book), or weakened kidneys.

- If sugar is consistently present in your urine, you will want to work on your diet and observe whether the changes you make has influenced its level. To do this, you need to reduce your consumption of sugar in all forms for three days. This includes eliminating fruits and fruit juices, any products containing sweeteners including all sweeteners, fruit juice, and bakery-type products—anything that is sweet or readily breaks down into simple sugars. Your diet should consist of whole grains, preferably rice, millet, and other grains; high-protein foods such as beans, nuts and seeds, hard cheese, fish, and poultry (organic whenever possible to avoid contaminants), and plenty of fresh vegetables. After three days, recheck your urine. If there is just a trace of sugar or none at all, you can most likely avoid further testing and continue on this type of diet with the addition of one or two pieces of fresh fruit daily. You can periodically check your urine to see if it is affected by the intake of sugary foods, and if it is negative when these are again eliminated from your diet. If the dipstick still shows a high sugar result in spite of your dietary efforts, a blood test may be warranted. Refer to the suggestions below for herbs that can be used along with dietary changes to improve kidney functioning and regulate blood sugar.

- Perhaps the most effective and yet gentlest herbal ally for nourishing and strengthening the kidneys during pregnancy is the humble nettle plant. This herb is reputed to restore health to damaged kidneys, improve the kidney filtration process, tonify the kidneys, regulate blood sugar, ease fatigue, improve the functioning of the adrenal glands and the thyroid, reduce stress, and provide a rich banquet of minerals. Taken daily, nettle can reduce both protein and sugar in the urine, reduce swelling and varicosities, alleviate low backache, urinary tract infections, circles under the eyes, damp feet, and other signs of compromised kidneys. A preventative dosage is 1 cup of nettle infusion daily, and a therapeutic dosage is up to a quart daily. I prepare a dark green nettle brew (more than once I've been asked, "What is that green stuff you are drinking, Aviva?")—à la Susun Weed, who told me she makes her nettle infusion so strong that the spoon stands up by itself in the cup—by steeping a handful of nettle herb in a quart of boiling water. I leave the herbs in the jar rather than straining them out, and I just sip off the top as the leaves gradually sink to the bottom over the course of the day. This drink has a flavor similar to a liquid chlorophyll supplement. For a milder brew, you can steep 4 tablespoons of nettle leaf in a quart of water for thirty minutes or up to two hours, and then strain out the herbs and drink the infusion. It will keep in the refrigerator overnight and is delicious with the addition of a dash of tamari soy sauce or umeboshi plum vinegar, a salty and sour Japanese seasoning available at health food stores. Nettle may also be obtained in freeze-dried form, which some claim to be highly effective (see "Resources").

URINARY INCONTINENCE

Involuntary leaking urine (urinary incontinence) can happen when you sneeze, cough, jump, or perform any physical exertion. It can vary in amounts ranging from a small dribble to a deluge wetting your pants. It is a common problem in America. Women who have already borne children are particularly susceptible to developing incontinence because the muscles of the pelvic floor stretch during birth. Further pregnancies will aggravate this tendency because pregnancy increases urination and because the uterus places a great deal of pressure on the bladder. Incontinence is not inevitable, however. In fact, it is quite preventable. In addition to urinary dribbling, you can also prevent uterine, bladder, and rectal prolapse (see "Further Reading" for an article I wrote on this subject), maintain long-term pelvic health, and improve your sexual experience.

The levator ani is a muscle group, commonly known as the pelvic floor, that forms a sling extending from the back of the pelvis to the front and supports all the pelvic organs and structures, including the uterus, bladder, vagina, urethra, and rectum. When the muscles forming this sling become weakened, they are less able to support these organs, and signs and symptoms of weakness begin to appear, one of the earliest and most common being urinary incontinence. At the first sign of this, do pelvic floor exercises to improve the tone of your muscles. If you wait until you have severe incontinence or prolapse of your organs, you will have to work much harder to improve tone.

Pelvic floor exercises, generally referred to as "Kegel exercises" after the physician who originally popularized them, is a nonsurgical method of healing urinary incontinence. With all due respect, I will refer to such exercises as "pelvic muscle exercises." Chapter 7 offers specific exercises that are beneficial for the prevention and healing of pelvic floor weakness, including incontinence. Follow these exercises each day. With commitment you will see improvement after a few weeks, even if you begin during pregnancy.

I have no internal recommendations for incontinence, although you may wish to try a sitz bath with astringent herbs such as witch hazel and nettle to help tighten the outer muscles and tonify your tissue.

URINARY TRACT INFECTIONS (UTIS)

The urinary tract consists of the kidneys, ureters, bladder, and urethra. Growing a baby places an additional load on these organs. Hormonal changes that soften the ureters, along with the weight of the womb upon them and the bladder, increase the likelihood of stasis, or stagnation, in your bladder or ureters, which breeds bacteria that can lead to infection.

Bladder infections (cystitis) can nearly always be treated at home with natural remedies. Beginning treatment at the earliest symptoms is optimal. Symptoms include extra-frequent urination (it's normally somewhat frequent during pregnancy), often accompanied by burning or pain ranging from subtle to severe; low abdominal tenderness just above the pubic bone; recurrent Braxton-Hicks contractions (the contractions normally occurring during pregnancy that you may or may not have noticed); flulike feelings; in some cases, vaginal bleeding ranging from mild to severe. A kidney infection (pylonephritis) is evidenced by fever, chills, backache, and a worsening of the previously mentioned bladder infection.

WARNING: *Left untreated, a bladder infection can easily become a kidney infection. Kidney infections can place the mother's health in danger, so the care of an experienced health professional should be sought immediately.*

Persistent UTIs can increase the risk of premature labor. You should always be screened for this if you are having a lot of premature uterine contractions or have a history of premature labor. If you experience persistent urinary tract infections, you will want to do more than address each individual bout; you will need to tonify your urinary organs but also improve your overall immunity. You may also want to have a vaginal culture for possible beta-strep infection, a bacteria that many women carry around with no symptoms, but which can lead to UTIs, premature labor, and neonatal infection. A high blood sugar level can also predispose you to UTIs, as can recent overconsumption of highly sweetened foods; refer to page 193 regarding sugar in your urine. You may not have sugar in your urine, but the dietary and herbal recommendations in that section will likely be useful. Consultation with a Chinese herbalist may provide help in preventing these repeated infections.

Refer also to "Vaginal Infections" for recommendations. Because the urethra (the entrance to the bladder) is located just above the entrance to the vagina and not far from the rectal opening, bacteria can easily spread to the bladder.

Many times women who have chronic urinary tract infections have underlying anger that seems to correlate with UTI recurrences. I've always gotten a chuckle out of the common expression for anger—"pissed off"—realizing that language arises from our subconscious mind as much as from our literal or analytic minds. Language can be revealing. Look within yourself about anger you may have, and if this registers, take the steps that will help you address and express your anger or resentment so you can resolve your problems without internalizing them as illnesses.

The following program has repeatedly assisted pregnant women in clearing up UTIs. It must be followed diligently.

- Dramatically reduce your intake of all sugars—sugar breeds bacteria.

- Be sure to urinate as soon as you feel the urge, and empty your bladder thoroughly. When you hold urine too long, it can serve as a breeding ground for bacteria. Too many women are accustomed to putting off urinating until they can no longer wait. This is an unnecessary and health-defeating habit based on not listening to our bodies and making external tasks more important than the body's needs. When you've got to go, go!

- Take echinacea root tincture, 1 drop per every 2 pounds of body weight every four hours until symptoms are gone, then 20 drops three times a day for a few more days to prevent recurrence. Echinacea is antimicrobial, it is an immune-system tonic, and it reduces inflammation.

- Cranberry juice, an old wives' remedy for UTIs, has been clinically demonstrated to be effective as an antimicrobial agent in the treatment of bladder infections. Eight ounces of unsweetened cranberry juice, or *diluted* cranberry juice concentrate, should be taken every four hours, along with four 8-ounce glasses of water each day, for a total of 64 ounces of fluid. This will dilute your urine, so that it is less burning. It also dilutes and flushes out the infecting organisms. A substance in cranberry juice prevents bacteria from adhering to the bladder lining.

One way my family enjoys cranberries is to blend 1/2 cup of frozen cranberries in the blender with 1 cup unsweetened apple juice and 2 cups water. We also put cranberries and fresh apples through our juicer for a refreshing, mildly tart drink very high in vitamin C. Take this high dosage for three to five days; then, when the infection is gone, continue to drink cranberry juice once a day for at least a few days.

- Take 500 mg of vitamin C four times each day for three to five days. Vitamin C encourages acidification of the urine, helping to kill bacteria and is also a reputable resource for helping the body resist and overcome infection.

Suzanne was experiencing insomnia, frequent urination, nausea, low backache, mild discomfort in her lower abdomen, and a slightly elevated pulse. She followed dietary and herbal protocols for the treatment of a urinary tract infection, and also began to take a relaxing nervine tea in the evening, including chamomile, lavender, and skullcap. Within 2 weeks all symptoms of the UTI had cleared up and she was sleeping restfully.

- Uva-ursi is a leathery-leafed bush that provides a medicine known to act on urinary tract infections, working specifically as an antimicrobial and gentle diuretic. In small quantities it is a highly effective, safe remedy for cystitis. It could also be used for mild kidney involvement, but that is best when accompanied by medical care. To prepare uva-ursi, place 4 tablespoons of the leaves in a quart jar; fill the jar with boiling water. Some herbalists say that this herb is more effective when steeped in cold water, and you can certainly do this, but I've found that hot water makes an effective remedy. Either way, remedies directed to the urinary system are most efficient when drunk at room temperature or slightly cool—hot herbal teas encourage perspiration, whereas cool teas encourage urination. Let steep for two hours, strain, and use. The dosage is 1/4 cup every four hours for subtle signs of a UTI, 1/2 cup every four hours for obvious symptoms, and 1 cup every four hours for a raging UTI. Do this until symptoms abate, decreasing the dosage as symptoms subside, but continuing to take 1 cup a day for up to ten days. Do not take uva-ursi for longer than this. For chronic UTIs, the effectiveness of the uva-ursi may be enhanced by taking two capsules of baking soda three times daily.
- Midwife and herbalist Sister Elizabeth Perdomo offers the following excellent advice for treating a pregnant mom with a UTI: Drink corn silk tea to relieve pain and soothe the entire urinary tract (steep 2 tablespoons of corn silk in a cup of boiling water for thirty minutes). Take a full bath in oatstraw infusion to relieve sore kidneys, bladder pain, and external tenderness. Drink a lot of water with lemon juice and use dandelion leaves as food or tea to flush the system. Chickweed eaten or taken as a tea helps with chronic bladder, kidney, and urinary tract distress. Burdock root or seed tinctures (25 to 30 drops in water three to four times daily) heals a weak, irritated urinary tract and supports the liver, kidneys, and lymph system. These latter recommendations (oatstraw, chickweed, dande-

lion, and burdock) can be used regularly throughout pregnancy as tonics.
- Wild yam is a urinary tract aid as well, reducing pain and inflammation. You can add it to any of the above remedies in a dose of 15 to 20 drops, two to four times daily depending upon the infection's severity.

VAGINAL INFECTIONS

Engorgement of the vulva with increased blood circulation and hormonal changes that alter the balance of vaginal acidity cause vaginal infections and heavy mucous discharges, a common complaint of pregnant women.

Drugs, such as Metranidazole, used to treat common vaginal infections such as candida (yeast) are often not safe for developing babies, so you would be wise to avoid them.

Some vaginal infections, such as chlamydia and beta-strep, can be asymptomatic (or at least some women may be unaware of the symptoms) yet pose a health threat to a baby born vaginally in the presence of these organisms. For example, chlamydia can lead to respiratory infections and blindness in newborns. While this is rare, you may choose to have vaginal cultures taken during your pregnancy to see if you have any such infections and discuss the findings with your midwife or another care provider. It may or may not be necessary to take precautionary steps before or during labor to prevent transmission of an infection to the baby, or you may be informed of specific symptoms to look for in your baby after birth.

WARNING: *If you suspect that you have gonorrhea or syphilis, especially evidenced by vaginal or vulvar lesions or discharge, or if you have had a positive test for either of these infections, seek medical treatment as soon as possible—before the birth of your baby. The risks of these diseases outweigh the risks of treatment.*

- Drink plenty of fluids, especially water. Lemon juice and herbal teas are also good.

- Wear cotton underwear or none at all. Synthetic fibers trap moisture in the crotch area and provide an excellent breeding medium for many organisms. You may even need to change cotton underwear by mid-afternoon if it gets damp from discharge or sweat.

- Wear loose-fitting cotton clothing; try not to wear pantyhose, especially those without a cotton panel in the crotch.

- Avoid all concentrated sugars, including honey, maple syrup, and corn syrup.

- Avoid caffeine, including coffee, caffeinated sodas, chocolate, and black tea.

- Don't use bubble bath, bath oils, bath salts, or strongly perfumed soaps in your bath or around your vulva.

- Use white, unscented toilet paper.

- Don't use any "feminine hygiene" or douche products.

- Practice excellent personal hygiene: Wipe from front to back after a bowel movement. Rinse your vaginal area with water (no soap) during the day, then pat dry, to reduce the likelihood of bacterial or fungal growth.

- Bacteria spread readily in heat and moisture. Dry yourself gently but thoroughly after bathing or swimming. Change out of wet swim clothes soon after swimming. Change undergarments and launder (with a mild detergent) frequently. Use 1 cup of white vinegar in the rinse cycle of your washer to remove soap residue, acidify garments, and disinfect and remove any remaining body fluids.

- Don't scratch your crotch. Scratching will further irritate the area and spread the infection.

- Avoid intercourse during the worst symptoms or if painful. Your partner may also need to be treated to prevent reinfecting you. Men can harbor asymptomatic infections that you then pass back and forth, and your attempts at eliminating the infection will be ineffectual.

- Use some form of natural lubrication during intercourse, such as almond or coconut oil. Urinate after sex and thoroughly rinse yourself off with warm water.

- Take 500 to 1,000 mg of vitamin C complex (with bioflavonoids) daily as a preventative or when infections occur.

- Eat plenty of live-culture plain yogurt each day to both prevent and treat vaginal infections. This is especially good when you are under stress or when you must take antibiotics. (Let your doctor know if you are prone to yeast infections *before* you take antibiotics.)

- Cut back on simple carbohydrates (starches and sugars, including processed flour and fruits and fruit juices).

- Eat nutritious meals that emphasize whole grains, vegetables, and high-quality protein foods. Reduce the amount of sweets in your diet while you are treating vaginal infections. Eliminate sweets altogether if you are prone to such infections. This includes reducing the amount of fruit you eat (get your vitamins and minerals from extra vegetables) and using rice, oats, millet, and other whole grains in place of yeasted breads whenever possible. These dietary changes alone can often clear up a yeast infection.

- Reduce stress in your life as much as possible. Get adequate rest. Infections thrive when your body is run down.

—Yeast Infections—

Candida albicans is the fungal organism that causes what is commonly known as a yeast infection. All women have this organism in their bodies, but various circumstances, such as the increased vaginal discharge that accompanies pregnancy (especially if you wear clothes that prevent adequate aeration of your vulva), changes in vaginal pH, increased consumption of carbohydrates, and stress and fatigue, can lead to the overgrowth of yeast. Symptoms of a yeast infection are itching and redness of the genitals; white, thick, yeasty-smelling discharge that may look curdy like cottage cheese (but might be slight); burning of the vulva; and painful intercourse. There may be frequent urination or even an attendant bladder infection caused by irritation of the urethra. Symptoms range from mild to severe, with itching and burning being the most noticeable.

If you have no history of yeast infection, the problem will likely clear up with no treatment at all as soon as the baby is born and can simply be kept under control with simple dietary and herbal treatments. If you have a history of yeast infections, continue treatment after birth if they persist. Occasionally, a woman who has a yeast infection may pass it on to the baby during birth. The baby may then develop oral thrush, which can cause digestive distress, and in turn pass it on to the mother's nipples, causing her mild to extreme discomfort and difficulty with breastfeeding. Therefore, you should at least try to minimize all yeast infections with natural remedies before the birth. For treatment of thrush in babies and on the breasts, refer to my book, *Natural Healing for Babies and Children*, listed in "Further Reading."

Treatment of a yeast infection includes close adherence to *all* the general and dietary guidelines on page 199, as well as the following internal remedies and your choice of external applications.

INTERNAL REMEDIES

- Chickweed, burdock root, dandelion root, and echinacea are among my favorite herbs for cooling and soothing all manner of damp, inflammatory conditions. They are perfectly safe for use during pregnancy. They may be used singly or in combination, as infusions or tinctures, short or long term. To prepare an infusion, place 1 ounce of any of these herbs, or a mix of equal parts, into a quart-size jar. Fill the jar with boiling water, cover, and steep for two hours. Drink 2 cups daily as needed. Or, if you prefer, take a total of 20 to 40 drops of any single tincture or combination two to three times daily depending upon the infection's severity.

- Drink 1 tablespoon of apple cider vinegar in water once or twice a day. It can help prevent and reduce yeast infections while adding extra B vitamins to your diet. Cranberries and cranberry juice also acidify the urine, preventing bladder infections which often occur in the presence of vaginal yeast infections.

- If your yeast infection seems related to your use of antibiotics, or if you also have gas regularly, your intestinal flora may have been overly reduced by the use of antibiotics, which can allow yeast to overgrow in your system. Eat 1/2 cup of live-culture yogurt daily to help restore your intestinal flora. Seaweeds such as kelp and dulse may also improve intestinal flora, and kelp is reputed to be excellent for reducing inflammation.

EXTERNAL REMEDIES

Choose a few of these suggestions to see what works best for you. Note that all of these remedies are for external use only.

- Live-culture, plain, unsweetened yogurt is perhaps one of the most effective remedies for treating yeast infections. Applied directly to the vulva it reduces inflammation, restores your pH balance, and also restores your normal vaginal flora while destroying the yeast. The best method I know for applying the yogurt is as follows:

1. An hour before you are ready to apply the yogurt, put about 4 tablespoons of it in a dish and let it come to room temperature. This is merely a comfort measure, but it is well worth it—very cold yogurt applied to your bottom will certainly cause you to catch your breath! Use a separate dish so you don't inadvertently contaminate the entire yogurt container.

2. Insert your index finger into your vagina and gently scoop out all the yeast you can (this is best done in the shower). Yeast likes to thrive on the vaginal walls and in the area up around the cervix. Do not attempt to scrape it out; merely get out what you can so that the lactobacillus and acidophilus cultures in the yogurt stand a better chance of overcoming the yeast.

3. Wash your hands thoroughly; then put 1 to 2 tablespoons of the yogurt onto your index and middle fingers. Smear this up inside your vagina.

4. Now apply the remaining yogurt to your vulva, the external genitals, getting it well into the creases.

5. Repeat this twice a day during an acute yeast infection, a couple of times a week if you are prone to yeast outbreaks.

- Apple cider vinegar makes a great rinse for the vulva and works like yogurt. Mix 1/4 cup vinegar in 3/4 cup of warm water and apply as you did the yogurt. Vinegar can sting considerably, especially if your flesh is raw or if you have been scratching, so it is best applied in a tub of warm water.

- One traditional remedy for yeast infections is to peel a clove of garlic very carefully so as not to nick it at all. Dip the clove in olive oil and insert vaginally. Repeat with a fresh clove each night for several days in a row. It may occasionally cause burning, but garlic is highly regarded for its antifungal properties. This treatment is not always effective.

- Black walnut bark can be made into an infusion that can be used as an antifungal rinse for your vulva (not a douche). To make the infusion, mix 1 ounce per 4 cups of water; boil for twenty minutes, and then strain. Rinse once a day during an active yeast infection. Use with care as it may stain clothing.

- Acidophilus, a live culture, can be used in capsules as a nightly suppository or in liquid form as a wash. You can also smear the liquid up inside of yourself as you did with yogurt. Acidophilus can acidify an overly alkaline vaginal environment and decrease the yeast population, although some women find that acidophilus aggravates the irritation, possibly because the vaginal environment is already overly acidic. In this case a baking soda rinse—2 tablespoons per cup of warm water—can be applied to your vulva and smeared inside of the birth canal.

- Slippery elm bark powder, marshmallow root powder, and comfrey root powder soothe irritated and inflamed tissue. Sprinkle the powder on your irritated vulva or rinse yourself with a tea of any of these (or a mixture of them), getting some up inside of yourself with your fingers. To prepare a tea, mix 1 tablespoon of herbal powder with 1 cup hot water, stirring well. You can also prepare an infusion with the whole dried herbs by boiling 4 to 6 tablespoons of the herbs in 4 cups of water for twenty minutes.

- The juice of the aloe vera plant is exceptionally cooling and soothing and mildly antiseptic as well. It can be scraped from the inside of fresh leaves or purchased at natural foods stores in the form of aloe vera gel and applied. In the case of an extremely irritated vulva, you can spread some of the gel onto a cloth menstrual pad and wear it throughout the day.

- A poultice or tea of fresh chickweed is a marvelous healing and anti-inflammatory application for a yeast infection. Chickweed is readily available as a wild herb, easy to recognize, and safe to use. It's one of my favorite healing herbs. Refer to a field guide for identification of this plant.

- Healing Salve can be applied to your sore vulva as a comforting ointment. To prepare, refer to "Herbal Preparations." in Appendix I. Include chickweed, plantain, and calendula in your salve.

- Yeast-Gard is a prepackaged homeopathic suppository that many pregnant women find highly effective for the treatment of persistent, difficult yeast infections. It is available at many regular drugstores and even at some supermarkets. Health food stores also carry it.

- You can also create your own boluses (suppositories) for persistent yeast infections. While it takes a little effort, they are well worth it and you can make a large supply at a time that keeps indefinitely in the refrigerator if well wrapped. Boluses are effective for soothing inflamed vaginal membranes and are mildly antifungal. Because it is safer not to douche during pregnancy, an herbal bolus is an excellent way to apply herbs up in the vagina. By varying the herbs, you can be use boluses after birth to heal hemorrhoids.

To prepare a supply, you will need 1/2 cup of either coconut oil or cocoa butter or a combination of both (these oils become hard when cold, holding their shape, but then soften when warmed), and approximately 3/4 cup of powdered herbs. A good combination would be equal parts of goldenseal powder, echinacea powder, and burdock root powder and 1/2 cup of slippery elm powder. Melt the oil in a small pot over low heat, but do not boil. When the oil is melted, turn off the stove. Add the herbal powders and stir thoroughly until the mixture forms a thick, sticky dough. Now put some slippery elm powder onto a cutting board and place your "dough" on it. Roll the dough into the shape of a long, thin log (like the clay "snakes" you made in kindergarten) about as thick as your index finger. Cut the roll into pieces about 1 1/2 to 2 inches in length, wrap in foil, and put into the refrigerator. They will be ready to use in a couple of hours.

To use, place one bolus up into your vagina each night before bed. The bolus will melt and can be a bit messy, so wear underwear with a pad or sleep on a towel. Repeat for a week.

—Trichomonas—

This infection, caused by a single-celled protozoa, often causes a yellow-green, foamy, fishy, foul-smelling discharge that usually burns and itches. The smell and color will be the main indication that you are dealing with "trich," though it can occasionally be present without these symptoms. It is usually spread through sexual contact, but can be contracted from hot tubs, sitting on moist towels belonging to someone with trich, or even toilet seats. Trich can inhabit the penis without causing any symptoms to the man, but will cause symptoms when spread to you, so male partners should also be treated.

Trich is considered difficult to cure, so your efforts to eliminate it must be very persistent. Medications for trich are strong and should be used only as a last resort. Flagyl (Metronidazole), the most commonly used drug for treating vaginal infections, is not safe for pregnant women or babies though it is regularly prescribed during pregnancy. The brochure included in the package cautions against use during pregnancy. If you absolutely must use a medication for a vaginal infection, ask your doctor for an alternative.

WARNING: *I am personally and strongly against the use of Flagyl for anyone who is pregnant. It is potentially carcinogenic, may damage the liver, and can affect the central nervous system.*

TREATING TRICHOMONAS

- To treat trichomonas, you must *completely* abstain from sex until the treatment is complete and the infection totally cleared up. This may take a month.

- *Treatment of men*: During this time your partner should also be receiving treatment. An excellent internal remedy for men is the following combination of herbs, which reduces what in traditional Chinese medicine is known as "damp heat" and eliminates infection: Mix together 1/4 ounce each of echinacea root, yellow dock root, gentian root, goldenseal, and bupleurum, and add 1/8 ounce each of wild yam root and marshmallow root. Prepare an infusion by boiling 1 ounce total of the mix in 5 cups of water for thirty minutes. Strain and drink 1/4 to 1/2 cup three times a day for ten days. Store the prepared tea in the refrigerator for no more than two days. Or take 60 drops of echinacea tincture, 30 drops of goldenseal tincture, and 20 drops of myrrh or calendula tincture four times a day for four weeks. Wash the penis twice a day with a solution of 1/4 cup apple cider vinegar and 3/4 cup water or thyme infusion. During this regimen, men can also take two cloves of garlic each day or the equivalent amount of garlic perles. To take raw garlic, chop it finely, put it into a teaspoon of honey, and, if you can, swallow without chewing, and chase with water. This will prevent nausea, headache, and bad breath, which sometimes occur with raw garlic.

- Because trichomonas requires an alkaline environment in which to thrive, your goal is to create an acidic vaginal environment. To do this you need to rinse yourself twice daily with apple cider vinegar—a solution of 1/4 cup vinegar to 1/2 cup water. Adding 2 teaspoons each of echinacea and calendula tinctures to the wash or replacing the water with 1/2 cup of thyme tea can help reduce the infection. All of these herbs have antibacterial and antifungal properties, making them excellent for use in all cases of vaginal infection.

- It may be advisable to use a mild douche if you are dealing with trich. Use 2 tablespoons of apple cider vinegar and 1 teaspoon each of echinacea, usnea and calendula tinctures per 2 cups of water. Repeat every day for ten days for maximum effectiveness.

WARNING: *Because there is the risk of a fluid embolism from air being forced into the uterus, it is absolutely essential that you apply the douche very slowly, gently, and low in the vagina.*

- Anne Frye recommends the following for treating trich: Douche daily (2 tablespoons white vinegar and 1 tablespoon activated charcoal powder to 1 quart water) for one week, every other day the next week, and twice weekly for the next two weeks. At the same time, place two to three garlic cloves in the vagina every three hours for the first three days of treatment, then once a day overnight for the next four days. During the third week use garlic suppositories every other day, then twice during the fourth week. As garlic is a bactericidal, take yogurt in conjunction with its use. After treatment is completed, place 1 to 2 teaspoons of yogurt into your vagina (use your index and middle finger or a vaginal applicator) daily for a week to prevent a secondary yeast infection.

- Drink water with lemon, or with 1 tablespoon of apple cider vinegar and 1 teaspoon of honey, or with cranberry juice concentrate every three hours throughout the day. Take 2,000 mg of vitamin C daily and 60 drops of echinacea tincture four times a day for up to four weeks.

- A final resort for eliminating trich is to insert 2 "00" capsules of boric acid (a pharmacy grade that is pure—check at the drugstore) into the vagina up near the cervix each night for seven days. Midwives across the United States use this home remedy with no obvious long-term side effects; however, it can cause temporary, but nonetheless mildly painful, burning sensations in the vagina. If you find it too uncomfortable, sit in a tub of water and discontinue the use of this remedy.

CAUTION: *Never take boric acid by mouth—it is toxic!*

—Vaginitis, Nonspecific—

Most of the other vaginal infections are lumped together under the term *nonspecific vaginitis*. They are not venereal diseases or caused by one of the organisms already mentioned. The microbes are not specifically identified. They can be treated by following all of the general guidelines for vaginal infections as well as the suggestions for treating trichomonas.

—Beta-Strep Infection—

BETA-HEMOLYTIC STREPTOCOCCUS, BETA-STREP, OR GROUP B STREP

Anywhere from 15 to 40 percent of all healthy women at any given time will be carriers of the organism known as beta-hemolytic streptococcus—or in short, beta-strep or group B strep. This organism, which is different from group A strep (which causes sore throats, for example), is also found on the bodies of more than 40 percent of all newborns. Of these newborns, only 1 percent will become ill from this bacteria Given the prevalence of this germ with the relatively low incidence of related disease, one might wonder why physicians and midwives would be concerned about its presence in a woman's vaginal canal prenatally. The reason is that the rate of complications (including paralysis from meningitis, kidney damage, and sight and hearing loss) and mortality to the baby is very high. It is estimated that as many as 2,000 babies in the U.S. die each year as a result of beta-strep infection.

Because it is simple to determine the presence of vaginal beta-strep with a vaginal culture, many doctors and midwives will request that you have a culture done at around 26 to 30 weeks pregnancy. If beta-strep is found, then your birth will be han-

dled differently. It is recognized that the risk of beta-strep infection for the baby grows in the presence of prolonged rupture of membranes—that is, the longer your bag of waters has been broken, the greater the risk. The greatest risk is considered to occur when the waters have been ruptured for over 24 hours; therefore, part of the management of your labor will be to get your baby to be born before 24 hours has passed, even if this necessitates a cesarean. The other aspect of labor management is to place the mother on antibiotics either prior to her due date, at the time the membranes rupture, or when the mother commences labor. Different doctors, hospitals, and midwives will all vary slightly in the length of time they allow a woman to labor before becoming aggressive in speeding along the birth, and their schedule for prescribing antibiotics may also vary.

There are advantages and disadvantages of routine prenatal screening for beta-strep, and there are possibilities for natural treatments that exist beyond waiting until a woman is due to begin labor to address the potential for infection. There are also practical and natural approaches to facilitating labor and monitoring the baby during labor and in the immediate postpartum, so that aggressive methods are rarely required. Here I will discuss the advantages and disadvantages of routine prenatal screening, as well as natural treatments you might wish to try if you do have vaginal beta-strep.

The primary advantages of prenatal testing for beta-strep are that if the organism is present you can approach your labor in a way that considers the optimal health of the baby. You can also do things prenatally that reduce the amount of the organisms, reducing the likelihood of your baby contracting the organism and becoming ill. The main disadvantage is that the standard accepted medical procedures for "managing" pregnant and laboring women with beta-strep can be unnecessarily invasive, especially considering the fact that this organism is a natural part of the vaginal flora for so many women, the vast majority of whom will have babies who don't become infected.

All practitioners who assist pregnant women face a double bind with beta-strep: because of its prevalence and potential risk it is too risky to ignore, but because of the prevalence of the organism and relative low incidence of problems, it is excessive to assume the worst for all women. Therefore the best approach may be to identity those women with the greatest risk, and to provide prenatal treatment that is natural to reduce the presence of the organisms.

WARNING: *Should the risk factors be high for the likelihood of neonatal infection, or should the fetus or newborn show any signs of infection, medical care should be sought immediately.*

Women who are at the greatest risk for having an active beta-strep infection that could be passed on to the baby include those with a history of urinary tract infections, persistent yeast infections, those who go into labor before 37 weeks, a bag of waters which ruptures prematurely, or membranes that rupture before contractions begin, women who had a fever before or during labor, those who had a previously strep-infected baby, and those who had a high beta-strep count earlier in the pregnancy. Not all these factors prove the present of beta-strep; however, if these symptoms have occurred and the presence of beta-strep is confirmed, you should try to reduce the bacterial count starting at about 32 weeks, and should have your labor, and especially your baby's heart during labor and in the hours after (these will usually rise in the presence of infection), monitored carefully.

GENERAL RECOMMENDATIONS

- A positive attitude toward your body, your sexuality, and your pregnancy, along with excellent nutrition can go a long way in promoting the strength of your immune system, and preventing and reducing any infections.

- Visualize your vaginal canal as pink and healthy, a nourishing place that your baby will pass through on his or her birth journey.

- Any vaginal infection, such as yeast, that causes tissue irritation can allow other organisms (such as beta-strep) to attack the damaged tissue. Therefore, follow all of the General Recommendations for vaginal organisms found at the beginning of this section.

- Be informed (read, research, ask questions, and consult your inner wisdom) about the risks, interventions, and issues surrounding beta-strep. Be sure that you understand whether you've had this test performed, and what your care provider's protocols are. Some midwives, for example, might not be aware of beta-strep, while others might immediately transport you to the hospital if your waters have been broken for longer than eighteen hours.

- Don't allow yourself to panic when a health care provider is nervous about beta-strep. Remember, while the risk to a small percentage of babies is high, the overall incidence of this infection compared to the incidence of its presence is very low. Do your best to reduce risk factors, but continue to trust your inner guidance regarding yourself and your baby.

- Refer to other relevant topics in this book if you are experiencing factors associated with beta-strep, for example, urinary tract infections.

- Overall, an excellent diet will keep you healthy and prevent organisms from proliferating in your vaginal canal. Refer to Chapter 5, Nutrition During Pregnancy, for a full discussion of this important aspect of your prenatal health.

- A prenatal vitamin and mineral supplement can provide nutrients that may be missing in your diet and can aid your body in creating a healthy environment that prevents a growth of unwanted organisms.

- As beta-strep infections may often occur in conjunction with persistent yeast infections, addressing the dietary factors that cause yeast to proliferate may assist you in reducing beta-strep.

HERBAL RECOMMENDATIONS

Ideally you will begin treatment at about 32 weeks, on confirmation of the presence of beta-strep in a vaginal culture, a urine sample that showed beta-strep, or a rectal sample (some doctors will do both a vaginal and rectal swab). Treatment will include taking herbs orally that strengthen your immune system and applying herbs vaginally that will restore your healthy vaginal flora, that will enable your body to reduce bacterial overgrowth, and also that will directly fight the bacteria. As you enter the last few weeks of pregnancy, from 37 weeks onward, since your baby is unlikely to be premature, most midwives will be willing to assist you at home if this is your plan. In the hospital, your baby will also be considered close to full term, and will not be treated prematurely in most circumstances. At 37 weeks you can therefore begin to use certain herbs both orally and vaginally that are sometimes considered labor stimulants, but which are nonetheless effective for reducing bacterial infections.

- At 32 weeks begin to take a supplement of 500 mg of vitamin C, and 1/4 cup of burdock root and echinacea root infusion. To prepare the infusion, steep 2 to 3 tablespoons of each of these herbs in 1 ounce of boiling water for two hours. Strain and take the above dose, storing the rest in the refrigerator for the next day.

- Eat a lot of fresh garlic every day. Here are several ways to do this:

Garlic Remedies

Chop a clove of fresh garlic and mix with a teaspoon of honey. Swallow this without chewing it. This can be done several times a day, preferably with a meal.

Make a garlic elixir by blending 1/2 cup of honey, 1/4 cup of apple cider vinegar, and half a bulb of fresh garlic in your blender until liquidy. Take 1 teaspoon up to twice a day. Adjust the taste as necessary with more or less of the honey or vinegar.

Chop fresh garlic onto a salad, or mix with olive oil to use as a dressing or dip French bread into this as a condiment.

Take garlic perles according to the dosage on the brand you purchase.

- Take 25 drops of astragalus tincture up to three times a day. You can also get dried astragalus in the herb department of your health food store and cook 2 strips into a pot of rice or soup. Remove the strips when done cooking and eat the rice or soup. Astragalus is an immune system tonic well known in the

Chinese pharmacopoeia, but also found growing in America.

- At 37 weeks you can begin to take 2 cups daily of thyme tea, made by steeping 1 teaspoon of dried, or 2 teaspoons of fresh thyme herb in a cup of boiling water. Cover while you steep, and let sit for ten minutes. Strain and drink. This can be sweetened lightly if you desire. Also begin to take small doses of goldenseal root, either in capsules (2 "00" capsules, twice a day) or as tincture (15 drops of tincture, four times daily). These herbs are both noted for their antibacterial properties.

- Beginning at 32 weeks, and continuing until the end of your pregnancy (**Warning: Discontinue if you have broken waters!**) take regular sitz baths (a bath filled to the height of your hips is sufficient for this) and rinse your vaginal and perineal area with a clean "peri-bottle" (available at a pharmacy or through Cascade Health Products) of the following herbal infusion and essential oil mixture. This will help to restore vaginal flora while reducing vaginal bacterial counts. Infuse equal parts of thyme, calendula, rosemary, and yarrow, 4 to 6 tablespoons of the herbal mix per quart of water, and steep for thirty minutes. Strain into a clean jar and add 1/4 cup of sea salt and 10 drops of essential oil of lavender. If you are taking a sitz bath, add the entire jar to the tub; if you are using a peri-bottle, fill the bottle and save the remainder as a refill. You can bathe as often as once daily, and can cleanse your vulva with the peri-bottle solution after each time you urinate. Spreading your labia apart with your fingers makes the peri-rinse more effective.

- After 37 weeks (and if your waters are not broken) you can begin to insert one capsule of goldenseal into your upper vaginal canal each night before bed. Goldenseal is a natural antibiotic. You can ask your midwife or other care provider to show you how to do this if you are uncomfortable trying it on your own, but all you need to do is push the capsule inside of your birth canal as far as you can reach. The capsule will dissolve, releasing the goldenseal. You may want to sleep in an old shirt and put a towel under you to protect the sheets should the goldenseal leak out.

- After 37 weeks, if your care provider agrees, you can use the above peri-bottle and sitz bath rinse as a very gentle douche. It is imperative that the douche be low and gentle, as a forceful douche can cause an embolism in the mother, which can be fatal. If you are uncomfortable with douching, spread your labia wide open, and irrigate your whole vulvar and perineal area quite thoroughly.

Remember that a healthy diet and a healthy sexuality—both your sense of yourself as a sexual being, and your relationship with your partner—are also important in preventing and healing vaginal infections. No amount of herbal remedies can compensate for these aspects of your life. Please give thought to these ideas and find ways to nourish your body as well as finding clarity, joy, and love in your sexual experience. Also, always remember that in healing any infection you are working to restore your body's natural balance and defenses, not just attacking organisms.

VARICOSE VEINS AND HEMORRHOIDS

Varicose veins occur when the valves that keep blood flowing one way through the vessels become weak, allowing blood to pool up in the veins and causing the veins to become lax and distended. This weakness of the valves may be due to diet, lack of exercise, or heredity. The hormonal changes of pregnancy can contribute to laxity of the

Jody had severe leg and vulvar varicose veins which had become very difficult during her second pregnancy. She also had perineal tearing at birth requiring stitches. Now in her third pregnancy, the varicosities were becoming a problem, and were looking extremely red and inflamed. She began a therapeutic dietary and herbal program to include foods high in bioflavinoids and rutin, nettles infusion and hawthorn tincture, and regular periods of rest as well as daily inversion on a slant board. Externally she applied compresses of witch hazel extract from the pharmacy. The inflammation completely subsided and while the varicosities were still obviously visible throughout the pregnancy, they remained unproblematic, and Jody gave birth at home with no difficulty. In addition, she had no perineal tearing with this birth.

valves. Pregnancy also predisposes women to congestion of blood in the lower body because the pressure from the heavy uterus reduces venous return from the legs and pelvis. Varicosities most commonly occur in the legs and feet, the vulva (vulvar varicosities), and the anus (hemorrhoids). They generally become more pronounced as pregnancy advances. Vulvar varicosities may or may not be noticeable until labor, but women usually notice large ones during pregnancy. A gentle birth and hot compresses applied to the distended veins usually prevent trauma to them. Occasionally, bleeding or a hematoma (an internal pooling of blood from a broken blood vessel) can result and may require medical care. Hemorrhoids usually become enlarged at the birth with the mom's pushing and may persist for a few days postpartum. Again, gentle pushing whenever possible will reduce their severity. Constipation during pregnancy aggravates hemorrhoids and should be treated because it can cause other health problems as well.

Natural remedies regularly taken and applied can effectively prevent and reduce varicose veins.

GENERAL RECOMMENDATIONS

- Follow all dietary and exercise suggestions, and use appropriate herbal remedies.

- Exercise can vastly improve circulation and must be a vital component in both the prevention and treatment of varicosities. By increasing your circulatory rate you are effectively removing stagnation in your blood vessels and directly reducing blood congestion, a primary factor in varicosities.

- Take a brisk walk for thirty minutes each day or ride a stationary bicycle for approximately that length of time.

Swimming is also an excellent form of exercise—as you swim, feel the water massaging your legs.

- Yoga postures and commonly known exercises such as leg lifts, lunges, and, if you can do them, shoulder stands can successfully strengthen your circulatory system and encourage venous return. Thumb through some of the yoga books listed in "Further Reading" for ideas.

- Vigorous pelvic tilting vastly improves pelvic circulation and venous return. This can be done for five to ten minutes daily. Stand with your feet shoulder-width apart, hands on your hips. Slowly tip your pelvis forward, then backward, gradually increasing your speed until you are swinging your hips forward and backward vigorously. You can also roll and rock your hips and make "figure eights" in belly-dancer fashion.

- Dance, dance, dance! Open to your creative flow as you exercise your legs, pelvis, heart, and spirit.

- In addition to exercising daily, you will want to spend at least twenty minutes, twice a day, with your feet elevated higher than the level of your heart. Putting your legs and feet up on two pillows as you recline is usually sufficient. If you are sitting at a desk, put your feet up on it!

- Don't sit in one place for any length of time because it encourages insufficient pelvic and leg circulation. Get up and walk around about once an hour for ten minutes to improve blood flow. You should do this on long car trips in your third trimester of pregnancy even if you don't have varicosities.

- Use support stockings if you have severe varicosities. If you put them on in the morning when you first get up from bed, they will be easier to get on and the most effective. You can dust a bit of slippery elm powder on your legs to help them slide on.

CAUTION: *Never massage varicose veins. Massage can dislodge clotted blood and lead to an embolism, a very dangerous situation. If you see signs of phlebitis (swelling, heat, pain, infection around the veins), seek the care of an experienced midwife or physician.*

- Visualizing your varicosities reducing in size may help you produce this result. Imagine your life flowing smoothly as you imagine the blood flowing smoothly through your veins. Let obstructions dissolve, and let yourself feel strong.

- Look at the emotional support you have. Are you getting the support you need, or are you afraid you won't have it after the birth? Allow yourself to ask for the help and support you need, and let go of the notion that you must be a superwoman.

DIETARY RECOMMENDATIONS

- A diet rich in healthful foods, especially a variety of whole grains, high-quality protein, and vegetables, will supply the nutrients you need for the maintenance of a healthy circulatory system.

- Vitamin C with bioflavonoids is vital for maintaining strength in the walls of blood vessels. Foods high in vitamin C include all citrus fruits, rose hips, dark green leafy vegetables, cherries, alfalfa sprouts, strawberries, cantaloupe, broccoli, tomatoes, and green peppers. In addition, a daily supplement of up to 2,000 mg of vitamin C with bioflavonoids can add to the integrity of the circulatory system. Bioflavonoids (vitamin P) are brightly colored substances that often appear in foods in conjunction with vitamin C. Sources of bioflavonoids include lemons, grapes, plums, black currants, grapefruit, apricots, buckwheat, cherries, blackberries, and rose hips. In citrus fruits they are more abundant in the inner skin (the white, pithy part) than in the juice. One of the main purposes of this vitamin is to increase the strength of the capillaries. One of the bioflavonoids, rutin, is specifically used to treat hemorrhoids and varicose veins, and is best taken in conjunction with vitamin C and a bioflavonoid complex. The best way to obtain rutin is to eat foods with a high bioflavonoid content.

- Vitamin E is also reputed for its beneficial action on the vascular system. It apparently works by dilating the blood vessels, thus directly facilitating the blood flow. Between 200 and 600 IU is considered a safe daily dosage during pregnancy, but *do not* exceed this amount.

CAUTION: *If you have heart or blood pressure problems, begin at 50 IU daily and work up to about 400 IU over a three-month period, gradually increasing the dosage each week. Also, if you have such problems, speak with your midwife or physician before taking this supplement.*

- Vitamin B complex is also necessary for healthy veins. Brewer's yeast, fortified nutritional yeast, whole grains, and organ meats contain substantial levels of B vitamins. B vitamins are also produced in our intestines to some degree when we have healthy intestinal flora. Alcohol, sugar, and antibiotics can damage intestinal flora, while an active-culture yogurt, eaten in small amounts on a regular basis, can help replenish and restore intestinal flora.

- I cannot overemphasize the importance of including dark leafy green vegetables in the diet on a daily basis. Salad greens like romaine, green or red leaf lettuce, and butter crunch lettuce, as well as greens which are tastier cooked, like kale, collards, mustard greens, dandelion greens, and turnip greens, all promote health and vibrancy and are particularly important for a healthy circulatory system.

This section is divided into two parts: herbs to be used internally and herbs to be used externally.

HERBS FOR INTERNAL USE

- The humble but highly nourishing nettle is by far the best herb for pregnant women with varicose veins. Because of its high mineral content and its ability to tonify the blood vessels, nettle makes a wonderful supplement and astringent brew for varicose veins. Women with severe varicosities may find that the blood vessels don't disappear completely, but will not develop into painful and swollen veins. Prepare an infusion using 1 ounce of herb to 1 quart of water, and steep for two hours. Drink between 1 cup and 1 quart daily depending upon the extent and severity of the varicosities.

- Other herbs that may be used for the vascular system include garlic, onions, oatstraw, calendula, hawthorn berries, motherwort, and dong quai. These should be used under the guidance of an experienced herbalist. Garlic and onions can be eaten as foods (see garlic oil on page 164 under "High Blood Pressure") and garlic can be safely taken in perles during pregnancy (Kwai and Kyolic are both reputable brands). You can add oatstraw to your nettle infusion (use about two-thirds nettle and one-third oatstraw), as well as 1 tablespoon of calendula.

- Kelp is a food-herb so high in trace minerals that it should be included in any program designed to strengthen the blood vessels. You can take 2 "00" capsules of kelp powder up to four times daily, or use kelp in food or as a tea.

- A deficiency of essential fatty acids may exacerbate varicose veins, so you may want to take 500 mg of one of these oils once a day: evening primrose oil, flaxseed oil, black currant oil, borage oil.

HERBS FOR EXTERNAL USE

- The primary aim of external therapies is to tonify the tissue and vessels and to maintain healthy circulation in the problem area while gently reducing obstructions in the blood vessels. To do this you will want to alternate the following applications at least once, but preferably twice, each day.

CAUTION: *You must not massage varicose veins. Massage could lead to the dislodging of a clot, which may result in a dangerous embolism.*

Astringent herbal application: Use witch hazel extract from the pharmacy or make your own (see Appendix I, "Herbal Preparations"). Soak a cloth in the extract, wring it out (save the liquid for future use), and wrap the affected areas with the cloth. In the case of vulvar and anal varicosities, apply the cloth as a compress. Leave it on for twenty minutes each time up to three times a day, whenever it is convenient for you. For an even more effective astringent, prepare your own infusion of these herbs in equal parts: witch hazel, bayberry bark, white oak bark, and calendula blossoms. Simmer a total of 2 ounces of this mix over a low heat (in a covered pot) for thirty minutes. Apply when cool enough to tolerate. This will keep refrigerated about three days if well strained.

Circulation-promoting herbal application: Dit Dat Jiao liniment, a Chinese herbal liniment intended for martial arts injuries, makes an excellent application for varicose veins. It reduces inflammation and bruising, and by promoting healthy circulation in the areas to which it is applied, helps to reduce and prevent blood clot formation. It can be gently rubbed into affected areas (but not on hemorrhoids) twice a day. It is most suitable for varicosities of the legs and feet. The recipe for this easy-to-make and worthwhile liniment is found on page 173. It has many applications beyond pregnancy, including bruises and injuries in which the skin is unbroken and for all muscle aches and tight muscles.

VOMITING, SEVERE
(*Hyperemesis gravidarum*)

This is a condition in which you are vomiting excessively and unable to keep much of anything down, causing you to lose vital nutrients and fluids and to become physically exhausted and emotionally drained. If severe, it can become a life-threatening, medical emergency in which you become clinically dehydrated with a mineral and electrolyte imbalance; it can also contribute to miscarriage. Treatment requires hospitalization, usually intravenous fluids to replace fluids, electrolytes, and nutrients as well as medication to control vomiting.

You must seek medical treatment for this condition, but you may be able to mitigate its severity with home treatment, preventing the problem from becoming serious. The following combination of therapies may help you avoid serious illness. It may take a few days to notice complete improvement, but you should see significant improvement within the first twenty-four hours. If you find no relief from these suggestions or if your condition worsens, seek medical care immediately.

GENERAL RECOMMENDATIONS

- Follow all of the general recommendations under "Morning Sickness."

DIETARY RECOMMENDATIONS

- Each time you throw up, drink a small amount of fluid. In addition, do this throughout the day. Even a quarter cup of liquid every fifteen to thirty minutes can help replace vital fluids. Also, try to eat a small portion of food after you vomit, to prevent clinical starvation.

- To keep your electrolytes in balance, drink Third Wind, Gatorade, or Recharge. Or, preferably, prepare the following drink by the quart and sip it throughout the day, up to every five minutes. Even if you vomit it up, you will still get some, and over the course of a few hours, it will often decrease the frequency of vomiting. This preparation, called "Rehydration Drink," is used worldwide as a remedy to prevent and offset dehydration and electrolyte imbalance, even in cases of severe vomiting and diarrhea in impoverished countries. It consists of 1 quart water, the juice of one lemon, 1 to 2 tablespoons honey, 1/4 teaspoon salt, and 1/4 teaspoon baking soda. You can replace the water and lemon with a half quart each of water and orange juice, if you prefer.

- If you are vomiting and unable to keep nourishment down, a nutritive enema is an effective method for infusing nutrients and fluids that can't be tolerated by mouth. This is an excellent technique that I've seen work several times. It can prevent the need for intravenous fluids in a hospital. To prepare the enema, mix 2 tablespoons of blackstrap molasses in 2 cups of warm spring water, and put the solution into your enema bag or bottle. Lying on your left side or on your hands and knees with your chest near the floor, slowly take the enema. If you are quite dehydrated, you may actually retain all the fluid; it will have been absorbed. This can be done up to twice a day during the acute phase of vomiting.

HERBAL RECOMMENDATIONS

- Take wild yam tincture by the dropperful, up to every two hours throughout the day, and, in addition, take ginger capsules every two hours. Try a few of the other herbal suggestions as well.

- A remarkably effective treatment for vomiting is to apply a warm salty pack to your stomach (*not* over your belly—just directly over your stomach). To do this, heat 1/2 cup of sea salt in a skillet for three minutes. Put the salt into a pillowcase—it will be very hot. Fold the pillowcase (or other suitable sack) into a small square or rectangular "pad" and apply. If it is too hot, wrap the pad in a towel before applying. This Japanese treatment sends penetrating warmth into the stomach, relaxing spasms and cold, and reducing the frequency of vomiting. Do it when you feel a bout of vomiting coming on, or if you have been vomiting repeatedly.

THE NATURAL PREGNANCY BOOK

Herbal Preparations

Preparing your own herbal products is both rewarding and cost-efficient. This section provides you with all of the information you need to begin this venture. In "Resources," later in the book, you will find companies that supply herbs and other products, such as jars, oils, and even decorative labels, that are useful in herbal product making. While you do not need fancy equipment or supplies for making or packaging most herbal products, get yourself a sturdy notebook for recording your recipes, successes, and failures, and be prepared to have friends, relatives, and even neighbors putting in requests for that special liniment or salve that you have created!

HERB GATHERING

Whether you plan to grow your own herbs, gather them from the wild, or purchase them, you are certain to find the process of making your own medicines fun and rewarding. In the long run, putting up a batch of iron tonic or belly massage oil that will last for months is less costly than buying vitamins or lotions. Although you may still need to buy packaged preparations, I think you will find yourself relying more and more on your home remedies. Making your own herbal preparations is empowering, giving you a new understanding of herbs.

—From the Wild—

Whenever possible, use herbs harvested from the wild in the area where you live. An uncultivated plant has more vitality than a cultivated one, just as wild animals retain more of their natural qualities than those living in zoos or in houses. Instruction in plant identification and harvesting is beyond the range of this book, but I encourage you to learn to identify a few local medicinals to enhance your connection with the plant world.

WARNING: *If you are going to use local wild plants, be absolutely certain that your plant identification is accurate. Mistakes can be fatal. Refer to "Further Reading" for a listing of field guides, and seek out the advice of botanists at local nature centers. Never pick plants that grow near roads, under power lines, or in any areas exposed to chemicals including fertilizers, pesticides, or toxic wastes. Choose healthy plants in clean, unpolluted areas.*

Don't pick all of the plants in one location. Leave enough growing to repopulate the area. Avoid endangered or rare plant species. Always offer your thanks to the plants and ask for their blessing and assistance in healing.

—In Your Garden—

Herb cultivation is a very broad field, one in which I am by no means an expert. I do know, however, that I experience the greatest joy when I am sitting in a garden filled with healing plants. Many herbs are not only useful but also beautiful, particularly when they are in bloom. Then the bees and butterflies will flock to your garden, and you will feel a new, profound connection to the plant world.

When you grow your own herbs, you will develop a greater understanding of them. You will see how they change through the seasons and what conditions cause them to thrive, and you learn to recognize their scent and appearance.

The initial investment in seeds or starter plants can vary. A small garden well cared for can provide you with enough herbs to make small amounts of a few remedies. A large garden could potentially provide you with all the herbs you could want and some to spare for friends or for sale. Many herbs are prolific, so even a small plant, tended well, will yield a plentiful harvest over time. Perennials return year after year, so if your budget is limited, go with these instead of annuals. Not at all herbs grow in every climate or location, so consult books and local gardening stores to determine exactly what can be raised where you live. Books by the Rodale Press tend to be informative and interesting. They are usually available at garden shops. Mountain Rose Herbs (see "Resources") sells a variety of medicinal herb seeds.

PURCHASING HERBS

It is preferable to obtain organic, wild-crafted plants or at least organically cultivated plants. Preparations such as capsules and tinctures should likewise be prepared from organic herbs. Many inorganic herbs are fumigated with fungicides and insecticides during storage, and some are even irradiated. Check your sources. All herbs and herb products should have a fresh smell, and their color should resemble that of the fresh plant. Herb freshness will affect the potency and therefore the effectiveness of your treatments. A moldy, dusty odor indicates that the herbs are not fresh. Look closely for insects; one infested batch of herbs can let tons of bugs loose in your home. They can then get into other herbs in your pantry as well as your food.

PREPARING HERBS

Seeing different herbs turn water, alcohol, and oils into lovely shades of gold, red, orange, green, and brown is nothing short of magic. Preparing one's own remedies adds a special potency to the medicines: that of love and care.

Common supplies are required for making everything from teas to salves in your kitchen: glass jars of varying sizes with lids, glass or stainless-steel pots, a sharp knife, a small funnel, a mesh strainer, a vegetable grater, measuring spoons, and a cutting board. Water, vegetable oil, vodka, and beeswax complete the list once you have the herbs you need.

Some preparations cannot be made easily at home. These include essential oils, which require special equipment for extraction, and herbs that must be powdered finely with a special grinder. If you wish, try experimenting with a coffee grinder to see if you achieve a powder that is satisfactory.

If you plan to use your own preparations as primary medicines, you will want to look through this book and plan ahead. Tinctures take weeks to prepare, for example, so you will need to have these on hand, since if you need a tincture today you can't wait. Keep in mind that most herbal preparations such as oils and tinctures will keep for up to a few years (oils must be kept refrigerated), so if you prepare small batches of medicines at a time, you will find that little gets wasted.

Throughout this book I've made every effort to give specific measurements for preparations in the form of teaspoonfuls, tablespoonfuls, and ounces. For convenience, I sometimes have listed recipe ingredients in parts. You can translate these to any measure you are using. For example, if you are using tablespoons, 1 part would be 1 tablespoon, 2 parts would be 2 tablespoons, and a half part would be about 1/2 tablespoon.

Choosing an appropriate measurement for these recipes allows you to determine the amount of preparation you want to make.

—Forms of Preparation—

Water, alcohol, and oil are the most common bases used (*menstruum* is another word for a base or solvent). Some herbalists also use

vinegar but since it is not suitable for all herbs, I reserve it for steeping fresh culinary herbs.

WATER BASES

The Earth, plants, and our bodies are primarily made of water, so our bodies accept water-based solutions easily. These include teas, infusions, decoctions, and syrups. Infusions and decoctions are used for baths, washes, and compresses as well as internal use.

Tea is the most basic herbal preparation. To make a tea, steep 1 teaspoon to 1 tablespoon of a dried herb in 1 cup boiling water for up to twenty minutes. Herbs with a lot of volatile oil content are easily extracted this way and so should be covered during steeping to prevent loss of their oils. Peppermint, catnip, lemon balm, chamomile, fresh ginger, lavender, and seeds such as fennel and anise are in this category.

Infusions are medicinal-strength teas. More herb material is steeped longer in slightly more water than is usual for a tea. The result is a darker, stronger-tasting, more potent brew. Pint- and quart-size canning (Mason) jars are the best vessels in which to make infusions.

To make an infusion, steep 4 to 6 tablespoons of chopped, dried herb or twice that of chopped, fresh herb in either a quart or pint jar filled with boiling water for anywhere from a half hour to eight hours. The steeping time and the amount of water correspond to the intended strength of the remedy and upon the part of the plant being used. The general recommendations are as follows:

Roots: Use 1 ounce dried root to 1 pint of boiling water; steep for eight hours.

Bark: Prepare as for roots.

Leaves: In general, when using delicate leaves or those rich in essential oils, use 1 ounce of dried leaves or 2 ounces of fresh leaves to 1 quart of water and steep for one to two hours. Thick leaves (such as uva-ursi) require steeping for up to six hours. Leaves used for nutritional purposes (such as nettle) should be steeped for up to eight hours.

Flowers: As these are delicate, steep 1 ounce of dried flowers in 1 quart of boiling water for a maximum of one hour.

Seeds: In general, you first gently crush the seeds with a mortar and pestle and then steep them for up to a half hour. Usually 1/4 to 1/2 ounce of seeds per pint of water is sufficient.

Generally the dosage of an infusion ranges from 1/4 to 1 cup, two to four times daily. Sometimes an infusion is sipped throughout the day.

Decoctions are concentrated infusions. This makes for a strong brew that is taken in smaller dosages. A decoction is an excellent way to take herbs when it is difficult to tolerate large amounts of a strong-tasting preparation. The method is especially suited for nutrient roots such as yellow dock and dandelion because you can get concentrated doses of minerals without having to drink cupfuls of beverage. Leaves, flowers, and seeds are rarely decocted as their constituents can be damaged by boiling.

To prepare a decoction, make an infusion and steep it for up to eight hours. Strain the liquid into a saucepan (discarding the used plant material), and simmer it until it is reduced to one-quart to one-half of the original amount. Take care not to boil off all the liquid. Reducing a pint of liquid by one-half (down to a cup) takes approximately an hour. Pour into a glass jar, let cool to room temperature, and then refrigerate.

When unsweetened, decoctions last in the refrigerator for up to three days. Two tablespoons of honey per 1/2 cup of liquid or about 2 tablespoons of brandy per cup of liquid can extend the life of a decoction for up to three months when kept refrigerated.

Dosage is usually 1 teaspoon to 1 tablespoon, two to four times daily.

Syrups are easy to make from a decoction. Syrups have two main advantages over decoctions: you will more readily take a small amount of a sweet-flavored medicine than any amount of an unpalatable one; the large amount of sweetener in the syrup preserves the preparation so that you can keep it in the refrigerator for a longer time than a sweetened decoction. Simply sweeten your decoction by adding an equal amount (by weight) of sweetener. One cup of a decoction is 8 ounces, so a decoction of this amount would require 8 ounces of sweetener. I use 1/4 to 1/2 cup of honey per cup of liquid and find this adequate; honey is considered to be twice as sweet as sugar. Add the sweetener to your hot decoction, bring to the boiling point while stirring, and then immediately pour into clean jars. Cool to room temperature, label, and refrigerate. Dosage is similar to a decoction but of course will vary from herb to herb.

Herbal baths are a rejuvenating ritual and are useful for all sorts of complaints: sore muscles, injured skin, exhaustion, irritability, congestion, and fever, to name a few. Be very careful to avoid burns from overly hot water.

A *foot bath* is given in a basin of water wide enough for the feet and deep enough to reach at least above the ankles. Add a quart of herbal infusion to enough hot water to fill the basin.

A *sitz bath* requires a quart of decoction or a couple of quarts of infusion placed in a shallow tub with enough water to reach hip level.

A *full bath* can be made two ways. You can to fill a cotton cloth or sock with at least an ounce of herbs and fasten the closed cloth to the faucet so bathwater runs through it while the tub is filling. Squeeze the sack now and then to wring out the tea. This will make a mild but pleasant herbal bath. You can also prepare a couple of quarts of herbal infusion or decoction and then strain these into the tub.

If you keep the door to the bathroom closed, the aroma of the herbs and any volatile oils will fill the air, adding to the relaxing effect of the bath. Herb baths are a nourishing gift to yourself during pregnancy. Floating herb flowers directly in the tub makes for a fun bath, but use a screen of some sort to keep the plant material from clogging the drain.

Poultices and compresses are ways of applying herbs externally to specific areas of the body. You can quickly make a poultice by mashing, bruising, or even chewing fresh herbs into a pulpy mass and applying it to the affected area. You can also make one by mashing fresh or dried herbs (dried herbs need to be moistened with warm water first), and spreading the material on a thin cotton cloth, which is then applied to the area. A hot-water bottle can be placed over the herbs or cloth to retain the warmth. Poultices are used for stings, bites, localized infections, wounds, boils, abscesses, swellings, and tumors.

To make a compress, soak a cloth in a hot infusion or decoction, wring out the excess liquid, and apply the cloth to the area. Replace the compress when it cools by dipping again into the hot infusion or decoction. As with a poultice, a hot-water bottle placed over the preparation retains heat.

Washes are just what they sound like: You wash the area with an infusion or decoction. For example, you might want to use an eye-wash for conjunctivitis or as a wash for a skin infection such as ringworm. Washes are an effective and simple external remedy.

ALCOHOL BASES

Alcohol is used for making tinctures, which are concentrated alcohol extracts of herbs. It is a valuable menstruum because certain plant substances can be extracted only by alcohol. Tinctures are concentrated, quick acting, and convenient (they can easily be transported in a small bottle), and they have a shelf life of many years. Because they are so concentrated, only a few drops are needed, making them particularly convenient for those who can't easily prepare infusions or decoctions. They are not, however, used when the nutritional aspects of herbs are being sought. For this, one should use teas, infusions, decoctions, and syrups.

The amount of alcohol ingested when taking tinctures is fairly insignificant, but if you are concerned, many tinctures can now be purchased in a glycerine base, which has no alcohol and lends a slightly sweet taste.

Making tinctures at home is fun and much less expensive than buying them. Because tinctures made with fresh plant material are superior to those made from dried herbs, obtain fresh herbs for your homemade tinctures. The best alcohol to use is 100-proof vodka, which is 50 percent alcohol and 50 percent water. Grain alcohol (almost 200 proof) or brandy can also be used. Brandy is nice for use in tinctures that will be given to very young kids because it is sweet and mildly warming, and it lacks a sharp alcohol taste.

Making tinctures: If you have gathered the herbs yourself, clean them by picking out damaged parts and brushing dirt off roots. Do not wash above-ground plant parts.

Roots, stems, and bark need to be chopped. Place about 2 ounces of plant material in a pint jar. Fill the jar to the top with alcohol to lessen the possibility of spoilage. Cap the jar tightly and label it with the name of the herb, alcohol content, and the date. Store where it won't be exposed to direct sunlight, and give it a gentle shake every few days. If you see the liquid level going down, top off the jar with some more alcohol.

The moon, which exerts ongoing effects on the Earth, including the level of oceans and the growth of plants, as well as our own internal regulatory mechanisms, including our hormones, is also said to influence tincture making. It may therefore be beneficial to honor the effects of the moon by allowing our tinctures to work for at least one complete moon cycle, going from one new moon to the next, or preferably for a full six weeks, from one new moon to the full moon six weeks later.

After two to six weeks, strain the alcohol tincture from the plant material. This usually requires some vigorous wringing of the herbs in cheesecloth or cotton muslin to extract as much of the liquid as possible. Pour your tincture into well-labeled glass jars or tincture bottles (the jars need not be filled to the top) and store in a cool, dark place such as a pantry or the refrigerator.

Dosage of a tincture depends on the herbs used, the condition being treated, and the person's age and weight. Usually between 5 and 25 drops are taken four times a day. Store tinctures out of reach of children as an overdose might make them sick. Tinctures remain good for a minimum of two to three years.

Making liniments: These are tinctures prepared for external use in the treatment of muscle and ligament trauma. They tend to contain herbs that act as local stimulants (for example, angelica, cinnamon, wintergreen, cayenne, calendula) in order to bring deep warmth to the affected area and disperse blood congestion to reduce bruising. The alcohol (use vodka or other 100-proof alcohol) makes them quick absorbing and penetrating. Prepare as for tinctures, or add essential oils to an alcohol base. Apply by rubbing enough into the skin to cover the sore or bruised area. Do not use on broken skin.

OIL BASES

Herbal oils, salves, and ointments can be made at home. Essential oils are highly concentrated plant extracts that cannot easily be made at home and are rarely used internally because their strength can be fatal. I have occasionally suggested the use of essential oils in this book as external remedies, and caution you to store them out of the reach of children.

Herbal oils are vegetable oils in which herbs have been infused. This is different from essential oils, which are derived by extracting large volumes of concentrated, active chemical ingredients from plants. Herbal oils are used in the treatment of sore muscles, sprains, aches, infections, and irritated skin, as well as for massage. Many herbal oils mentioned in this book can be used on broken skin, although arnica oil cannot.

To make an herbal oil, fill a clean and totally dry jar with dry herbs. Now fill the jar to the brim with oil. Almond, olive, and sesame oils are the most commonly used, but any vegetable oil is acceptable. Store at room temperature in partial sunlight for one to four weeks. Some herbs, such as garlic and rosemary, will keep well in oil for the longer time span, while other herbs, particularly the more delicate plants and plant parts such as chickweed and rose petals, will begin to spoil after a week. Hot weather will cause the plants and oil to spoil more quickly, whereas plants extracted in a cool environment will keep longer before you decant them. Direct light and heat should be avoided. Infuse and store on a surface that will not be damaged by any oil seepage that may occur. At the end of the given time period, strain well and store in a cool, dark place or refrigerate. Oils will keep for up to a year or more, and are considered good as long as they have not turned rancid. A rancid oil has a peculiar smell that is distinctly different from either the smell of the fresh oil or the plant being steeped. If you suspect that your oil has turned, discard it and begin anew.

Salves are used for healing skin injuries: wounds, burns, stings, rashes, sores, and the like. Salve can be made a few different ways, all of which are effective. This first method is preferable because it requires less time than the others, thereby retaining more of the subtle properties of the herbs. Prepare an herbal oil from your desired ingredients; then pour it into a small pot. To this add grated beeswax, 1 tablespoon per ounce of oil. Heat over a low flame until the wax is melted. To test for readiness, put a small amount onto a teaspoon and place it in the refrigerator. After a minute it will harden to its finished consistency. Salve should be firm and solid but not so hard that it won't melt into your skin. If the consistency is correct, pour your salve into small jars, cool to room temperature, cover, and store. If your salve is too soft, add more beeswax; if it is too hard, add more oil.

A second method is to place about an ounce of herbs and a 1/3 cup of oil in a small pot. Simmer for two hours on a *very low* flame with the pot covered. Add a bit of oil if necessary, and watch carefully to avoid scorching.

After cooking, strain the herbs well through a cotton cloth or cheesecloth, squeezing as much of the oil as possible out of the plant material. You may need to let the oil cool before this can be done. Clean the pot and dry it (discarding the used plant material); then pour the oil back in, adding a couple tablespoons of grated beeswax. Melt this over a low flame, stirring constantly. Check for readiness as in the first method; then bottle and store.

Another method requires less watching. Mix 4 ounces of oil, 1 ounce of herb, and 1/2 ounce of beeswax in an ovenproof pot. Cover the pot and bake the mixture for about three hours at 250° F. Strain through cheesecloth, bottle, and store.

Salves will keep for a couple of years if stored in the refrigerator, about a year if not. To extend the life of your salve to the full two years, add 1 teaspoon of vitamin E oil or 1 to 2 tablespoons of an herbal tincture per 4 ounces of salve (while still warm, before bottling). Any herbal tincture will work, as it is the alcohol that helps preserve it, but to increase the healing qualities of your salve, use a tincture with either skin healing or antimicrobial properties. Echinacea and calendula tinctures make good choices for use in herbal salves.

Ointments are prepared exactly like salves, but less beeswax is used in order to obtain a softer product. Cutting the amount of beeswax by half should yield a desirable consistency.

When you experiment in your kitchen pharmacy, above all enjoy yourself. Of course it is best not to be wasteful, but don't worry if you make a mistake and have to discard something. Compost piles are very forgiving. Try to be patient and learn from your mistakes. Be persistent; the rewards are worth it!

Common and Latin Names for Herbs in This Book

Many plants may have the same common name, and any given plant may have a number of common names. A plant's Latin name (also known as the "botanical" or "horticultural" name) is its internationally recognized name. When purchasing herbs, check their Latin names to ensure that you are using the correct plants in your herbal preparations.

Alfalfa: *Medicago sativa*

Anise: *Pimpinella anisum*

Astragalus: *Astragalus membranaceus*

Bayberry: *Myrica cerifera*

Bethroot: *Trillium erectum*

Black cohosh: *Cimicifuga racemosa*

Black haw: *Viburnum prunifolium*

Black walnut: *Juglans nigra*

Blessed thistle: *Cnicus benedictus*

Blue cohosh: *Caulophyllum thalictroides*

Borage: *Borago officinalis*

Bupleurum: *Bupleurum falcatum*

Burdock: *Arctium lappa*

Calendula: *Calendula officinalis*

Catnip: *Nepeta cataria*

Chamomile: *Anthemis nobilis; Matricaria chamomilla*

Chasteberry: *Vitex agnus-castus*

Chickweed: *Stellaria media*

Cinnamon: *Cinnamomum zeylanicum*

Cleavers: *Galium aparine*

Comfrey: *Symphytum officinale*

Cramp bark: *Viburnum opulus*

Dandelion: *Taraxacum officinale*

Dong quai: *Angelica sinensis*

Echinacea: *Echinacea angustifolia*

Elder: *Sambucus nigra*

False unicorn: *Chamaelirium luteum*

Fennel: *Foeniculum vulgare*

Fenugreek: *Trigonella foenum-graecum*

Flax seed: *Linum usitatissimum*

Gentian: *Gentian officinalis*

Ginger: *Zingiber officinale*

Ginseng: *Panax quinquefolium*

Goldenseal: *Hydrastis canadensis*
Hawthorn: *Crataegus oxyacantha*
Hops: *Humulus lupulus*
Irish moss: *Chondrus crispus*
Kudzu: *Pueraria lobata et thunbergiana*
Lady's mantle: *Alchemilla vulgaris*
Lady's slipper: *Cypripedium pubescens*
Lavender: *Lavandula officinalis*
Lemon balm: *Melissa officinalis*
Lemon grass: *Cymbopogon citratus*
Licorice: *Glycyrrhiza glabra*
Liferoot: *Senecio aureus*
Lime (linden) blossom: *Tilia europea*
Lobelia: *Lobelia inflata*
Marshmallow: *Althaea officinalis*
Meadowsweet: *Filipendula ulmaria*
Motherwort: *Leonurus cardiaca*
Myrrh: *Comiphora molmol*
Nettle: *Urtica dioica*
Oatstraw: *Avena sativa*
Parsley: *Petroselinum crispum*
Partridge berry: *Mitchella repens*
Passion flower: *Passiflora incarnata*
Peony: *Paeonia* spp.
Peppermint: *Mentha piperita*

Plantain: *Plantago major*
Red clover: *Trifolium pratense*
Red raspberry: *Rubus idaeus*
Rehmannia: *Rehmannia glutinosa*
Rose: *Rosa canina*
Rosemary: *Rosmarinus officinalis*
Sage: *Salvia officinalis*
Sarsaparilla: *Smilax officinale*
Saw palmetto: *Serenoa serrulata*
Shepherd's purse: *Capsella bursa-pastoris*
Skullcap: *Scutellaria laterifolia*
Slippery elm: *Ulmus fulva*
Spearmint: *Mentha viridis*
St. John's wort: *Hypericum perforatum*
Thyme: *Thymus vulgaris*
Usnea: *Usnea barbata*
Uva-ursi: *Arctostaphylos uva-ursi*
Valerian: *Valeriana officinalis*
Vervain: *Verbena officinalis*
White oak: *Quercus alba*
Wild yam: *Dioscorea villosa*
Witch hazel: *Hamamelis virginiana*
Wood betony: *Betonica officinalis*
Yarrow: *Achillea millefolium*
Yellow dock: *Rumex crispus*

Herbs and Herbal Supplies, Books, Support and Information Groups, Educational Programs, and Additional Health Supplies

Catalogs and brochures are available from most of the companies in this resource list. Write or call for further information.

BULK HERBS, HERBAL PRODUCTS, BOOKS, AND SUPPLIES

Avena Botanicals
20 Mill Street
Rockland, ME 04841
207-594-0694

Deb Soule grows and prepares her own medicinal preparations from herbs especially for women. The mail-order catalog offers more than 150 tinctures.

Bushy Mountain Bee Company
800-BEESWAX

Not an herb supplier, but a great source of pure beeswax for making salves.

Cascade Health Care Products
141 Commercial Street NE
Salem, OR 97301
800-443-9942

A complete line of health products for pregnant women and midwives as well as many for babies and kids; good source of moxibustion supplies. The Birth and Life Catalogue (Imprints) offers a comprehensive selection of books on prenatal health, pregnancy, midwifery, and herbs. Their Moonflower catalog offers herbs, nutritional supplements, and homeopathic remedies.

Frontier Cooperative Herbs
P.O. Box 299
Norway, IA 52318
800-669-3275

Bulk herbs and health and beauty products at wholesale prices.

Herb Pharm
P.O. Box 116
Williams, OR 97544
800-348-4372

The highest-quality tinctures available from a company that takes extraordinary pride in its products and values its customers.

Maine Seaweed Company
P.O. Box 57
Steuben, ME 04680
207-546-2875

Excellent sea vegetables harvested with complete respect for the health of the ocean.

Mountain Rose Herbs
P.O. Box 2000
Redway, CA 95560
800-879-3337

Beautiful catalog of bulk herbs, jars and tins, books, and pre-made formulas; also very nice products for use in women's rituals, such as candles, oils, and special art objects that are woman affirming.

Mountain Spirit
P.O. Box 368
Port Townsend, WA 98368
360-385-4491

Herbs, spiritual tools, and books. This is a great source for smudge sticks.

Penn Herbs
603 North Second Street
Philadelphia, PA 19123
800-523-9971

A good source for hard-to-find powdered herbs.

Sage Mountain Herb Products
P.O. Box 420
Barre, VT 05649

Offers herbs products formulated by Rosemary Gladstar Slick, a highly experienced herbalist. All of Rosemary's products, as well as her new book *Herbal Healing for Women*, are highly recommended.

Wish Garden Herbs
1308 Kilkenny Road
Boulder, CO 80303
303-665-9508

A home business that supplies high-quality and hard-to-find herb tinctures, especially for mothers and midwives.

CHINESE HERBS, BOOKS, AND SUPPLIES

Some of the companies listed above also sell these products, but the following carry a wide range of Chinese herbal and medical supplies.

Brion Herbs
9250 Jeronimo Road
Irvine, CA 92718
714-587-1238
East Coast: 800-283-5191

This is the distributor of Sun Ten Herbal Formulas, an excellent Chinese herbal product that is freeze-dried and easy to give to kids.

Herbalist and Alchemist
P.O. Box 553
Broadway, NJ 08808

Herbalist David Winston provides dried Chinese herbs by mail-order, as well as a full line of Western herbs and formulas. He has also written lovely booklets that accompany his catalog, which explain the indications for using many of the herbs he sells.

The Herb Shoppe
4372 Chris Greene Lake Road
Charlottesville, VA 22901
804-973-1700

Paul Olko keeps a large variety of of both Western and Chinese herbs and patent products in stock for mail order.

Redwing/Meridian
44 Linden Street
Brookline, MA 02146
800-873-3946 or 800-356-6003

A great source of lay and technical books on traditional Chinese medicine as well as herbs.

SUPPORT AND RESOURCE ORGANIZATIONS

A.L.A.C.E. (Association of Labor Assistants and Childbirth Educators)
P.O. Box 382724
Cambridge, MA 02238
617-441-2500

Boston Women's Health Information Center
240A Elm Street
Somerville, MA 02144
617-625-0271

This organization is an excellent informational resource on a wide variety of women's health issues and illnesses, provides well-written educational packets, and produced the important book, *The New Our Bodies, Ourselves*.

Citizens for Midwifery
P.O. Box 82227
Athens, GA 30608-2227
316-267-7236
http://www.cfmidwifery.org

This organization serves as the national clearinghouse for consumer groups supporting midwifery and educates the public about the advantages of midwifery care.

Doulas of North America
1100 Twenty-third Avenue East
Seattle, WA 98112

This organization offers training in the postpartum support of new mothers.

I.C.A.N. (International Cesarean Awareness Network)
April Kubachka
1304 Kingsdale Avenue
Redondo Beach, CA 90278
310-542-6400
Fax: 310-542-5368

International Childbirth Education Association
P.O. Box 20048
Minneapolis, MN 55420
612-854-8660

Offers excellent catalog of books on pregnancy, birth, and related topics. Also a resource center for this information.

La Leche League International
9616 Minneapolis Avenue
Franklin Park, IL 60131
708-455-7730

An international organization with numerous locally placed "League leaders," women trained to support and educate women who want to breastfeed. Ardent supporters of breastfeeding and mother-child relationship.

Menstrual Health Foundation
P.O. Box 1775
Sebastopol, CA 95473
707-302-2744

Dedicated to empowering women during the years from menarche through menopause, and providing products and publications.

Midwives Alliance of North America
P.O. Box 175
Newton, KS 67114
316-283-4543

This is a national midwifery organization dedicated to women's freedom and reproductive health, with members all over the globe. A good contact if you are trying to find or become a midwife.

Women to Women
1 Pleasant Street
Yarmouth, ME 04096
207-846-6163

Dr. Christiane Northrup, a holistic obstetrician-gynecologist and author of *Women's Bodies, Women's Wisdom*, runs this women's health clinic with other women practitioners, as well as produces several audio cassettes on topics relevant to women's health.

EDUCATIONAL RESOURCES AND MAGAZINES

Ancient Arts Midwifery Institute
P.O. Box 788
Claremore, OK 74018

The institute's three-year home-study course provides a well-respected academic foundation in the science of midwifery.

Avena Institute
20 Mill Street
Rockland, ME 04841
207-594-0694

Deb Soule, a woman-centered herbalist and author of *The Roots of Healing*, heads an herbal teaching center and herbal products business. On-site classes also include organic gardening, herb walks, and herbal animal care.

Birth Gazette
42 The Farm
Summertown, TN 38438
615-964-3798

Published and edited by Ina May Gaskin, author of *Spiritual Midwifery*, this magazine offers a range of topics on pregnancy and birth, including current issues and events and interviews with midwives and others in the field of midwifery and childbearing health.

Center for Midwifery and Herbal Studies
Aviva Jill Romm
2275 Mountain Road
Alpharetta, GA 30201
770-667-0867

I provide herbal and midwifery education and consultation in the Southeast. My goals are to empower families to take a more active role in their healthcare, preserving and passing on the traditions of midwifery and herbalism, and promoting Earth awareness and social change—all of which are intimately connected to our health. Ongoing classes in midwifery care, pregnancy, birth, parenting, and herbal healthcare for women and children are available. All classes are approached with respect for both ancient, traditional wisdom and scientific knowledge.

Compleat Mother
P.O. Box 209
Minot, ND 58702
701-852-2822

In its own words, "the magazine of pregnancy, birth, and breastfeeding." Very honest and uncompromising.

The Doula Magazine
P.O. Box 71, Dept. MT
Santa Cruz, CA 95063

This magazine includes articles on pregnancy, birth, parenting, natural health care, toddlers, and more. Always a nurturing read.

HerbalGram
P.O. Box 210660
Austin, TX 78720

An excellent and informative magazine that keeps abreast of scientific studies in phytotherapy.

Herb Companion
201 East Fourth Street
Loveland, CO 80537

This is a very readable magazine for those interested in growing, cooking, and learning about herbs. Lovely photos and a variety of herbal topics.

Homeopathic Educational Services
2124 Kittredge Street
Berkeley, CA 94704
207-594-0694

Offers a comprehensive catalog for those interested in homeopathy.

Hygieia College
P.O. Box 111
Junction, UT 84740
801-527-3738

Jeannine Parvati Baker is the founder of this program, which is "a college in the original meaning, that is in a grove of trees, which is a state of mind…." Lessons are in womancraft, herbalism, and the art of midwifery. Baker is the author of a number of books, including *Hygieia: A Woman's Herbal* and *Prenatal Yoga and Natural Birth*, and a coauthor of *Conscious Conception*.

Journal of Family Life
72 Philip Street
Albany, NY 12202
518-432-1578

Midwifery Today
P.O. Box 2672
Eugene, OR 97402
503-344-1422

A magazine for midwives and others involved with pregnancy and birth. Many pregnant women find it very informative.

Mothering Magazine
P.O. Box 1690
Santa Fe, NM 87504
800-984-8116

Perhaps the oldest of the alternative parenting magazines in the United States, *Mothering* seeks to honor and celebrate pregnancy, birth, parenthood, and children.

Mother's Underground
4825 North Meade Avenue, # 2
Chicago, IL 60630

"Wise women sharing knowledge and herstories." A beautiful magazine supportive of mothers, daughters, pregnancy, and birth.

New Mexico Herb Center
122 Tulane SE
Albuquerque, NM 87106
505-265-0795

Founded by Tierona LowDog, this herbal training center and clinic is committed to promoting both the art and science of herbalism, as well as affordable health care. It offers a variety of programs in clinical herbalism as well as herbal consultation by phone and at the center.

Sage Mountain
P.O. Box 420-M
East Barre, VT 05649

Rosemary Gladstar Slick, founder of the California School of Herbal Studies, is a pioneer woman herbalist and author of numerous booklets on herbs for women, men, and children. She offers a correspondence course in herbal studies.

Therapeutic Herbalism
David Hoffman, M.N.I.M.H.
2068 Ludwig Avenue
Santa Rosa, CA 95407

David, a highly respected medical herbalist, offers an herbal training program that is at once comprehensive, scientifically sound, and holistically oriented.

Wise Woman Center
Susun S. Weed
P.O. Box 64-M
Woodstock, NY 12498
914-246-8081

Susun Weed, the author of *Healing Wise*, *Wise Woman Herbal for the Childbearing Year*, and *Menopausal Years*, offers workshops and apprenticeships at her home and travels internationally on speaking engagements.

Dr. George Wootan
P.O. Box 270
Hurley, NY 12443
800-635-2126

Dr. Wootan teaches an excellent weekend course called "Pediatrics For Parents," which you can sponsor where you live. It is highly recommended. Dr. Wootan is the author of *Take Charge of Your Child's Health*.

Further Reading

MENSTRUAL HEALTH AND FERTILITY AWARENESS

Baker, Jeannine P., F. Baker, and T. Slayton. *Conscious Conception.* Sevier, Utah: Freestone Publishing, 1986.

Dharmananda, Subhuti. Treatment of Infertility and Miscarriage with Chinese Herbs. Portland, Oregon: Institute for Traditional Medicine and Preventive Health Care, 1989.

Francia, Luisa. *Dragontime: Magic and Mystery of Menstruation.* Woodstock, NY: Ash Tree Publishing, 1991.

Guay, Terrie. *The Personal Fertility Guide.* New York: Beaufort Books, 1986.

Nofziger, Margaret. *A Cooperative Method of Natural Birth Control.* Summertown, Tennessee: Book Publishing Co., 1979.

_____. *The Fertility Question.* Summertown, Tennessee: Book Publishing Co., 1982.

Shuttle, Penelope, and P. Redgrove. *The Wise Wound.* New York: Grove Press, 1986.

Taylor, Dena. *Red Flower: Rethinking Menstruation.* Freedom, California: The Crossing Press, 1988.

Winstein, Merryl. *Your Fertility Signals.* St. Louis: Smooth Stone Press, 1990.

PREGNANCY

(see also "Birth")

Baldwin, Rahima. *Special Delivery.* Berkeley: Celestial Arts, 1986.

Bing, Elizabeth, and Libby Colman. *Making Love During Pregnancy.* New York: Bantam Books, 1977.

Cohen, Nancy W. *Open Season.* New York: Greenwood, Bergin, and Garvey, 1991.

Cohen, Nancy W., and Lois Estner. *Silent Knife.* New York: Greenwood, Bergin, and Garvey, 1983.

Corda, Murshida. *Cradle of Heaven: Psychological and Spiritual Dimensions of Conception, Pregnancy, and Birth.* Lebanon Springs, NY: Omega, 1987.

Davis, Elizabeth. *Heart and Hands: A Midwife's Guide to Pregnancy and Birth.* Berkeley: Celestial Arts, 1987.

Goldsmith, Judith. *Childbirth Wisdom from the World's Oldest Societies*. New York: Congdon and Weed, 1984.

Grossinger, Richard. *Embryogenesis*. Berkeley: North Atlantic Books, 1986.

Huxley, Laura. *The Child of Your Dreams*. Rochester, Vermont: Inner Traditions, Destiny Books, 1992.

Kitzinger, Sheila. *The Complete Book of Pregnancy and Childbirth*. New York: Alfred A. Knopf, 1983.

————. *Education and Counseling for Childbirth*. New York: Schocken Books, 1979.

Miller, Johnathan, and D. Pelham. *The Facts of Life*. New York: Penguin USA, Viking, 1984.

Peterson, Gayle, and L. Mehl. *Pregnancy as Healing, vols. 1 and 2*. Berkeley: Mindbody Press, 1984.

Schwartz, Leni. *Bonding Before Birth*. Boston: Sigo Press, 1991.

Stukane, Eileen. *The Dream Worlds of Pregnancy*. New York: Quill, 1985.

Verny, Thomas, and John Kelly. *The Secret Life of the Unborn Child*. New York: Dell Publishing, 1981.

HERBS FOR PREGNANCY

Gardner, Joy. *Healing Yourself During Pregnancy*. Freedom, California: The Crossing Press, 1987.

McIntyre, Anne. *The Herbal for Mother and Child*. Rockport, Massachussetts: Element Books, 1992.

Moskowitz, Richard. *Homeopathic Medicines for Pregnancy and Childbirth*. Berkeley: North Atlantic Press, 1992.

Romm, Aviva. *Natural Healing for Babies and Children*. Freedom, California: The Crossing Press, 1996.

Romm, Aviva. "Healing a Uterine Prolapse." *The Birth Gazette*. Vol. 10, No. 3, Summer, 1994.

Weed, Susun. *Healing Wise*. Woodstock, New York: Ash Tree Publishing, 1989.

————. *Wise Woman Herbal for the Childbearing Year*. Woodstock, New York: Ash Tree Publishing, 1985.

NUTRITION

Ballantine, Rudolph. *Diet and Nutrition*. Honesdale, Pennsylvania: Himalaya International Institute, 1978.

Brewer, Gail S., and Tom Brewer. *What Every Pregnant Woman Should Know: The Truth About Diet and Drugs in Pregnancy*. New York: Penguin Books, 1977.

Colbin, Annemarie. *Food and Healing*. New York: Ballantine Books, 1986.

Dufty, William. *Sugar Blues*. New York: Warner Books, 1975.

Eisenberg, Arlene, H. E. Murkoff, and S. E. Hathaway. *What to Eat When You're Expecting*. New York: Workman Publishing, 1986.

Galland, Leo. *Superimmunity for Kids*. New York: Delta Books, 1988.

Kirschmann, John, and L. Dunne. *Nutrition Almanac*. New York: McGraw-Hill, 1984.

Kushi, Michio, and Aveline. *Macrobiotic Pregnancy and Care of the Newborn*. New York: Japan Publishing, 1983.

Luke, Barbara. *Maternal Nutrition*. Boston: Little, Brown and Co., 1979.

Phillips, David. *Guidebook to Nutritional Factors in Foods*. Santa Barbara, California: Woodbridge Press, 1979.

EXERCISE AND MASSAGE

Baker, Jeannine P. *Prenatal Yoga and Natural Birth*. Berkeley: North Atlantic, 1986.

Chi-uh. *Yoga with the Unborn*. Mill Valley, California: Whatever Publishing, 1980.

Leboyer, Frederick. *The Art of Breathing*. Great Britain: Element, 1983.

————. *Inner Beauty, Inner Light: Yoga for Pregnant Women*. New York: Alfred A. Knopf, 1978.

Markowitz, Elysa, and H. Brainen. *Baby Dance: A Comprehensive Guide to Prenatal and Postpartum Exercise.* Englewood Cliffs, New Jersey: Prentice Hall, 1980.

Noble, Elizabeth. *Essential Exercises for the Childbearing Year.* Boston: Houghton Mifflin Co., 1982.

Olkin, Sylvia. *Positive Pregnancy Through Yoga.* Garden City, NY: Avery, 1991.

Rush, Anne K. *Getting Clear: Body Work for Women.* New York: Random House, 1982.

Stillerman, Elaine. *Mother Massage.* New York: Dell Publishing, 1992.

BIRTH

Arms, Suzanne. *Immaculate Deception.* New York: Bantam Books, 1975.

Ashford, Janet I. *The Whole Birth Catalog.* Trumansburg, NY: The Crossing Press, 1983.

Baird, Jan. *Childbearing: The Classic Series.* Childbirth Graphics, 1985.

Baker, Jeannine P. "Deep Ecology of Birth." Monroe, Utah: Freestone Publishing, 1991.

Dick-Read, Grantly. *Childbirth Without Fear.* New York: Harper and Row, 1979.

Gaskin, Ina May. *Spiritual Midwifery.* Summertown, Tennessee: Book Publishing Co., 1980.

Goer, Henci. *Obstetric Myths Versus Research Realities: A Guide to the Medical Literature.* Westport, Connecticut: Greenwood, Bergin, and Garvey, 1995.

Hazell, Lester. *Commonsense Childbirth.* New York: Berkley Books, 1976.

Hobbs, Valerie. *Complications of Labor and Delivery.* Ann Arbor, Michigan: Informed Homebirth and Parenting, 1982.

————. *Herbs for Women: A Guide for Lay Midwives.* 1981.

Kitzinger, Sheila. *Birth at Home.* New York: Penguin, 1979.

Klaus, Marshall, and John Kennell. *Bonding.* New York: Penguin USA, Plume, 1983.

Koehler, Nan. *Artemis Speaks: VBAC Stories and Natural Childbirth Information.* Occidental, California: Jerald R. Brown, 1985.

Leboyer, Frederick. *Birth Without Violence.* New York: Ballantine, Fawcett, 1990.

Linden, Zur. *When a Child Is Born.* New York: Thorsons, 1984.

Milinaire, Caterine. *Birth.* New York: Harmony Books, 1974.

Nilsson, Lennart. *A Child Is Born.* New York: Dell Publishing, Delacorte Press, 1982.

Noble, Elizabeth. *Childbirth with Insight.* Boston: Houghton Mifflin Co., 1983.

Panuthos, Claudia. *Transformation Through Birth.* South Hadley, Massachussetts: Greenwood, Bergin, and Garvey, 1984.

Peterson, Gayle. *Birthing Normally.* Berkeley: Mindbody Press, 1984.

Ray, Sondra. *Ideal Birth.* Berkeley: Celestial Arts, 1986.

Sears, William, and Martha. *The Birth Book.* Boston: Little, Brown, and Co., 1994.

Sousa, Marion. *Childbirth at Home.* Englewood Cliffs, New Jersey: Prentice Hall, 1976.

Star, Rima Beth. *The Healing Power of Birth.* Austin: Star Publishing, 1986.

Wagner, Marsden. *Pursuing the Birth Machine.* Camperdown, Australia: ACE Graphics, 1994.

WOMEN'S HEALTH

Airola, Paavo. *Every Woman's Book.* Phoenix: Health Plus Publishers, 1983.

Boston Women's Health Collective. *The New Our Bodies, Ourselves.* New York: Simon and Schuster, 1984.

Brooke, Elizabeth. *Herbal Therapy for Women.* London: Thorsons, 1992.

Dreifus, Claudia, ed. *Seizing Our Bodies: The Politics of Women's Health.* New York: Vintage Books, 1977.

Federation of Feminist Women's Health Centers. *A New View of a Woman's Body*. New York: Touchstone, 1981.

Flaws, Bob. *Free and Easy: Traditional Chinese Gynecology for American Women*. Boulder: Blue Poppy Enterprises Press, 1986.

————. *A Handbook of Traditional Chinese Gynecology*. Boulder: Blue Poppy Enterprises Press, 1987.

Gladstar, Rosemary. *Herbal Healing for Women*. New York: Simon and Schuster, 1993.

Harrison, Michelle. *A Woman in Residence*. New York: Penguin, 1982.

Madaras, Lynda, and Jane Patterson. *Womancare: A Gynecological Guide to Your Body*. New York: Avon Books, 1984.

Marieschild, Diane. *Motherwit*. Trumansburg, New York: The Crossing Press, 1981.

Mendelsohn, Robert. *MalePractice: How Doctors Manipulate Women*. Chicago: Contemporary Books, 1982.

Nissim, Rina. *Natural Healing in Gynecology*. New York: Pandora Press, 1986.

Parvati, Jeannine. *Hygieia: A Woman's Herbal*. Monroe, Utah: Freestone Collective Books, 1978.

Roberts, Helen, ed. *Women's Health Matters*. New York: Routledge, 1992.

Walker, Alice, and P. Palamr. *Warriot Marks: Female Genital Mutilation and the Sexual Blinding of Women*. New York: Harcourt Brace and Co., 1993.

CHILD CARE

Konner, Melvin. *Childhood*. Boston: Little, Brown and Co., 1991.

La Leche League. *The Womanly Art of Breastfeeding*. New York: Plume, 1981.

Liedloff, Jean. *The Continuum Concept*. Reading, Massachussetts: Addison-Wesley Publishing Co., 1977.

Lorie, Peter. *Wonder Child*. New York: Fireside Books, 1989.

McClure, Vimala Schneider. *Infant Massage*. New York: Bantam Books, 1989.

Mendelsohn, Robert. *How to Raise a Healthy Child in Spite of Your Doctor*. New York: Ballantine Books, 1984.

Montagu, Ashley. *Growing Young*. New York: McGraw-Hill, 1981.

Mothering Magazine. *Becoming a Father: Family, Work, and Self*. Santa Fe: John Muir Publications, 1990.

Schultz, Karen. *A Theosophical Guide for Parents*. Ojai, California: Parents Theosophical Research Group, 1984.

Thevenin, Tine. *The Family Bed: An Age-Old Concept in Child Rearing*. Garden City, New York: Avery, 1992.

Vissell, Joyce, and Barry. *Models of Love: The Parent Child Journey*. Aptos, California: Ramira Press, 1986.

Wallerstein, Edward. *Circumcision: An American Health Fallacy*. New York: Springer Publishing Co., 1980.

West, Melissa G. *If Only I Were a Better Mother*. Walpole, New Hampshire: Stillpoint Publishing, 1992.

Wootan, George. *Pediatrics: A Course for Parents*. Hurley, New York: George Wootan, 1986.

GENERAL HERBALISM

Audubon Society. *Field Guide to North American Trees*. New York: Alfred A. Knopf, 1980.

Bairacli-Levy, Juliette de. *Nature's Children*. New York: Pantheon Books/Schocken Books, 1971.

Bear, Walking Night, and S. Padilla. *Song of the Seven Herbs*. Summertown, Tennessee: Book Publishing Co.

Beinfield, Harriet, and E. Korngold. *Between Heaven and Earth: A Guide to Chinese Medicine*. New York: Ballantine Books, 1991.

Bennett, Jennifer. *Lilies of the Hearth*. Ontario, Canada: Camden House Publishing, 1991.

Birzneck, Ella. *Dominion Herbal College Manuals I, II, and III*. Burnaby, B.C., 1962.

Conrow, Robert, and A. Hecksel. *Herbal Pathfinders*. Santa Barbara, California: Woodbridge Press, 1983.

Cruden, Lorien. *Love Is Green: An Herbal for Parents*. Port Townsend, Washington: Pan's Forest Herb Co.

Cummings, Stephen, and D. Ullman. *Everybody's Guide to Homeopathic Medicines*. New York: St. Martin's Press, 1984.

Dharmananda, Subhuti. *Chinese Herbology*. Portland, Oregon: Institute for Traditional Medicine and Preventive Health Care, 1989.

————. *Your Nature, Your Health: Chinese Herbs in Constitutional Therapy*. Portland, Oregon: Institute for Traditional Medicine and Preventive Health Care, 1986.

Elliot, Doug. *Roots: An Underground Botany and Forager's Guide*. Old Greenwich, Connecticut: Chatham Press, 1976.

————. *Woodslore and Wildwoods Wisdom*. Union Mills, North Carolina: Possum Productions, 1986.

Flaws, Bob. *Turtle Tail and Other Tender Mercies: Traditional Chinese Pediatrics*. Boulder: Blue Poppy Enterprises Press, 1985.

Foster, Steven, and J. Duke. *Eastern/Central Medicinal Plants*. Boston: Houghton Mifflin Co., 1990.

Frawley, David, and V. Lad. *The Yoga of Herbs*. Santa Fe: Lotus Light, Lotus Press, 1986.

Gabriel, Ingrid. *Herb Identifier and Handbook*. New York: Sterling Publishing Co., 1979.

Gardner, Joy. *Healing the Family*. New York: Bantam Books, 1982.

————. *The New Healing Yourself*. Freedom, California: The Crossing Press, 1989.

Gibbons, Bob. *How Flowers Work: A Guide to Plant Botany*. Dorset, England: Blandford Press, 1984.

Gibbons, Euell. *Stalking the Healthful Herbs*. Putney, Vermont.: Alan C. Hood & Co., 1966.

Grieve, Maude. *A Modern Herbal, Vols. 1 & 2*. New York: Dover, 1971.

Haas, Elson. *Staying Healthy with the Seasons*. Berkeley: Celestial Arts, 1981.

Hoffman, David. *The Holistic Herbal*. Scotland: Findhorn Press, 1983.

Hsu, Hong-yen. *Major Chinese Herbal Formulas*. Oriental Healing Arts Institute, 1980.

Hylton, William, ed. *The Rodale Herb Book*. Emmaus, Pennsylvania: Rodale Press, 1974.

King, Kurt. *Herbs to the Rescue: Herbal First Aid Handbook*. Hamilton, Montana: Higher Ground Publications, 1991.

Kloss, Jethro. *Back to Eden*. Loma Linda, California: Back to Eden Books, 1981.

Kushi, Michio. *Macrobiotic Home Remedies*. New York: Japan Publications, 1985.

Lee, Deborah. *Exploring Nature's Uncultivated Garden*. Takoma Park, Maryland: Havelin Communications, 1989.

Meunick, Jim. *The Basic Essentials of Edible Wild Plants and Useful Herbs*. Merrillville, Indiana: ICS Books, 1988.

Moulton, Le Arta. *Herb Walk*. Provo, Utah: Gluten Co., 1979.

Mowrey, Daniel. *The Scientific Validation of Herbal Medicine*. Cedar Run, New Jersey: Down the Shore Publishing, Cormorant Books, 1986.

Muramoto, Naboru. *Healing Ourselves*. New York: Avon Books, 1973.

Peterson, Lee Allen. *A Field Guide to Wild Edible Plants, Eastern/Central*. Boston: Houghton Mifflin Co., 1977.

Riggs, Maribeth. *Natural Child Care*. New York: Harmony Books, 1989.

Rose, Jeanne. *Jeanne Rose's Herbal Book*. New York: Grosset and Dunlap Publishing, 1976.

Santillo, Humbart. *Natural Healing with Herbs*. Prescott Valley, Arizona: Hohm Press, 1987.

Scott, Julian. *Natural Medicine for Children*. New York: Avon Books, 1990.

Tierra, Lesley. *The Herbs of Life*. Freedom, California: The Crossing Press, 1992.

_____. *Planetary Herbology*. Santa Fe: Lotus Light Publications, Lotus Press, 1988.

Tierra, Michael. *Chinese Planetary Herbal Diagnosis, Prts. 1 and 2*. Santa Cruz, California: East West Herb Course, 1986.

_____. *The Way of Herbs*. Santa Cruz, California: Orenda/Unity Press, 1980.

Tierra, Michael, and Lesley Tierra. *Master Course in Herbology*. Santa Cruz, California.

Tyler, Varro. *Herbs of Choice: The Therapeutic Use of Phytomedicinals*. Hudson, NY: Anthroposophic Press, Hawthorn Press, 1994.

Weiss, Rudolf. *Herbal Medicine*. Gothenburg, Sweden: AB Arcanum, 1988.

PREGNANCY-RELATED HISTORY AND ANTHROPOLOGY

Achterberg, Jeanne. *Woman as Healer*. Boston: Shambhala Publications, 1991.

Dunham, Carroll. *Mamatoto: A Celebration of Birth*. New York: Penguin USA, Viking, 1991.

Ehrenreich, Barbara, and Deidre English. *Witches, Midwives, and Nurses: A History of Women Healers*. New York: Feminist Press at the City University of New York, 1973.

Gelis, Jacques. *History of Childbirth: Fertility, Pregnancy, and Birth in Early Modern Europe*. Boston: Northeastern University Press, 1991.

Liedloff, Jean. *The Continuum Concept*. Reading, Massachussetts: Addison-Wesley, 1985.

Litoff, J. B. *The American Midwife Debate*. New York: Greenwood Press, 1986.

Mitford, Jessica. *The American Way of Birth*. New York: Dutton/Signet, 1992.

Sorel, Mary C. *Ever Since Eve*. New York: Oxford University Press, 1984.

Ulrich, Laurel Thatcher. *A Midwife's Tale*. New York: Vintage Books, 1990.

Vincent-Priya, Jacqueline. *Birth Without Doctors*. London: Earthscan Publications, 1991.

WOMEN'S STUDIES AND SPIRITUALITY

Davis, Elizabeth. *Women's Intuition*. Berkeley: Celestial Arts, 1989.

Dinnerstein, Dorothy. *The Mermaid and the Minotaur*. New York: Harper and Row, 1976.

Eisler, Rianne. *The Chalice and the Blade*. San Francisco: Harper and Row, 1987.

Griffith, Susan. *Woman and Nature*. New York: Harper and Row, 1978.

Louden, Jennifer. *The Woman's Comfort Book*. New York: Harper Collins, 1992.

Merchant, Carolyn. *The Death of Nature: Women, Ecology, and the Scientific Revolution*. San Francisco: HarperSanFrancisco, 1980.

Noble, Vicki. *Shakti Woman*. San Francisco: HarperSanFrancisco, 1991.

_____. *Uncoiling the Snake*. San Francisco: HarperCollins, 1993.

Plant, Judith, ed. *Healing the Wounds: The Promise of Ecofeminism*. Philadelphia: New Society Publishers, 1989.

Rich, Adrienne. *Of Woman Born: Motherhood as Experience and Institution*. New York: W.W. Norton & Co., 1986.

Stukane, Eileen. *The Dream Worlds of Pregnancy*. New York: Quill, 1985.

Verny, Thomas, and John Kelly. *The Secret Life of the Unborn Child*. New York: Dell Publishing, 1981.

COOKBOOKS

Colbin, Annemarie. *The Natural Gourmet*. New York: Ballantine Books, 1989.

Katzen, Mollie. *Moosewood Cookbook*. Berkeley: Ten Speed Press, 1977.

Kushi, Aveline. *Complete Guide to Macrobiotic Cooking*. New York: Warner Books 1985.

Galland, Leo. *Superimmunity for Kids*. New York: Bantam Books Doubleday Dell Books, 1988.

Goldbeck, Nikki, and David Goldbeck. *American Wholefoods Cuisine*. Woodstock, New York: Ceres Press, 1983.

McCartney, Linda. *Home Cooking*. New York: Arcade Publishing, 1989.

Robertson, Laurel, Carol Flinders, and Bronwen Godfrey. *Laurel's Kitchen*. New York: Bantam Books, 1982.

TEXTBOOKS AND TECHNICAL REFERENCE BOOKS

Bates, Barbara. *A Guide to the Physical Examination*, 3d ed. Philadelphia: J. B. Lippincott Co., 1983.

Buckley, Kathleen, and Nancy W. Kulb. *Handbook of Maternal Newborn Nursing*. New York: John Wiley and Sons, 1983.

Cavanagh, Dennis, Ralph Woods, Timothy O'Connor, and Robert Knuppel. *Obstetric Emergencies*. Philadelphia: Harper and Row, 1982.

Frye, Anne. *Holistic Midwifery: A Comprehensive Textbook for Midwives in Homebirth Practice. Vol. 1, Care During Pregnancy*. Portland, Oregon: Labrys Press, 1995.

_____. *Understanding Lab Work in the Childbearing Year*. New Haven, Connecticut: Labrys Press, 1990.

Garrey, Matthew, A. D. T. Govan, Colin Hodge, and R. Callander. *Obstetrics Illustrated*. New York: Churchill Livingstone, 1980.

Jensen, Margaret D., Ralph Benson, and Irene Bobak. *Maternity Care: The Nurse and the Family*. St. Louis: Mosby, 1981.

Klein, Susan. *A Book for Midwives*. Palo Alto, California: Hesperian Foundation, 1995.

Olds, Sally, Marcia London, and Patricia Ladewig. *Maternal Newborn Nursing*. Menlo Park, California: Addison-Wesley, 1984.

Pritchard, Jack, and Paul MacDonald. *William's Obstestrics*. New York: Appleton-Century Croft, 1976.

Reeder, Sharon, Luigi Mastroianni Jr., and Leonide Martin. *Maternity Nursing*. Philadelphia: J. P. Lippincott Co., 1983.

Taber, Ben-Zion. *Manual of Gynecologic and Obstetric Emergencies*. Philadelphia: W. B. Saunders Co., 1984.

Tortora, Gerard, and Nicholas Anagnostakos. *Principles of Anatomy and Physiology*. New York: Harper and Row, 1984.

Varney, Helen. *Nurse Midwifery*. Boston: Blackwell Scientific Publications, 1980.

Werner, David. *Where There Is No Doctor: A Village Health-Care Handbook*. Palo Alto, California: Hesperian Foundation, 1977.

Index

A

abdomen
  feelings of fullness in, 19, 75, 91-92
  pain in, 54, 139, 148, 162
  See also eating disorder
abortion, 36, 37, 148. *See also* deformity
abuse, 22, 119-120. *See also* relationships
aerobics, 73. *See also* exercise
affirmations, 12-13, 24, 116. *See also* visu-
    alizations
AFP. *See* prenatal testing
alcohol, 19, 22, 59. *See also* caffeine
allergies, 10, 63, 67
amniotic fluid, 19-20, 144
anemia
  B12 deficiency, 133
  discussed, 132-136
  folic acid anemia, 132
  herbal remedies, 66, 69, 71, 153
  iron deficiency, 133-136
  nutritional remedies, 54, 59, 94
  prenatal testing for, 35, 37
  See also fatigue; iron
anger, 22, 42, 150, 197. *See also* feelings;
    irritability
antacids, 167. *See also* digestion
antibiotics, 57, 179, 200. *See also* infection
anxiety, 21, 24, 85-86
  discussed, 169-170
  herbal preparations for, 68, 69, 103
  recognition of, 12-13, 39, 95, 97-99,
    114, 142, 150, 159, 165, 175, 182
  visualization for release of, 87, 116
  See also feelings; mood swings
appetite, 53, 67, 68. *See also* eating disor-
    der; hunger
art, 13, 25, 117-118, 151
attitude, 9-12, 17, 23, 89, 143. *See also*
    affirmations

B

baby, 5, 28, 83
  communication with, 21, 22-25, 117,
    128, 175
  dreams about, 14, 17-18, 23, 98, 117
  drugs affecting, 19, 22, 183, 198, 202,
    203
  massage for, 23, 24, 115, 187
  mother's attitude affecting, 17, 21, 25
  movement of, 18, 19, 20, 22, 73, 74,
    97, 122
  prenatal testing risks to, 5, 8, 17-18,
    35-38
  sensitivity in womb, 6, 84
  supplies for after birth, 106-107
  visualization of, 18, 97
  See also birth weight; growth of baby
Bach Rescue Remedy, 152
backache, 12, 70, 74, 83, 91, 93, 103
  discussed, 136-138
baths, 67, 68, 86, 99, 114, 141, 144, 146,
    152, 161, 170, 173, 175, 189, 199
belly mask, 111-112
birth
  body preparation for, 104-105
  breech birth, 27, 150
  discussed, 142-143
  in the caul, 117
  home birth, 4, 6-8, 28, 39, 162
  hospital birth, 4, 7-8, 29, 31, 39, 165
  natural, 4, 6, 17-18, 28
  physical requirements of, 73
  premature, 20-21, 42, 54, 63
  See also baby; Cesarean section; labor
birth canal, 86, 91. *See also* pelvis
birth defect. *See* deformity
birth weight, 42, 46, 50, 51, 58, 162, 189,
    193. *See also* growth of baby; weight
    loss
black cohosh, 102, 166, 179
bladder. *See* infection; urination

(continued)

bleeding, 148, 154, 175-181, 192, 208
  after sex, 91, 138
  discussed, 138-141
  remedies, 47, 133
  See also hemorrhage
blood clotting, 50, 55, 83. *See also* hemor-
    rhage
blood pressure, 27
  nutrition affecting, 55, 67, 69, 102, 103
blood pressure. *See also* heartbeat; hyper-
    tension
blood purification, 66, 69, 83, 160
blood sugar level, 12, 34, 42, 50, 51, 53,
    66, 67, 102, 103, 151, 152, 157, 183,
    185, 189, 194.
  See also mood swings
blood type, 35
blue cohosh, 102-103, 179
body
  cultural definition, 9, 72-74, 187
  feelings and fears about, 12-13, 40, 99,
    115-116, 120, 149, 159
  messages from, 10-13, 25, 42, 48-49,
    151
  preparation for birth, 104-105
  relation to mind and spirit, 10, 15
body awareness, 6 12, 14-15
body-centeredness, 9-13, 115
bones, 93
borage, 65
bowel movements, 10, 51, 65, 91, 146,
    155-156. *See also* constipation; elimi-
    nation
brain, 10, 19, 51, 54, 102. *See also* nervous
    system
bran muffins, 147
breastfeeding, 5, 15, 28, 133
  anxieties about, 13, 105
  education about, 39, 41, 90
  nipples, 89, 93, 105-106, 141
  nutritional requirements, 50, 53, 93
  See also nutrition

breasts, changes in, 12, 19, 89-90, 97, 141, 184, 187
breathing techniques, 39, 75, 86
burdock, 66-67, 157, 159, 160, 161, 171

C

caffeine, 12, 46, 65, 135, 137, 139, 147, 157, 160, 164, 170, 185, 199
calcium requirements, 47, 48, 49, 52, 58, 59, 60, 66, 93, 157, 169
carbohydrates
    deficiency, 51, 190
    requirements, 51-52, 57
    See also nutrition; whole grains
cervix, 8, 13, 91, 139, 141
    friable cervix, 138
    incompetent cervix, 174
Cesarean section (C-section), 28, 37, 39, 158, 159, 204
    compared to vaginal birth, 6, 34
    See also birth
chamomile, 67, 103, 140, 153, 166, 170, 186
children, 6, 15
    affect of on pregnant mother, 59, 73, 85, 95, 96, 97, 98, 107, 121-123, 143, 150
    involvement in pregnancy, 33, 122-123
    See also family
chills, 68
chocolate, 12, 46, 51, 59-60, 137, 139, 157, 160. *See also* sugar; sweets
chromosomal abnormality, 38. *See also* deformity; prenatal testing
cigarettes, 19, 22, 59
circulatory system, 14, 68, 82, 83, 163, 165, 210. *See also* blood
colds. *See* illness
colostrum, 89
coltsfoot, 65
comfrey, 53, 65
communication
    between mother and baby, 21, 22, 23-25
    between parents, 98
    talking to baby, 23-24, 142
conception, 14, 17-19
confidence, 8, 18, 24, 28, 32, 88, 98, 116
constipation, 12, 85, 136, 137, 157, 184
    discussed, 146-148

remedies, 47, 53, 54, 58, 62, 71, 190
    See also bowel movements; elimination
contractions, 91, 92, 102, 144, 157, 196
    herbs stimulating, 65, 69, 166, 178-180
corn silk tea, 198
cramp bark, 103, 137, 140, 176
cramping, 14, 72, 175
    discussed, 138-141, 172-173
    remedies, 54, 55, 67, 103
    See also miscarriage
crying, 12, 20, 96, 114, 150-151. *See also* feelings; mood swings
cultural stereotypes
    about pregnancy, 5-6, 15, 38, 105, 149-150
    affecting health, 9-10, 14-16, 40, 114-118
    body definition by, 9, 12-13, 72-74, 90, 91-92
cystic fibrosis, 37

D

dairy products, 50, 52, 53, 54, 55, 57, 163. *See also* nutrition
    avoidance of, 58-59, 135, 139, 147, 155, 169-170
    yoghurt, 54, 55, 139, 147, 167, 185, 199-201, 203
dance, 14, 73, 208. *See also* exercise; movement
dandelion, 67, 69, 135-137, 148, 152, 154, 157, 168, 171, 186
daydreams, 99. *See also* dreams
death
    anxiety about, 98-99
    as medical event, 10
    trauma of, 21
    See also fetal demise; infant mortality
decision making, 5-6
deformity
    acceptance of, 17
    Down's syndrome, 36, 37
    dreams about, 24, 98
    nutrition affecting, 52, 54
    prenatal testing for, 36, 37, 38
dehydration, 151, 157, 184, 185, 192. *See also* fluids
depression, 12, 38, 83, 85, 96, 149, 150

affecting baby, 22
    as cause of overweight, 42
    exercise affecting, 14, 72
    remedies, 47, 50, 51, 53, 54, 68, 151
    See also fatigue; feelings
diabetes, 31, 34, 194. *See also* blood sugar
diarrhea, 52, 133, 143
    herbal remedies, 63-64, 68, 146
    remedies, 54
    See also dehydration
diet diary, 43-48, 44, 45-47. *See also* journal
diet. *See* eating habits
dieting. *See* eating disorders
digestion
    aids to, 62, 65, 66, 67, 68, 71, 73, 81
    changes in during pregnancy, 91, 184
    difficulties with, 52, 53, 54, 74, 75, 85, 146
    See also eating disorders; heartburn
dilation and curettage (D&C), 177, 179. *See also* miscarriage
disease. *See* illness
dizziness, 35, 53, 132, 148
Down's syndrome, 36, 37. *See also* deformity
dreams, about pregnancy, 14, 17-18, 23-24, 98, 117
    See also visualizations
drugs, 4-6, 28, 34, 39
    harmful effects, 19, 22, 183, 198, 202, 203
    See also herbal remedies

E

eating disorders, 9, 11-12, 16, 42
    remedies, 53, 54
    See also digestion; heartburn
eating habits
    changes in, 16-17, 29, 48-49, 59, 91, 98
    problems of, 12, 40, 60, 95
    See also digestion; nutrition
echinacea, 144, 159, 160, 161, 175, 180-181, 197
eclampsia. *See* toxemia
education, 4-5, 7, 115, 122, 127, 150, 205
    childbirth education classes, 38-39, 42
eggs, 53, 54, 55, 56. *See also* nutrition; protein

hemorrhage, 132, 138-139, 148, 162, 189
  remedies, 56, 66, 69, 177, 179-180
  See also bleeding
hemorrhoids, 81
  discussed, 207-211
herbal remedies
  Calming Tea, 151
  Chamomile Tea, 170
  Constipation Remedy, 147
  Cramping Formula, 140-141
  Digestion Tea, 168
  Dit Dat Jiao, 138, 173, 210
  Feminine Nourishment Tea, 181
  Flower Oil, 138
  Garlic Lemonade, 145
  Garlic Remedies, 206
  Garlic-Onion-Ginger-Kudzu, 145
  Ginger Tea, 145
  Heartburn Tea, 168
  High Calcium Tea, 173
  Iron Tonic Syrup, 135-136, 148
  Kudzu Apple Juice, 145
  Kudzu Root Tea, 168-169
  late-pregnancy tonics, 104
  Liver and Kidney Wellness Formula,
    191
  Liver Strengthening Tea, 156
  Miscarriage Prevention Tea, 176
  Muscle Ache Oil, 138
  Nourishment Tea, 70
  Relaxation Tea, 157
  Slippery Elm Lozenges, 168
  Spirulina Smoothie, 191
  teas, 62, 70, 86, 146, 153-154
herbs
  avoidance in pregnancy, 63-69, 64, 145,
    146, 148, 152, 154, 156, 166, 168, 170
  carminative herbs, 140
  emmenagogic herbs, 63, 65, 69, 152,
    186
  use in pregnancy, 8, 14, 29, 40-41, 53,
    59, 62-63, 65-71, 91
  See also nutrition; specific herbs
herpes, 33, 66
  discussed, 158-161
  See also infection; sexually-transmitted
    disease
homeopathic remedies, 70, 142, 187
hops, 170
hormones

affecting body, 89, 93, 180, 184
affecting thoughts and feelings, 21-22,
  96
in foods, 57-58, 59, 65, 155
herbal regulation of, 53-54, 65, 67, 71
horror stories, 97, 98, 115, 150
housekeeping, 98, 121
hunger, 12, 42, 51, 96, 169, 185. *See also*
  digestion
hypertension, 31, 55, 69, 95, 103, 146,
  189, 192-193
  discussed, 161-166
  remedies, 164
  See also blood pressure
hypoglycemia. *See* blood sugar level
hysterectomy, 154

lemon balm, 68-69, 161, 165-166

lifestyle, affect on well-being, 10, 13, 32, 88, 115

light, response of baby to, 21

liver function, 65, 93, 171

liver tonics, 66, 67-68, 70-71, 155-156, 191

lordosis, 74, 136. *See also* backache; posture

love, 6, 17, 18, 21, 22-25, 97, 175. *See also* affirmations; relationships

lung maturity, 20-21, 37

M

macrobiotic diet, 57, 153. *See also* nutrition; vegetarianism

mammogram, 90

mask of pregnancy, 93, 132. *See also* skin conditions

massage, 8, 14, 16, 26, 29, 83-84, 139, 146, 153, 165, 171, 187

for baby, 23, 24, 115, 187

for breasts, 90, 105, 141, 188

cautions for, 173, 210

foot massage, 83, 173, 179, 189

vaginal massage, 104-105

See also touch

massage oil, 68

meat, 48-49, 50, 52, 54, 55, 56, 57, 58, 133, 134

cautions for, 35, 132, 155

chicken, 57, 58, 183, 187

fish, 52, 57, 58, 139, 146, 164

See also nutrition; protein

medication. *See* drugs

men

infection carriers, 199, 203

nutritional requirements for, 56

participation as partners in pregnancy, 3-4, 38, 39

prenatal care provided by, 27, 31, 34

view on pregnancy, 123-128

See also father

menopause, 10

menstruation, 19, 138, 148

herbal stimulation of, 63, 69, 181

relation of to pregnancy commencement, 18, 97

See also bleeding; hemorrhage

mental difficulties, 54, 94. *See also* feelings

metabolic disorders, 37

midwife, 27-31, 39, 83, 84, 95, 96, 150

certified nurse-midwife, 7

Certified Professional Midwife (CPM), 29

doula, 107

nurse-midwife, 30, 31, 34

See also prenatal care

midwifery, 6-8, 14

legality of, 28, 29, 30

minerals, 62, 66

calcium, 47, 48, 49, 52

discussed, 55-56

deficiency, 55, 133-136, 146, 157, 185, 190

iodine, 48, 56

iron, 48, 56, 133-136, 146, 157

lysine, 159-160

phosphorus, 48, 56

potassium, 56

sodium (salt), 49, 56, 60, 134, 163, 172, 188-189, 190

supplements, risks and benefits, 59, 134, 135-136, 146, 185-186

zinc, 48, 56

See also nutrition; vitamins

miscarriage, 4, 95, 97, 122, 139, 141, 154, 157

discussed, 174-183

herbal cautions, 63, 65, 67, 69, 145

nutrition affecting, 54-55, 67, 139

prenatal test affecting, 36

See also bleeding; cramping; emmenagogic herbs

mood swings, 85, 114, 122

discussed, 149-152

by trimester, 95-99

See also anxiety; feelings

mothers

communication with baby, 21, 22, 23-25, 74, 84, 117

connection to child, 15, 23, 97

involvement in pregnancy, 28, 38

sharing of experiences by, 11, 97-98

single, 95, 96, 123

massage for, 84

self-care provided by, 32

teenagers, 16, 190

motherwort, 69, 103, 151-152, 162, 166, 188

movement, 13-14, 72-73, 105

of baby, 18, 19, 20, 22, 73, 74, 97, 122

recommendations for, 75

bridge, 78

butterfly pose, 77

centaur, 78

forward bend with variation, 78

leg extensions, 79

leg lifts, 80

lumbar stretch, 80

pelvic rock, 79

standing twist, 76

yogic squat, 77

See also exercise

moxibustion, 142-143

muscle ache, 70, 75. *See also* backache

muscle tone, 73, 83. *See also* exercise; movement

muscles, changes in, 93

music, 75, 84, 86, 87, 144

response to by baby, 6, 20, 22, 23, 25

singing, 23, 25, 108

N

nasal congestion, 94, 155

natural food diets, 48, 57-59. *See also* nutrition; vegetarianism

natural food stores, midwifery resources available at, 29

nausea, 12, 35, 85, 91, 95, 96-97, 98, 143

affecting eating habits, 43

discussed, 183-187, 211-212

herbal remedies, 62, 67, 68

morning sickness, 43, 120, 153, 183-187, 211

nutrition affecting, 52, 54, 59

reduction of, 20, 83, 175-177

See also eating disorder; nutrition

negativity, 11-13, 22, 116. *See also* affirmations

nervous system tonics, 10, 54, 56, 63, 68, 69

nettle, 69, 103, 135, 137, 153, 157, 171, 191, 193, 195, 208, 210

neural tube defects, 54, 132. *See also* deformity

prenatal visits, 32-33, 123
    diet diary evaluation in, 43
    midwife, 30, 33
    nurse-midwife, 34
    obstetrician, 34
    schedules for, 27
prostate gland, 56
protein
    deficiency, 50, 134, 188, 190
    requirements, 48, 49, 50-51, 52, 57,
        58, 59, 60, 66
    in urine, 162, 189, 192-193
psychic experience, 14-15, 23, 117, 167

R

raw-food diet, 57. See also nutrition; veg-
    etarianism
reading to baby, 23-24
    See also communication
red clover, 53, 55, 56
red raspberry, 53, 55, 69, 140, 157
relationships
    affect of on baby, 22
    with father, 119-121, 124-125
    growth of during pregnancy, 3-6, 114
    with midwife, 29, 30, 33, 34
    stress in, 33, 38, 95, 96, 97-98, 120-121,
        143, 150, 182
    See also family; father
relatives. See family
relaxation
    benefits of, 16, 83, 84
    contemporary ignorance about, 40-41
    and exercise, 72, 74, 75
    herbal preparations for, 67, 68
    and nutrition, 101
    techniques for, 85-88
    vaginal muscles, 81
respiratory problems, 52-53. See also illness
responsibility
    acceptance of in self-care, 32
    denial of to pregnant women, 4-5, 8
rest, 16, 73-74, 85-88, 91, 153
    denial of with stimulants, 12, 13
    and nutrition, 101-102
    See also relaxation; sleep
Rh disease, 37, 38
Rh-factor, prenatal testing for, 35

rituals, 117-118, 150
    Blessingway, 107-111
rose hips, 70, 153-154
rubella, 35

S

St. John's wort, 70, 137, 152
sciatica. See backache
seaweed, 53, 55, 56, 68, 134, 139, 153, 155,
    157, 166, 191, 210
self-care, 7, 32, 33. See also prenatal care
self-criticism, compared to self-acceptance,
    12-13
self-empowerment, 114-118
self-image
    cultural stereotypes affecting, 9-11,
        72-74
    enhancement of, 14, 25, 187
    feelings and fears about, 12-13, 95,
        150-151
sex
    difficulties with, 34, 38, 83, 90, 99, 105,
        120, 181, 199, 202
    during pregnancy, 30, 90, 139
    exercise affecting, 81
    exercise combined with, 82, 105, 137
    nipple stimulation, 89
    See also intimacy; relationships
sexual differentiation, in baby, 19
sexual functioning, 56
sexual organs
    health of, 56, 81-82, 158-161
    sacredness of, 15
sexual sensitivity, 89, 90
sexually-transmitted diseases (STDs), 35,
    158-161, 198
shock, 148, 178
shortness of breath, 74-75, 95, 132, 148
sight, capacity of baby for, 21
singing, 23, 25, 108. See also music
skin conditions, 52, 53, 71, 93, 132, 134,
    146, 171-172
skullcap, 152, 170, 197
sleep, 10, 153
    denial of with stimulants, 12
    enhancement of, 73, 75, 83
    herbal preparations for, 67, 68
    and nutrition, 101

positions for, 165, 167, 188
    See also insomnia
smells, 90, 91, 93, 94, 183, 184
soda, 59, 135, 139, 164
sound
    changes in during pregnancy, 94
    response to by baby, 6, 20
soy products, 50, 54, 133, 144. See also
    nutrition
spatial awareness, 94, 133
spina bifida, 54, 132. See also deformity
spirit
    calming of, 68
    relation to mind and body, 10, 15
    role in nutrition, 40
spirituality, 8, 27, 108, 116-118, 175, 182
spirulina, 59, 66, 93, 132, 136, 146, 153,
    195
    Spirulina Smoothie, 191
stamina, 55, 73
stress
    affecting baby, 17, 21-22, 95
    affecting health, 42, 50, 95, 153, 156,
        162, 165
    causes for, 10, 41, 42
    discussion about with health care
        provider, 33
    of employment, 21, 22, 95, 143, 153
    normalcy of in pregnancy, 21
    nutrition affecting, 54, 56, 59, 69
    See also relaxation; tension
stretch marks, 90, 92, 171, 187-188
sugar, 12, 46, 51, 163, 197
    in urine, 27, 34, 35, 45, 47, 193-195
    See also blood sugar; sweets
support
    after birth, 106-107, 114, 182
    during pregnancy, 7, 22, 26-27, 28,
        32-33, 42, 89, 122, 125-126, 209
    See also relationships
sweets, 12, 45, 46, 47, 51, 59-60, 153,
    185, 193-195, 197. See also chocolate;
    junk food; sugar
swelling (edema), 53, 56, 162, 163,
    188-189, 193
swimming, 14, 73-74, 137, 208. See also
    exercise; movement

T

temperature sensitivity, 52, 57
tension, 10, 14, 95
   exercise for relief of, 72, 86
   herbal remedies for, 68
   in relationships, 120-121
   See also relaxation; stress
thoughts
   affect of on baby, 17, 21-22
   bodily response to, 10
   See also affirmations; visualizations
touch
   baby's requirement for, 19, 20, 23, 24, 83
   benefits of, 83
   changes in during pregnancy, 94, 169
   in natural childbirth, 14
   See also massage
toxemia, 31, 50, 56, 67, 146, 156, 162, 188, 193
   discussed, 189-191
toxins, 19, 57, 171
trauma, affect of on baby, 21-22

U

urinary tract, 62, 66
urinary tract infection, 35, 162, 192, 205
   affects of, 12, 139
   discussed, 196-198
   remedies, 53, 67, 74, 91, 103
   See also infection
urination, 12, 20, 82, 84, 86, 90-92, 98, 169, 195-197. *See also* elimination
urine
   ketones in, 194
   protein in, 162, 189, 192-193
   sugar in, 27, 34, 35, 45, 47, 193-195
   testing, 27, 34, 35, 45, 139, 162, 191-195
uterine prolapse, 67, 72, 81, 91, 196
uterus, 15
   changes in during pregnancy, 91-92
   embryologic development in, 18-19
   herbal tonics for, 62, 67, 69
   non-invasive measurement of, 35
   relaxation of, 86
   self-awareness of, 8

See also pelvis
uva-ursi, 198

V

valerian, 152, 166
varicosities, 69, 83, 173. *See also* cramping
   discussed, 207-211
vegetable oil, 52
vegetables, 41, 47, 48, 49, 50, 51, 53, 54, 55, 56, 58, 155, 171, 209
vegetarianism, 48-49, 54, 57-59, 183. *See also* nutrition
vernix, 20, 21
visualizations, 74, 75, 87, 118, 138, 142, 155, 156, 175, 179, 205, 209. *See also* affirmations
vitamins, 62, 66
   deficiency, 52, 53, 54, 132, 133, 190
   folic acid, 54, 93, 132-133
   overdose, 52, 54-55
   relation to fats, 52
   supplementary, 59
   vitamin A, 48, 52-53
   vitamin B1, 48, 53, 59, 185-186, 209
   vitamin B2, 48, 53
   vitamin B6, 48, 53-54
   vitamin B12, 48, 54, 133
   vitamin C, 48, 54-55, 135, 139-140, 144, 160, 176, 180, 197, 209
   vitamin D, 48, 52, 55
   vitamin E, 48, 52, 55, 105, 140, 172-173, 176, 188, 209
   vitamin K, 52, 186
   See also minerals; nutrition
vomiting. *See* nausea

W

walking, 14, 75, 86, 99, 136, 165, 208. *See also* exercise; movement
water, 50, 163-164, 171. *See also* fluids
weight loss, 51, 65, 95. *See also* eating disorders; overweight
whole grains, 45, 46, 48, 49, 50, 51-52, 53, 54, 56, 58, 155
wild yam, 70, 103, 157, 186-187, 198, 211
"womanplace", 117-118
womb. *See* uterus

women, 4-5, 11, 14, 27. *See also* mothers
women-centeredness, basis for in pregnancy, 5-6
women's wisdom, reclamation of, 14-16

Y

yellow dock, 71, 135-136, 148, 154, 157, 160
yoga, 8, 14, 72, 73, 74, 86, 142, 146, 153, 159
yoni, 15, 81, 104

Books on Health and Healing from The Crossing Press

NATURAL HEALING FOR BABIES AND CHILDREN

By Aviva Jill Romm

Foreword by William Sears, M.D.

This is an indispensable volume for parents seeking safe and effective ways to promote and maintain their child's health. Using a wide range of herbal and other natural remedies, Aviva Jill Romm—midwife, herbalist, and mother of four—presents her expertise in a form that is comprehensive and user-friendly.

"Just the kind of book I like to have around the house to refer to when my children are ill. Aviva Romm's book is like having a wise woman neighbor to call in times of need."

—Peggy O'Mara, *Mothering*

$16.95 • Paper • ISBN 0-89594-786-2

HEALING YOURSELF DURING PREGNANCY

By Joy Gardner-Gordon

A guide to a healthy pregnancy from conception to nursing. Natural alternatives for most conditions associated with pregnancy including toxemia, insomnia, yeast infections, stretch marks and more.

"This book contains a high level of practical information compiled by a holistic teacher with much clinical experience. I wish I'd known about Gardner's book during my pregnancies. Now I recommend it to my friends."   —*Alive, The Canadian Journal of Health and Nutrition*

$12.95 • Paper • ISBN 0-89594-251-8 • Over 25,000 in Print

THE HERBS OF LIFE
HEALTH & HEALING USING WESTERN & CHINESE TECHNIQUES

By Lesley Tierra, L.Ac., Dip. Ac.

"An outstanding herb book."   —Rosemary Gladstar

"Directions are especially clear with a good bibliography and resource guide. A nicely done addition to the popular literature."   —*Library Journal*

"A concise and highly readable book on herbal healing." —*The Herb Quarterly*

$16.95 • Paper • ISBN 0-89594-498-7 • Over 25,000 in Print

THE NATURAL REMEDY BOOK FOR WOMEN

By Diane Stein

This bestseller includes remedies for fifty common problems using natural healing methods. Also includes a helpful resource guide.

"A must-read for women." —*Booklist*

$16.95 • Paper • ISBN 0-89594-525-8 • Over 60,000 in Print

Look for these books in your local bookstore or order from The Crossing Press at 1-800-777-1048
Visit our Web site on the Internet at: www. crossingpress.com

GOOD FOOD: THE COMPLETE GUIDE TO EATING WELL

By Margaret M. Wittenberg

"An exceptionally well-organized, up-to-date, and easily accessible treatise on food and nutrition. Wittenberg has transformed what is too often a confusing mishmash of facts and figures into a clear, conversational format. She delineates a direct connection between food and quality of life."

—Susan Jane Cheney, food writer/columnist

$18.95 • Paper • ISBN 0-89594-746-3

HEALING WITH CHINESE HERBS

By Lesley Tierra, L. Ac., Dip. Ac.

Expert practitioner Lesley Tierra shows how certain tonic herbs have been used by the Chinese for over 4,000 years to increase vitality and strengthen the body's natural functions, often relieving so-called incurable conditions.

"An impressively cogent and authoritative book that will make the great healing potential of Chinese herbalism accessible to all."   —David Hoffman, M.N.I.M.H.

"From the preparation of seasonal soups and nourishing congees to the formulation of time tested herbal remedies, this work is a delightfully concise, practical guide for applying the energetics of disease prevention and cure. A true gift."   —James Green, herbalist and author

$14.95 • Paper • ISBN 0-89594-829-X

POCKET HERBAL REFERENCE GUIDE

By Debra Nuzzi, Master Herbalist

100,000 in Print! Includes the therapeutic uses of over 140 medicinal plants and natural remedies for more than 100 health problems.

"The remedy to help a person quit smoking may be worth the price of the book itself."

—*Canadian Journal of Herbalism*

$6.95 • Paper • ISBN 0-89594-568-1

POCKET GUIDE TO AYURVEDIC HEALING

By Candis Cantin Packard

Focusing on dietary and life-style recommendations specific to the three constitutional types (doshas), this guide enables readers to take an active role in their own wellness and healing processes.

$6.95 • Paper • ISBN 0-89594-764-1

POCKET GUIDE TO NATUROPATHIC MEDICINE

By Judith Boice

Combining the best of conventional medical wisdom with effective natural therapies, this guide offers an introduction to naturopathic philosophy as well as techniques and home remedies for common ailments.

$6.95 • Paper • ISBN 0-89594-821-4

Look for these books in your local bookstore or order from The Crossing Press at 1-800-777-1048
Visit our Web site on the Internet at: www. crossingpress.com